T0226132

CONTENTS

ACKNOWLEDGEMENTS

I am very grateful to my friends Alan Massey and Tony Payne for reading various chapters and commenting on them. Alan's interpretation on the evolution of early man (Chapter 5), and Tony's comments on various aspects of classical history and correction of my Latin and Greek were invaluable and greatly appreciated.

I would also like to thank my children, Alexander and Rhiannon, who inspired this project and my wife, Susan, who has proof read everything I have written, and encouraged me during the numerous occasions when I wondered if I had started more than I could finish.

Prologue

Human history has been influenced by many diseases over the last four or five millennia, and probably even longer. Our ancestors may not have known the cause of these epidemics, but they were only too well aware of the devastating effects of contagious diseases, such as the Black Death, smallpox, and cholera on their societies.

Scientific advances over the last two centuries, especially the introduction of immunisation and antibiotics, have made us very complacent about the effects that a major epidemic would have on our communities. However, our perception of contagious diseases is starting to receive a sharp shock. The demographic effects that HIV and AIDS are already having on certain countries are becoming obvious, and the recent heightened awareness of bird flu and the lethal potential of biological weapons has disturbed many people. In addition, over the last three or four decades, a number of "new" diseases have appeared which have the potential to become major epidemics.

An examination of diseases, such as cholera, also makes us realise just how fragile the infrastructure of our society is, especially in the "developed" countries, and how difficult it would be to cope if that infrastructure were compromised in any way.

A study of infectious diseases is important to students of both history and biology (in its widest sense), and is also crucial as a predictor of possible future events that might influence our society. This book therefore studies how diseases evolved, the human response to these diseases, and the influences they have had on our history and society.

A number of diseases are examined; it is obviously not a comprehensive list, but these specific diseases have been selected for two reasons. Firstly, they have had a significant influence on human populations, civilisations and societies, and secondly, they represent a range of diseases caused by different types of micro-organisms and transmitted by a number of different mechanisms.

Although the diseases described are divided into separate chapters, it should be appreciated that in many cases it is impossible to disentangle the effects of one disease from those of another. Obvious examples are the effects of malaria and yellow fever on the building of the Panama Canal, and more recently, the inter-relationship of HIV/AIDS and tuberculosis.

Having read through the finished version of what I have written, and being a fan of the TV series, Dad's Army, I am not quite certain of whether to take the advice of Corporal Jones, *"don't panic, don't panic"*, or to accept the prophesy of Private Fraser, *"we're doomed, I tell ye, we're all doomed"*.

Chapter i

Introduction

The course of human history has been influenced by many diseases over the centuries. These changes may have caused the death of a key individual at some important point[1], or the destruction of an army at a siege or during the critical stage of a campaign. Diseases also caused the massive demographic changes in the Old World resulting from The Plague of Justinian in the sixth century, the Black Death in the fourteenth century, and smallpox and measles in the New World in the sixteenth century.

In this book, the term disease will mean a communicable or infectious (contagious) disease, that is, a disease that can pass from one person to another either directly, via some inanimate object, or by means of a vector such as an insect. It will not include genetic diseases or diseases caused by factors such as a dietary deficiency or poison.

With a few exceptions, the effects of infectious diseases are not widely discussed in history textbooks, indeed in many cases they are totally ignored. One major exception is the Black Death in Europe, which started in the mid-fourteenth century, and killed approximately one third of the population leading

---

[1] As the Bible puts it "Woe unto thee o land when thy king is a child" (Ecclesiastes 10, 16). The classic example in English history is the death of Henry V, at the age of thirty-five, from dysentery in 1422, leaving a six month old son, Henry VI, on the throne. The lack of strong government during his minority, and the periods of madness suffered by Henry VI later in life, ushered in the most violent and bloody phase of the War of the Roses (1455-85).

to major social and economic changes. This is considered in Chapter 9.

Many infectious diseases are related intimately to various aspects of human history and behaviour, for example, smallpox (Ch 10) is effectively the history of vaccination and immunisation, cholera (Ch 12) is the history of water purification and sewage treatment, whilst tuberculosis (Ch 11) initiated the process of pasteurisation in milk and similar products.

A DEFINITION OF SOME IMPORTANT TERMS

Some specialist terms used in microbiology are not found in everyday language, and a definition of these at an early stage is useful.

Micro-organisms are generally defined as organisms which are so small that it is necessary to use a microscope to see them. This includes organisms such as the bacteria, fungi, protozoa, algae and metazoa (many-celled organisms) covered in Chapter 4. Whilst viruses can also be seen using a sufficiently powerful microscope, they are not, strictly speaking, micro-organisms as they cannot exist as separate entities.

MICROBIAL NOMENCLATURE

It is obviously important to have standardised names for micro-organisms so that doctors, microbiologists and bacteriologists throughout the world know when they are dealing with the same organism. Micro-organisms are subdivided into groups using two names; the first of these is the genus or generic name, whilst the second is the species or specific name[2]. This is known as the Linnaean or Binomial

---

2   Biological organisms such as animals are divided into groups; initially the groups are large with only a small number of characteristics in common; as the groups get smaller, the number of common characteristics increases. Initially these characteristics were those visible to the naked eye, now they include the genetic similarities. The group known as a genus may be defined as a group of related species. The definition of a species is more problematical; in fact, Darwin considered that the concept of a species was *"attempting to define the indefinable"*. There are now numerous definitions

system of classification after the Swedish biologist Karle von Linné (1707-1778, also known as Carolus Linnaeus[3]). He initially trained as a doctor, but his main interest was in botany. There had been a number of attempts to classify living organisms before Linnaeus, but in 1735 he published *Systema Naturae,* which is generally agreed to be the starting point for a logical classification of biological organisms, even although it was initially only applied to animals and flowering plants[4]. The system is somewhat artificial, but has been so successful and simple to use that it has never been successfully replaced, although there have been several attempts to do so. Linnaeus was obviously proud of his system; one of his favourite comments is reputed to have been *"Deus creavit, Linnaeus disposuit"* (God created it, Linnaeus organised it).

The basic problem for Linnaeus was to encapsulate in two words the important characteristics of a newly discovered species, whether it be animal, plant or bacterium. As the biologists put it, *"Nomen est numen"* (the name is the knowledge); the names are either Latin or Latinised Greek, and frequently describe some anatomical feature of the organism. Classic examples in microbiology are the bacteria *Staphylococcus aureus* and *Streptococcus pyogenes.* In the first example, the organism resembles bunches of grapes when seen under the microscope (staphule is the Greek word for grapes,

---

of species, but in organisms such as animals, a definition frequently used is a group of related organisms capable of breeding successfully to produce fertile offspring. This definition cannot be applied to micro-organisms, and the microbial species is defined as a group of organisms showing common characteristics, many of these characteristics being their biochemical properties or their ability to carry out certain reactions.

3   This was common at the time as it was thought that a Latin sounding name added to the professional gravitas.

4   There are questions over the originality of Linnaeus's work. Many of the theories in *Systema Naturae* were developed in partnership with Peter Artedi, a fellow student at Uppsala, but Linnaeus took sole credit after Artedi drowned. Even the binomial system had been used previously by the brothers Gaspard and Johann Bauhin (over one hundred years earlier), Linnaeus just simplified it.

whilst kokkus means berries). In the case of *Streptococcus,* the bacteria appear microscopically as short chains (strepto is Greek for a twisted chain), and *pyogenes* is derived from a word meaning to produce pus, thus, the twisted chain of berries producing pus. If two micro-organisms are in the same genus, then they are closely related as in *Staphylococcus aureus* (the golden staphylococcus, so-called because it produces a bright yellow colour when grown), and *Staphylococcus epidermidis* (the staphylococcus found on skin).

The two names are always written in italic script as shown above, with the generic name beginning with an upper case letter, and the specific name beginning with a lower case letter. The first time the name of a micro-organism is used in an article it is written in full, but subsequently, a shortened version may be used, e.g. *Staph. aureus,* as long as no ambiguity is introduced[5].

Further subdivisions of a microbial species into varieties, strains and serotypes may take place for medical reasons. These divisions tend to be technical, and are not required in the present context.

Although the Latinised version of names can be unwieldy at times, it is the most reliable and precise way of conveying information. It comes into its own for naming plants, when there are frequently a large number of local vernacular names for one plant, for example, the common cowslip (*Primula veris*) is known by a number of different regional names in England. There are obviously problems in the use of Latin names, as Latin is no longer the *lingua franca* of the educated classes, but it does have the major advantage of being a dead language[6]. Any attempt to use an extant language would no doubt lead

---

5   Journalists seem to have considerable difficulty in understanding these simple rules. The misuse of the name *Clostridium difficile* during the continuing hospital "super-bug" crisis is a case in point.

6   Certain rules are applied to the naming of any new species. If the name of a person is used it must end in "i" or "ae". If the word is not a name, it must be a word that can be translated into Latin. Religious names and words are not allowed.

to many acrimonious discussions about which language was used[7].

Biological protocol requires that the earliest recorded name is used. This can be a serious nuisance when an organism has been known by one name for decades, and then gets renamed as the result of some piece of obscure historical research. One of the main microbiological problems is the naming of the fungi (Ch 4). In a number of cases, the fungus exists in two states, a perfect or sexual state, and an imperfect or asexual state. Historically, these two states may not have been recognised as being the same species, and would have been given two different names. This can cause considerable confusion when it is later realised that they are just two different forms of the same organism.

Further problems can occur when modern research such as genetic analysis shows that a group of micro-organisms that had been considered to be a single genus for many years, can in fact be split into two or more genera.

THE INTER-RELATIONSHIP BETWEEN A MICRO-ORGANISM AND HOST

The relationship between a micro-organism and its host organism is an extremely complicated one known as symbiosis (living together), and can range across a wide spectrum of interactions. At one end is a situation in which the micro-organism and host are totally dependent on each other, each derives some benefit from the association, and they are incapable of an independent existence. This situation is called mutualism, and one of the best examples are the micro-organisms known as lichens, which are the growths frequently found on old gravestones in churchyards. Lichens are a combination of fungi and algae living together, neither of which is capable of living alone; the fungus forms a thallus (network of threads) which give protection to the algae carrying out photosynthesis

---

7   One can just imagine the howl of outrage from the French if English was used, and a similar howl from the Americans if any language other than English prevailed.

(utilisation of the light energy of the sun). In return, the fungus gets a constant supply of surplus sugars from the algae. In practical terms, lichens are valuable indicators of pollution (especially levels of sulphur dioxide to which they are extremely sensitive), as their maximum possible age is known from the date on the gravestone.

The micro-organism may be parasitic on its host, that is, the host organism is providing food and lodging for the micro-organism. In many cases, the host does not realise that the micro-organism is present as no disease is caused, and no recognisable symptoms occur. In cases where the host becomes ill, the micro-organism/host relationship has progressed to the pathogenic state in which the micro-organism causes a disease, and in extreme cases kills the host organism. If the parasite kills the host then it must find another host, but if the host resists the infection totally, then the parasite has a different problem as discussed later in this chapter.

The host/parasite relationship is a very finely balanced one, and is easily changed from the parasitic into the pathogenic state by small alterations in the life-style of the host. The most common of these are increasing age, pregnancy in females, a poorer diet or the presence of another disease causing a debilitated state. The status of any given disease can also change significantly from person to person; a relatively trivial disease in a fit, healthy, young adult can easily be life-threatening in an old person, a young baby, or an individual whose immune state has been compromised, either by the use of drugs, or by an immuno-suppressive disease such as AIDS.

One such example is the yeast *Candida albicans;* this is frequently found in the human gut, as a commensal (from Latin "[to eat] at the same table") organism, where it causes no problems. In many women it invades the vagina where it may cause the condition known as thrush that is frequently associated with changes in body chemistry caused by pregnancy, menstruation or the menopause. In people who are immunologically impaired however, it can invade the tissues causing candidiasis, which results in abscesses throughout the body, and is fatal in over forty per cent of cases.

Plague, Endemic, Epidemic, Pandemic and Epidemiology

The word plague, which occurs frequently in the terminology of disease, is used very loosely in non-medical texts, and also in some medical texts, to describe any epidemic disease killing a large number of its victims. The Latin word "*pestis*" which was used in medieval times to describe the Black Death (*Pestis magna* [The Great Pestilence]), is generally translated as plague, and when the Black Death was assigned to bubonic plague in the nineteenth century (Ch 9), the situation became very confusing. The terms epidemic and plague are now regarded as more or less synonymous, particularly in non-specialist texts.

The term plague will be used in this book to describe bubonic plague. In cases where the disease is commonly known as a plague, for example, the "Plague of Athens", it will be made obvious in the text whether or not it could be assigned to bubonic plague.

An endemic disease is one which is always present within a certain geographical area or community. Many infectious endemic diseases are the so-called childhood diseases, which are always present at a relatively low level (e.g. chickenpox), and which kill only a small number of people. The presence of an endemic disease implies that the population and the disease have reached equilibrium; however, some diseases, which many people in the developed world may regard as relatively trivial childhood diseases (e.g. measles), are major killers in developing countries. Measles is estimated to kill about two hundred thousand people every year, most of them children in underdeveloped countries. Even common childhood diseases, such as chickenpox, may be fatal if they attack a person who has a poor immune response, or if there is a secondary bacterial infection.

Epidemic (the word is derived from the Greek words *epi* [upon] and *demos* [the people]) is used to describe a disease which is occurring at a higher than normal rate, within a given area or community, and during a given time period. This requires knowledge of both the number of cases and the size of the community. Many infectious diseases producing distinctive symptoms (e.g. cholera) move from endemic to epidemic status, both quickly and in large numbers. The phrase, "a higher than normal rate" implies that if an epidemic disease is present in a community for a number of years, the base line of measurement will change, and over time the disease will be downgraded from epidemic to endemic status.

Pandemic describes a disease that is passing from person to person on a large scale in several countries simultaneously. One common mistake encouraged by hyped-up press reports is that pandemics always kill large numbers of people. This is not correct, whilst some pandemics may kill large numbers, others do not.

The origin of the science of epidemiology lies in a study of population statistics and mortality rates, and unlike most other aspects of medicine, epidemiology is concerned with group health and dynamics, rather than the health of a specific individual[8]. Basically epidemiology asks three questions, who becomes ill, why do they become ill and how are the figures changing over time? The answer to these questions is not always as straightforward as it might seem. Consider two populations; last year, population A had two cases of HIV per 1,000 people, population B had 200 cases per 1,000. This year, population A has four cases of HIV, population B has 300. Which population is in the more serious state? Most people

---

8   One major problem with epidemiology is that it is not a politically correct subject and the application of epidemiological principles, even although they might be scientifically and factually correct, frequently raise howls of outrage from the politically correct brigade.

would no doubt answer B. The epidemiologist however, might argue A, on the grounds that a rise from two to four is a rise ·of 100%, whereas in B, the rise has been from 200 to 300, a rise of only 50%. This of course, makes the assumption that no-one in group B has died of AIDS in the last year. If they have, some statistician might make a case for adding them to the total of 300, so that one was comparing like with like, and re-calculating the results. A third statistician might argue that special formulae applied to the statistics of small numbers should be used for population A[9].

Starting in 1532, each parish in England was required to publish Bills of Mortality regularly which stated the cause of death, and in 1662, John Graunt wrote, "*Natural and Political Observations on the Bills of Mortality*" listing the numbers who had died from each disease. These Bills of Mortality and the statistics associated with them became, over time, the basis of the actuarial rates worked out by life insurance companies.

MORBIDITY AND MORTALITY

Two terms frequently confused during epidemics are the morbidity rate, which is the number of people who catch the disease after exposure to it, and the mortality rate which is the number of people who die from the disease once they have caught it.

Even the most serious epidemics and pandemics do not kill the entire population. People range from being completely resistant to a disease to totally susceptible to it; resistance and susceptibility are very complex and involve numerous genes (Ch 7). The survival of the host species depends on some individuals being more resistant to the disease than others, and the morbidity and mortality rates being less than 100%.

---

9   As the great politician, Benjamin Disraeli said, "*there are lies, damned lies and statistics*". The blunt fact is that one set of results can be made to tell several different stories, depending on how the epidemiologist/statistician manipulates them. How the results are manipulated frequently depends on whether the researcher involved is trying to raise funds for some pet project or has a political agenda.

These more resistant members of the host species will survive the pandemic, and produce offspring who will frequently inherit parental resistance. Over a period of time, a larger and larger percentage of the host species will become resistant to the disease. Infectious diseases giving long-term immunity to those who survive, and which return to a community at intervals, will usually become downgraded to a childhood disease over a number of generations.

Progress of a Disease

The sequence of events during a simple disease transmitted directly from person to person, and not involving a vector, such as an insect, is shown in Figure 1.1.

Figure 1.1

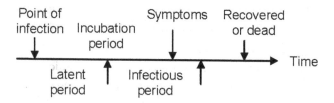

The latent period is the time from the point of infection to the time at which a person becomes infectious, and one important point shown in the diagram is that the patient becomes infectious before the symptoms appear. The incubation period is the time from the point of infection to sufficient organisms being present in the victim to produce symptoms. This period is not fixed, it will depend on the size of the infectious dose an individual has received, and the state of health and immune response of the individual at the time of infection.

The incubation period may vary significantly from disease to disease; in the case of smallpox it is only about ten days, and it is relatively easy to trace people who have been in contact with, or exposed to, the infected individual. In other cases such as HIV, the patient may be infectious for years before the symptoms (AIDS) appear, making it extremely difficult to trace the contacts of an infected individual, and hence control the spread of the disease.

In Figure 1, the infectious period is shown as ending before the victim recovers or dies. This is not always correct, in some cases the infected person may become a carrier (see later), and remain infectious for a considerable period, even life, and in certain diseases, such as smallpox, a corpse may remain infectious for a considerable time after death. There are a number of apocryphal stories from the eighteenth century claiming that entire villages succumbed to smallpox when the graves of individuals who had died of smallpox were opened thirty years after they had been buried. None of the sources are reliable but scientists take sensible precautions when exhuming the body of a person known to have died of an infectious disease, especially smallpox.

The number of susceptible contacts infected by each infectious person is known as the transmission number, and this determines the speed with which an epidemic will peak and also the length of the epidemic. When the epidemic is growing, the transmission number is more than one; once the transmission number falls below one, the epidemic starts to subside. As the susceptible members of the population catch the disease, they either die or become immune, and the epidemic eventually runs out of susceptible people to infect. The transmission of a disease will also depend on social factors such as the density of the population (whether the community is rural or urban); the behaviour of communities such as schools, universities, prisons and army barracks will differ significantly from the behaviour of the general community.

HERD IMMUNITY AND CHILDHOOD DISEASES

Herd immunity describes the immunity of a community to an infectious disease, and is based on the immunity of a large percentage of the individuals in that community. The percentage of immune individuals needed to provide the herd with immunity will vary from disease to disease; it can also vary within the same disease (for example, diphtheria), depending on the density of the population.

Herd immunity may be natural or can be induced by immunisation; some individuals within a community are naturally resistant to certain diseases due to their genetic makeup. In the case of induced immunity, it is not necessary to immunise all the animals in a herd; if a sufficiently large percentage are immunised, although there may be the occasional case of infection, the disease cannot get a foothold because the susceptible animals are too far apart. For the disease to spread there must be a susceptible population large enough to overcome herd immunity.

Figures of seventy per cent immune individuals have been suggested as necessary to provide herd immunity against polio, whilst for highly infectious diseases such as influenza and measles, the corresponding figure is ninety to ninety-five per cent. The immunity of the herd is constantly challenged and boosted by re-infections, especially in the case of childhood diseases such as chickenpox, rubella (German measles) and mumps. In the case of more serious infections such as measles or smallpox, the weakest will be killed, and the immunity of the rest will be increased. Herd immunity will be high immediately after an epidemic, but will then start to fall due to population movements and the birth of new susceptible children.

The immunity of the community to a specific disease does not depend totally on the immunity of individuals, it can also depend on the exposure of the community to the disease. For example, the vast majority of individuals in the UK are not immune to yellow fever, but yellow fever does not normally occur in the UK, because the mosquito carrying the disease cannot survive in the British climate. Although there have been a few small outbreaks of yellow fever in England in the past, it is unlikely to become epidemic in the UK, even if introduced by some infected individual arriving from an area where yellow fever is endemic. This situation may change if global warming continues apace.

Many of the diseases transferred directly from human to human become childhood diseases, and one bout of infection frequently immunises the individual for life. However, when childhood diseases attack a population without herd immunity, they can cause epidemics that frequently kill young adults and cripple the entire society. The effect of this is extremely serious; in terms of the survival of a society or community, the death of an old person is usually not a great loss as they have returned the investment society made in them. The loss is only serious in a non-literate society, in which the old person was the depository of community knowledge, and has not had time to hand that knowledge on to an apprentice or acolyte. Whilst the death of a child is unfortunate and tragic for the immediate family, society as a whole has not made a major investment in a young child; in terms of the whole society a single child is easily replaced, and the deaths of a small number of very young children generally has very little demographic impact on a large community. However, the death of a young adult is serious, it destroys the providers and the next breeding generation before they have started to repay the investment society has made in them. If sufficiently large numbers of young adults die in an epidemic, the effect on a society can be devastating, as events in much of sub-Saharan Africa are demonstrating at the present moment with AIDS (Ch 18).

VIRULENCE

The virulence of a micro-organism is an important concept in any study of disease and has two features. It involves the ability of the micro-organism to invade the host, and also the severity of disease produced in the host. Virulence can be measured by the lethal dose (known as the LD_{50}); this is the number of micro-organisms necessary to kill 50% of the animal species attacked by the pathogen. Inbred animals in the laboratory show a much lower LD_{50} than animals that have not been inbred, indicating a more uniform susceptibility to the disease in the former. This has important implications when the spread of diseases such as smallpox and measles in the Americas in the sixteenth century is considered. A similar situation occurred when Europeans penetrated the Pacific in the eighteenth and nineteenth centuries. The genetic reasons for this are discussed later (Ch 7). Virulence is influenced by the age, sex, genetic background, behaviour, nutritional and physiological state of the host, as well as previous exposure to the disease. It can also be influenced by the route of infection, a fact used in the variolation process against smallpox (Ch 10).

THE "CARRIER" STATE

The concept of "carrier" is also an important one in medical microbiology. A carrier can be defined as a person who harbours, or carries, the micro-organism responsible for causing a disease, without developing the disease or displaying any of its symptoms. The carrier state is frequently found in people after they have suffered from an infection, but it normally only lasts for a few weeks before the micro-organism is eliminated from the body. In a small number of individuals, and certain diseases however, it can persist for years, or indeed life.

The classic example is a lady known to history as "Typhoid Mary". Mary Mallon was an Irish cook employed in a number of households in New York State during the early part of the twentieth century. Following an outbreak of typhoid in a family in Long Island, Major Soper of the US Medical Corps traced Mallon through an employment agency. He found there had been outbreaks of typhoid (enteric fever) in about seven houses where she worked over a period of approximately a decade, and investigations showed her to be the source. Typhoid was a major epidemic disease at this time with a death rate of approximately ten per cent of those infected. Mallon refused to accept that she was the cause of the problem, and although she was offered an operation to remove her gall bladder, which is known to be the reservoir of the bacterium, *Salmonella typhi,* (the causative organism of the disease), she declined the operation. She was forcibly quarantined (in 1907, for three years), in an isolation hospital on North Brother Island, off the coast of Manhattan, after refusing to give up the job of cooking. The case caused major public interest and Mallon sued for release on the grounds of *habeas corpus* on a number of occasions, but was refused each time. A new Health Commissioner was appointed in 1910, and one of the first acts of the new administration was to release Mallon, after she promised not to cook or handle food again, and to visit the Health Department at regular intervals for checks. She disappeared virtually immediately, changed her name and started cooking again in restaurants, hotels and private homes causing a series of outbreaks of typhoid that included at least forty-seven confirmed cases and three known deaths. She finally got a hospital job causing a large number of cases amongst the medical staff.

A satirical verse publicising the situation appeared in Punch.

> *"In the USA (across the brook)*
> *There lives unless the papers err*
> *A very curious Irish cook*
> *In whom the strangest things occur.*
> *Beneath her outside's healthy gloze*
> *Masses of microbes seethe and wallow*
> *And everywhere that Mary goes*
> *Infernal epidemics follow".*

Mallon was finally recaptured and remained imprisoned in the isolation hospital, where she lived in solitude until her death in 1938.

It has been estimated that approximately three per cent of patients recovering from typhoid become carriers in the absence of antibiotics; the organism survives in the gall bladder and is continuously secreted into the gut. This example demonstrates how certain diseases can flare up at intervals for no immediately apparent reason. The case of Mallon also raises the important question of how much right the state has to restrict the freedom of a non-criminal individual[10]. This question has become extremely pertinent recently with the imprisonment of HIV+ve individuals found guilty of deliberately infecting their sexual partners. It is a problem that is not going to go away, and is probably only going to be a matter of time before there is a major clash between human rights campaigners and public health officials attempting to enforce quarantines.

An even more extreme situation occurred in England; between 1907 and 1992 over forty women were held in Long Grove Mental Asylum in Epsom. All of them were typhoid carriers and were considered to be a danger to public health so were held in isolation in secure units. Over a period of time many deteriorated mentally to the point that they would have been incapable of surviving if released. The unit finally closed in 1992, when the last few patients were moved to other institutions, and the records were destroyed.

Isolation hospitals were a common feature of many British cities prior to antibiotics, and children suffering from diseases such as scarlet fever or diphtheria in the 1920s and 30s were collected by the fever-van, which was frequently horse-drawn and transported to a hospital usually on the outskirts of town. The families were not allowed to visit, each child was allocated a hospital number, and parents could only read about the progress of their offspring in the local paper each evening. Any belongings of the infected child were destroyed, including

10   Public health has been described as a fascist discipline in which it is occasionally necessary to violate the rights of the individual to protect society as a whole, *"the greatest good of the greatest number"* principle.

clothing and bedding, which was a serious financial blow for poor families.

More extreme historical examples of this type of state intervention are seen with the enforcement of quarantine for both shipping and individuals. The forcible confinement of families to their homes during the Black Death, even although only one member of the family may have had the disease, virtually guaranteed that every member of the family would be exposed to it over a long period, and probably succumb to the infection.

A second common example of the carrier state is found in a member of the Herpes virus group, the *Varicella-zoster* virus that causes chickenpox and shingles. Contrary to widely held public opinion, granny does not catch shingles from grandchildren who have caught chickenpox at school, rather granny passes the virus to children where it manifests itself as chickenpox, and they take it to school. This highly infectious childhood disease frequently reappears as shingles in the elderly, who have been carrying the virus for years. It is carried in the nervous system of certain individuals following a childhood infection of chickenpox, and reappears in the infectious form in older people as their immune system weakens. It solves the problem of how this highly infectious virus can propagate itself in a relatively small community in which everyone rapidly becomes immune. Chickenpox flares up at regular intervals, frequently infecting whole classes of children in their first year at school, and in countries such as the UK, most children are probably immune to it by the age of seven. Even if the entire child population is infected with chickenpox and becomes immune, shingles reappears in the elderly, and infects new susceptible children (i.e. the ones born after the last epidemic) at some later date.

The mildness of the disease and the period of latency of shingles suggest that it is a viral disease that has afflicted humans for a very long time in evolutionary terms, unlike many viral diseases that appear to be relatively recent acquisitions. The strategy used by this virus is interesting because this method of transmitting the disease would allow it to survive in relatively small hunter-gatherer groups, whereas most other childhood diseases need large numbers of potential victims, and therefore needed urban conditions, before they could become effective human diseases.

THE PROBLEMS

There are many problems that arise when studying diseases in history. The modern epidemiologist has a large number of techniques at his/her disposal, including microbiology, autopsy, biopsy, molecular biology, serology and statistics to name just a few. Even with all of these techniques available, there are still some diseases such as Ebola and Marburg disease, whose behaviours are not fully understood.

None of these techniques were available to doctors in historical times, and historically most diseases were generally described under one of three headings, poxes, fluxes and fevers (which were also known as agues). Poxes were basically any disease causing a rash on the skin (they might be subdivided, e.g. smallpox or the Great Pox [syphilis]). Fluxes were gastrointestinal diseases (and could also be further characterised, for example, the bloody flux [dysentery]). The term "fever" had much the same meaning as it has today, in that it produced a high temperature and shivering, and fevers were also subdivided into various categories, such as quotidian (every day) or tertian (every third day). After the introduction of Jesuits bark (quinine) to Europe (Ch 16), Francesco Torti produced an engraving known as the Fever Tree (*Lignum febrium*). This showed a tree whose branches on the left side were alive and covered with leaves, and whose branches on the right side were dead and bare. The left side represented those fevers that could be treated with Jesuits bark and those on the right fevers that could not.

This process of lumping everything under a small number of headings can make it very difficult to distinguish between historical accounts of diseases producing similar symptoms. Even as late as the early nineteenth century, many physicians thought that there was only one, or at most a few different forms of fever, and that different presentations were caused by differences in the victim such as age, race and gender, or by extraneous factors, such as temperature and climate.

Problems are also caused by different diseases being given the same name at various times in history. The most extreme example of this occurring is probably the disease known today as ergotism. This is caused by poisoning by the ergot fungus (*Claviceps purpurea*) which is found growing on rye and other cereals, especially after wet, severe winters. This killed large numbers of people in France and Germany in the Middle Ages, and epidemics were common in Russia until well into the twentieth century[11]. The disease is complicated by the fact that it can present itself in two forms, depending on which of the four main alkaloids (toxic chemicals) are present in the fungus when it is ingested. One form produces gangrene of the extremities, whilst the other produces convulsions as some of the alkaloids are related to the psychotic drug, lysergic acid diethylamide (LSD). Some authors consider it to have been responsible for the behaviour leading to the Salem witch trials in America in 1692.

It is frequently known historically by the name St Anthony's Fire, but was also called Ignis Sacer (sacred fire), Saints fire, evil fire, holy fire and Devil's fire. To further complicate the situation, the Roman physician Celcus (25BC-50AD) grouped the gangrenous form with numerous other skin afflictions, whilst more recently the name St Anthony's Fire has been used to describe erysipelas, a bacterial infection of the skin.

---

11   In the Middle Ages, preparations of the fungus were used to promote abortions in young women who had become pregnant without benefit of clergy. Chemicals derived from the fungus are still used today to control heavy bleeding after childbirth.

Another example is the term elephantiasis, which has been used historically to describe certain types of leprosy (Ch. 11), but in modern medicine is used to describe the condition caused by filarial worms (Ch 4) transmitted by mosquitoes and other insects. Leprosy was also known as leontiasis by the Romans and a number of later writers, because of the perceived lion-like features in the early stages of the disease. Leprosy was another example of diseases being lumped together, as the term is derived from a Greek word (*lepra*), used to describe any skin condition producing scales.

A modern day example of this problem is the term typhus (derived from a Greek word meaning stupor). For a number of centuries, it was very difficult to distinguish between typhus and typhoid, both of which produce similar symptoms, although typhus is carried by lice (Ch 13), and typhoid is a bacterial disease of the intestine transmitted by polluted drinking water or contaminated food. These are distinguished in English, but in some European languages, the term *Typhus abdominalis* means typhoid, and *Typhus exanthematicus* means typhus. Unfortunately, both get abbreviated to, or translated as, typhus.

Relatively few epidemic diseases leave traces on skeletal remains and even in those that do, the signs are frequently ambiguous. Infectious diseases taking months or years to kill their victims may produce bone lesions; for example, lesions due to tuberculosis or leprosy are frequently reported in skeletal tissue. Neolithic skeletons have been reported containing bone deformities that indicate TB of the spine. Lesions on skeletal tissue dated to before 1493 and claimed to have been caused by syphilis (Ch 14) are also found, but the pathology of these is doubtful in many cases, and could have been caused by any one of several related diseases. Epidemic diseases such as influenza, smallpox, bubonic plague, typhus and cholera that kill their victims quickly, within a few hours or days, produce no skeletal pathology.

Recent advances in technology have allowed the extraction of deoxyribonucleic acid (DNA) (Ch 4) from human bones found in ancient graves, and the tentative identification of microbial DNA linked to certain diseases. In many cases, however, the condition of the bones has been extremely poor, resulting from serious contamination by soil micro-organisms. Under these conditions, the reliability of results linking the body to a specific disease is questionable. The technique also makes the crucial assumption that the microbial DNA entered the skeletal system and therefore can be extracted from it.

Another major problem when reading contemporary reports, is that when a new disease strikes the human population, the symptoms are frequently much more severe than they are after several centuries of human exposure to it. Therefore, historical descriptions of a disease may differ significantly from the modern day pathology of the same disease; syphilis (Ch 14) is a classic example of this situation.

It can also be very difficult to assess what is new. Descriptions of diseases improve as one travels through history, and the apparent appearance of new diseases in the fourteenth to eighteenth centuries may have been artificial reporting phenomena, caused by the improvement of medical knowledge due to information being written down instead of being passed on orally.

With a few exceptions such as The Black Death in the fourteenth century, and to a lesser extent cholera in the nineteenth century, any Old World epidemic that changed the course of history tends to have occurred before the end of the first millennium AD, with relatively little contemporary written record being available. Even when there are contemporary accounts of an epidemic, a question arises over their reliability. For example, our only primary source of information relating to the Plague of Athens (Ch 8) is Thucydides (*ca* 460-400BC) who actually suffered from the disease. However, Thucydides wrote his "*History of the Peloponnesian War*" approximately a quarter of a century after the events took place. In addition, even the most reliable contemporary authors were not trained in objective scientific assessment, and their accounts were frequently highly subjective, and more often than not tinged with religion or superstition in some shape or form.

Over the last thousand years or so, the population of the Old World has been exposed to many diseases causing high levels of herd immunity; as a result it has become highly disease experienced and hence many epidemics have been terminated relatively quickly. Historians, therefore, tend to disregard contemporary accounts of the massive death tolls caused by disease in the first millennium AD as exaggeration and legend. This tendency has been exacerbated by the effectiveness of mass immunisation and public health programmes during the twentieth century, which has changed disease patterns significantly. The widespread use of antibiotics and chemotherapy since 1945 has also contributed to this popular disbelief of the devastating effects of a pandemic on a non-immune population.

During the twentieth century, there was one major pandemic, influenza (Ch 15) that killed millions, and also a less widespread epidemic of typhus (Ch 13). Both occurred immediately after World War I, and their effect tended to be lost in the aftermath of that war. In addition, whilst influenza is a major epidemic disease killing large numbers, the effects of it on any one individual are much less visual and spectacular than those of diseases such as bubonic plague or smallpox, and hence the general public usually ignores or disbelieves the large-scale effects of a major flu epidemic.

People also tend to disregard how quickly information can be forgotten and vanish; a classic example of this problem is seen in the epidemic disease diphtheria, in which a membrane frequently closes up the throat and causes rapid death by choking in young children. During the first few decades of the twentieth century, any junior and relatively inexperienced doctor in Europe or the USA, would have recognised diphtheria instantly, and been prepared to carry out an emergency tracheotomy on a child, using the kitchen table as an operating table and working by candlelight, if necessary. Due to mass immunisation programmes against diphtheria, it is now probable that many junior doctors in Western Europe or North America would not recognise a case of diphtheria until it was too late for surgical intervention. Even if they did, most would certainly not be prepared to carry out a tracheotomy without the support of a surgical team in a well-equipped operating theatre. Diphtheria however, has not disappeared, there have been a large number of cases in the former Soviet Union since its disintegration, and any relaxation of the immunisation programme against this disease would almost certainly result in its resurgence in Western Europe. Indeed, figures in Western Europe including Britain, suggest that immunisation against a number of serious diseases including diphtheria and measles is falling to a dangerously low level.

Several maladies are also known historically whose symptoms cannot be matched to those of any present day disease. The *"Sweating disease"* is mentioned frequently in English history of the sixth and seventh centuries but the description is very vague. The *"Sweats"* or *"English Sweats"* are also documented widely between 1485 and 1551, but this disease is unknown today. Whether the disease described in the earlier period is the same one as that described later is debatable. The fifteenth century version is generally assumed to have been brought to England by French mercenaries used by Henry VII at the Battle of Bosworth in 1485, the last great battle in the Wars of the Roses, a series of dynastic struggles fought in England from 1455-1485. It has been postulated that it killed Prince Arthur[12], the elder brother of Henry VIII thus changing the course of English history as, until this happened, Henry's intended career had been the Church, which is rather

---

12   This is not the only theory, it has also been suggested that he died from tuberculosis.

ironic considering what he later did to the Catholic Church in England. The disease known as "Sudor Anglicus" was first described by John Caius (after whom Gonville and Caius College, Cambridge is named)[13] in 1552, shortly after it had disappeared, and is one of the earliest monographs known that is devoted to a single disease. It appears to have attacked mainly the upper classes producing a fever and profuse foul smelling sweat followed by death, frequently within a matter of hours. If a person survived more than 24 hours, they usually recovered. It caused five major epidemics between 1485-1551, but then disappeared and has not been seen since.

The phrase "upper classes" used in the previous paragraph illustrates another problem facing the historian. Historically, it is probable that many diseases are only mentioned when they attacked members of the ruling classes, such as a member of the aristocracy or a senior member of the church; any effect on the peasant population was largely ignored in contemporary literature. This would have been compounded by the fact that only the ruling class, the merchant class and clergy were literate[14].

The identity of the *"Sweats"* has been hotly debated as the disease was reported to have a number of unusual features, in addition to only attacking the upper classes. It does not appear to have created immunity as Cardinal Wolsey apparently suffered from several attacks. It also only occurred in England, there were no reported outbreaks in Scotland and very few in Wales or Ireland. It is alleged to have killed English people in continental Europe, but did not attack foreigners in England. The most serious epidemic occurred in 1528-9, which again stopped at the Scottish border, but unusually this time it caused an extensive epidemic in northern, but not southern, Europe. As a result, the Catholics referred to it as *"God's judgement on Martin Luther and the Protestant faith"*. This tendency to

---

13   His original name was Keys, but he Latinised it to Caius.

14   One epidemic in Ireland, whose identity is not known, is recorded as killing *"many nobles and infinite numbers of the meaner sort"*.

blame *"the other lot"* (whoever the other lot might be) for various epidemics, is a recurring theme throughout history, and is frequently accompanied by extreme violence towards the minority group perceived to be the cause of the epidemic.

Suggestions for the identity of the Sweats include a virulent form of influenza which is unlikely, as flu is spread by droplet infection (Ch 6), and it is difficult to understand how such an epidemic could have been restricted to one social class. Dr Caius had noted the susceptibility of the English upper classes to the disease and blamed it on some aspect of their diet. One recent suggestion is that it may have been caused by a hanta virus that produces similar symptoms to those described. This virus is carried by rodents such as mice, and is passed on when their droppings contaminate human food. This is a somewhat more likely explanation, as it is easy to envisage the upper classes and their servants eating certain types of food not available to the general peasantry.

All the attacks also occurred in the summer, leading to the suggestion that it might have been carried by an insect vector. There are some similarities between the Sweats and a disease known as relapsing fever, which is caused by spirochaetes carried by lice and ticks. This suggestion would also explain the recurrent attacks and the apparent lack of immunity developing, although again it is difficult to understand how this method of transfer would have been restricted to a single social class.

The disease polio shows a similar pattern in that, unlike many epidemic diseases, it attacks the middle classes and the better-off. These have a lower immunity than poorer people, who have come into contact with gastro-intestinal viruses more frequently, and therefore have a higher level of immunity. Polio was uncommon around 1900, with only a few hundred recognised cases, but by 1950, as public health measures improved, 60,000 new cases were occurring every year in the USA. Unlike many diseases, it did not get milder as time progressed, but the symptoms became more serious. Paralysis in an individual depended on whether the virus reached the Central Nervous System, in what quantities, and the damage done. The virus became a problem in advanced nations as the poverty levels fell, but there were relatively few cases in under-developed nations, as most children were immune by the age of three.

Polio is probably one of the first diseases that can be positively identified. Egyptian tomb paintings, dated to the Eighteenth Dynasty (*c*1580-1350BC), show an individual known as Roma, with the withered leg and the down-wards flexed foot that are characteristic of polio. Both Hippocrates and Galen describe clubfoot, and Galen distinguished between children born with a clubfoot and those who acquired it (through polio).

CHAPTER 2

The Early Development of Medicine

INTRODUCTION

The history of any science cannot be arranged in an orderly manner travelling in one direction only, and medicine is no exception. The practice of medicine evolved in many different parts of the world over a number of millennia, and took varying directions depending on the culture involved. Over time, theories and practices were accepted, expanded, fused or discarded as different societies came into contact with each other and exchanged ideas.

The excavation of a number of Neolithic graves in different areas shows that early man possessed the surgical skill to carry out trepanning of the skull, and the examination of skeletons indicates that some of the patients survived a sufficient length of time to allow the wound to heal. Trepanning was probably carried out in an attempt to exorcise demons, that is, to cure problems such as epilepsy and migraines. Skeletons from Neolithic graves in Europe, one as early as 4,900 BC, show that amputations were also carried out successfully using flint tools. The evidence for trepanning and amputations would suggest that soporific or hallucinogenic plants may have been used to subdue the patient.

If Neolithic people had this skill in surgery and were also able to prevent such a wound becoming infected, it is reasonable to suppose that they were aware of the curative properties of various plants and herbs for a variety of conditions. Much of this knowledge may have come from the observation of animals eating certain plants. The modern great apes certainly appear to be aware of the curative properties of some plants for problems such as intestinal worms. No doubt there would have been a process of trial and error attended by many mistakes and some fatalities.

Cave paintings in France and Spain dated to around 25,000 BC, show dancing figures dressed in animal skins and horns, some of whom appear to be acting as magicians or shamans. It is probable that any use of plants or herbs for medicinal purposes, by such shamans, would have been accompanied by ritual music, magic and sorcery[15].

One of the best examples of the early use of plants comes from the Monte Verde site in Chile. This archaeological site has been dated to about 10,500 BC, and is in an excellent state of preservation due to being sealed beneath a layer of peat bog. Numerous plants have been found at the site, including eighteen different ones that have medicinal properties and are still used by the local people to treat skin problems and chest infections. About half the plants were local, about half came from the coast about 50 miles away and one came from over 400 miles to the north. This would indicate that the group either ranged over a considerable area or that there were well developed trade routes even at this early date. Only those portions of the plants having medicinal properties were found, suggesting that this was their sole purpose.

Many ancient cultures invoked the supernatural, such as gods, to explain the causes of disease, the implication being that the diseased person had upset a deity or transgressed a ritual in some way. A typical example occurs in the opening book of the Iliad, when the Greek army is attacked by an epidemic caused by arrows fired by the god Apollo, as a punishment for the ill treatment of one of his priests; "[Apollo] *fired an arrow at men and hit them. The funeral pyres burned everywhere and did not stop*". The same symbolism is found in the Bible; "*I will heap*

---

15   Graves from later periods, that have been identified as belonging to shamans, frequently contain plants producing hallucinogenic drugs such as mescaline.

calamities upon them and spend my arrows against them. I will send famines, pestilence and plagues" (Deuteronomy 32, 23).

Apollo was considered by the Greeks to be the God of both Healing and Epidemics. Curiously he is also the God of Mice, and carvings of mice have been found in a number of his temples, leading one to speculate whether the early Greeks had made the connection between rodents and disease. Strabo had certainly made the connection by the first century BC stating, *"Pestilential diseases often ensue from mice"*.

The result of the belief that the gods sent disease, was that in many cultures of antiquity, medical treatment was part of a religious process with priests acting as doctors. Spells, talismans and amulets were widely used to fend off poisons, witchcraft, malignant demons, evil spirits and diseases.

In addition to their uses in medicine, humans have used plants and their extracts for several thousand years at least, for hunting, dyeing, inducing hallucinations, murder, suicide and judicial executions. It was frequently thought that the plant would give a sign for its use, for example, if the seed was heart shaped, it would be used to treat heart disease, if ear shaped it would treat earache. The effect of many of these plants depends on the dose administered and numerous plants generally considered poisonous may also have medicinal properties. For example, the alkaloid curare, produced by plants such as *Strychnos toxifera* is used in hunting, as it causes paralysis leading to asphyxiation. However, it is also used as a muscle relaxant during surgery. Other plants might be safe to use externally, but not internally, an example is the foxglove (*Digitalis purpurea)* that is poisonous if taken by mouth, but poultices of it are used to treat skin complaints.

As Shakespeare wrote in Romeo and Juliet,
> *"O mickle is the powerful grace that lies*
> *In herbs, plants, stones and their true qualities*
> *For naught so vile that on earth doth live*
> *But to earth some special good doth give*

. . . .

. . . .

> *Within the infant rind of this weak flower*
> *Poison hath residence and medicine power"*.

EGYPTIAN AND MIDDLE EASTERN MEDICINE

Possibly the earliest evidence of medicine is a seal from the city of Lagash in Mesopotamia, dated to about the fourth millennium BC, which is stamped with a deity thought to be the god of pestilence. Many authors claim that the first physician who can be identified is Imhotep (*ca* 2650BC), the chancellor, grand vizier and court physician of the Egyptian Pharaoh, Djoser of the Third Dynasty (*ca* 2686-2181BC). Imhotep was the architect of the step pyramid, the first of the stone pyramids at Saqqara, and the oldest stone pyramid in the world. Whilst he was obviously a polymath of great distinction, there is no contemporary evidence that definitely shows Imhotep was a physician. His tomb has not been discovered, but he was reputed to be the author of various medical texts, and is frequently shown in statues holding a scroll of papyrus. He became revered in Egypt as a demigod of medicine within a hundred years or so of his death, circumstantial evidence suggesting that he may have been a physician of some renown. He was later deified as the God of Wisdom and Medicine[16], and some authors link him to the later Greek God of Medicine, Asklepios.

The first recorded doctor is Hesy-ra, a doctor of the Third Dynasty, who would have been a near contemporary of Imhotep. His tomb has been found near that of Djoser, and it contained a number of stelae (stone slabs), one of which proclaims him to be *"chief of dentists and doctors"*. There is also evidence of women doctors at a very early stage, one tomb dating to the Fifth or Sixth Dynasty, refers to Peseshet with a text that has been translated as the *"lady director of the lady*

---

16   Hollywood also turned him into "The Mummy" in the film of that name!

physicians". Numerous other Egyptian doctors from the Old, Middle and New Kingdoms (Ch 5)[17] are known by name, and it is obvious that in many cases, the necessary learning was passed from father to children. In at least one case from the Middle Kingdom, the doctor also carries a further title that has been translated as "magician".

The practice of mummification meant that the Egyptians had a thorough knowledge of human anatomy that many other cultures probably lacked; in addition, the use of various resins and unguents in the mummification process gave them a wide chemical knowledge. Mummification has also given us a considerable amount of information about Egyptian diseases, and it is obvious that tuberculosis (Ch 11), bilharzia (Ch 19) and various types of worms were serious problems.

About twelve Egyptian medical papyri have been found, the two most important being the Ebers' papyrus and the Edwin Smith papyrus. The Ebers' papyrus dates to around 1550 BC, and was acquired by George Ebers in Thebes in the mid-nineteenth century. The papyrus is the longest medical one known, and appears to be a copy of several earlier papyri copied in a random manner. A number of plants known to have pharmacological properties are mentioned, along with spells for their use, and claims that some of the medicinal preparations had first been prepared by various gods.

A second papyrus, the Edwin Smith papyrus, is a treatise on surgery and the treatment of wounds, the description of some of these strongly suggesting that they are battle wounds. It has also been dated to around 1,550 BC, but some authors consider that the style of writing suggests that it is a copy of a much earlier work dated to around 3,000 BC. It would appear that surgeons would refuse to treat any patient they thought was not going to survive (and hence could not be blamed for being unsuccessful). The Smith papyrus is more or less free

---

17   Many of the existing medical papyri are thought to have been written during the Middle Kingdom (*ca* 2040-1795 BC) and the rest during the New Kingdom that dates from *ca* 1550-1069 BC.

of magic, and takes a very practical approach to dealing with injuries such as broken bones and dislocations. Papyrus was an expensive commodity and it was common to use the back as well as the front. The back of the Smith papyrus contains descriptions of medical problems not related to those on the front, and these rely heavily on magic. Unfortunately, neither the Smith nor Ebers papyri can be traced to the tomb(s) from which they were removed.

The Egyptians had a large collection of herbal preparations and minerals used to treat a wide variety of conditions ranging from arthritis to worms. The hieroglyphic names of a few cannot be translated, but over sixty per cent were drugs still in use in the early twentieth century for identical or very similar complaints.

Egyptian doctors in antiquity had an international reputation, and several instances are known of other rulers requesting one to be sent to their court. In the Odyssey, probably written around 800 BC, Polydamna, the wife of an Egyptian known as Thon, gave Helen of Troy a drug reputed to wipe grief and sorrow from the memory.

In the mid-fifth century BC, the Greek writer Herodotus, who travelled through Egypt, wrote that every court physician was in charge of a single illness. Medicine was frequently administered in beer, wine or honey, presumably to cover the taste, and many of the cures also involve advice over rest and diet that are not very different from modern day practices. He also stressed that Egyptian doctors were reluctant to consider the advances made by doctors of other nationalities, by this time the Greek medical schools such as Cos were thriving.

A major university was founded in Alexandria during the fourth century BC. A number of important scholars who studied there included Archimedes, Euclid and Ptolemy the astronomer, and it is known that medical students were required to train for four years. Both the university and its library were destroyed in the civil war of the late third century

AD at the time of Roman Emperor Aurelian. A daughter library was also destroyed in 391 AD by Christians, as part of a campaign against paganism.

About 280 BC, an Egyptian scribe, Manetho, was commissioned to write an Egyptian history by the Pharaoh Ptolemy II, and a considerable amount of our information is due to him. It is however, difficult to distinguish between fact and fiction, especially when he refers to the early pharaohs, as he is obviously quoting from earlier documents that have been lost.

The most important doctor of the Ptolemaic period was Herophilus of Chalcedon, a Greek doctor from Cos, who was born around 325 BC, but who practised in Alexandria under the patronage of Ptolemy I and II. He carried out dissections on the bodies of executed criminals, and also possibly vivisection on live criminals, making major advances on the structures of the brain, eyes, intestines and reproductive organs. Although his writings have not survived, both Galen and Celsus refer to him, and his name is still commemorated today, being used to describe certain anatomical features of the brain.

By the Middle Ages, the phrase *"learned in the wisdom of the Egyptians"* implied the possession of great knowledge. However, although they had a substantial and effective pharmacopoeia, much of Egyptian medicine included ritual magic and incantation and the Egyptians never managed to separate medicine from the priesthood.

In the eighteenth century BC, Hammurabi, King of Babylon, wrote the code of laws for which he is famous, which included the statement, *"I brought health to the land"*. Doctors were paid a fee for curing a patient, the actual amount depending on the status of the patient, irrespective of the problem. It also prescribed punishment for an unsuccessful physician. A doctor who killed a patient could have his hand amputated, however, if the patient was a slave the doctor only had to replace him. It is obvious that the medical profession was highly regulated and well organised even then, and was also involved with the priesthood.

The Babylonian God of Pestilence and Destruction, Nergal, was a mosquito-like insect, which given the number of diseases that mosquitoes can transmit, was not a bad guess for the second millennium BC. The Philistines also had a God of Pestilence, Beelzebub, Lord of the Flies, who is mentioned in the Bible (II Kings 1), again a good guess for the period.

Thousands of clay tablets dated to around 650 BC have been found from the reign of Ashurbanipal, King of Assyria, and are the remains of a large library at Nineveh, the first in the Middle East. A considerable number of these tablets are scientific and medical texts, listing several hundred recognisable herbs and drugs, many of which are known to possess therapeutic properties. In common with the Egyptian pharmacopoeia, a considerable percentage of these drugs appeared in early twentieth century pharmacopoeia, including such old favourites as castor oil, turpentine and mustard. It is reasonable to suppose that if the Assyrians were aware of castor oil, which is derived from the seeds of the castor bean plant (*Ricinus communis*), they were also aware of the poison ricin, which remains in the pulp after the oil has been extracted. The Assyrians were certainly not averse to using poison, in the sixth century BC they are recorded as contaminating the wells of enemies with ergot (Ch 1). Ricin is one of the most powerful poisons known, on a weight for weight basis, it is several times more poisonous than cobra venom, and can kill by ingestion, injection or inhalation. It was used by the Bulgarian secret service in London in 1978, to assassinate the Bulgarian dissident, Georgi Markov, by injecting him with a ricin pellet on the tip of an umbrella.

A university and medical school were founded in Gondeshapur by Khosrow I, who ruled the Sassanid Empire in Persia from 531-579 AD. He reputedly sent the physician Burzoe to India to obtain Sanskrit medical texts, which became the basis of the medical training in Persia (legend claims that he also brought the game of chess back with him). It was mainly through Gondeshapur that much of the Greek and Roman ideas reached the Muslims, after they conquered Persia, in the seventh and eight centuries AD.

CHINESE AND INDIAN MEDICINE

The earliest Chinese medical texts have been dated to the second and third millennia BC. One of the best known is the *Nei Ching,* which legend says was written by Huang Ti, the Yellow Emperor, in the third millennium BC. The present version, the *"Yellow Emperor's Classic of Internal Medicine"* was probably written between the third and first centuries BC. One of the diseases mentioned is a fever occurring at regular intervals and associated with an enlarged spleen, which is highly suggestive of malaria. A major problem relating to the study of Chinese medicine in antiquity is that although a number of medical documents exist, very few have been translated into a western European language. Many documents were also destroyed by the orders of the Emperor, Qin Shi Huangdi[18], (the builder of the Great Wall and the founder of China) at the end of the third century BC.

Chinese medicine is based on the balance of Yin (female) and Yang (male) elements of the body, and the role of the physician was to control the level and balance of these. In the early stages especially, treatment was irreversibly intertwined with ancestor worship, and propitiating them with sacrifices. Demons and evil spirits were blamed for sickness and required ritual exorcism and it has been suggested that the origin of acupuncture was the killing of demons, which had entered the body, with needles that represented symbolic spears and swords[19].

---

18   Of Terracota Warrior fame.
19   One modern attempt at explaining acupuncture speculates that it stimulates the release of chemicals known as endorphins in the brain. These mimic the behaviour of pain suppressing compounds such as morphine and its derivatives.

An Imperial University was founded in 124 BC and taught medicine as one of the subjects. Hospices and hospitals appeared around 500 AD, and in the seventh century AD, an Imperial medical school was started and qualifying examinations were introduced. The first known Chinese pharmacopoeia was produced in the eighth century AD, and medicine developed very strongly in the direction of herbal remedies and drugs. Surgery played a small part and only developed to a rudimentary level; surgeons were considered inferior to physicians. The only operation routinely practised was castration, which was used widely to produce large numbers of court eunuchs. Numerous medical documents describing drugs have been found in tombs of the period 200 BC-100 AD, and in 1596 AD, Li Shih Chen collected numerous papers and published a pharmacopoeia of fifty-two volumes. This contained more than 11,000 drugs and prescriptions. Several of the drugs mentioned have made their way into Western medicine, including the use of chaulmoogra oil for the treatment of leprosy. However, the most important modern day medicine to emerge from traditional Chinese herbal treatments is an extract of sweet wormwood, used for centuries as a treatment for malaria. A study of this extract has led to the production of the potent anti-malarial drug, artemisinin (Ch 16) in recent years.

In India, several different types of medicine developed, the earliest records being the sacred texts known as the Vedas, especially the Athavaveda, which probably dates to the second millenium BC. Vedic medicine mentions a number of recognisable problems such as fevers, coughs, leprosy and diarrhoea, and recommends various herbal remedies for their treatment.

Later texts known as the Carake-Samhita and Susruta-Samhita, named after the physicians they are associated with, appeared in the first millennium BC. Much of the later Indian medicine was based on the versions of these texts written between about 100-700 AD, which are closely intertwined with philosophy and religion. A number of recognisable diseases are mentioned, including pulmonary tuberculosis, smallpox and malaria. Many of the treatments used herbs and their extracts from indigenous plants, and also mineral medicines based on sulphur and arsenic. These were frequently administered with prayers, whilst malignant demons were invoked to explain the causes of many diseases. Personal hygiene was also recognised as important, as were dietary measures. Herbal treatments are also mentioned in a number of Hindu treatises on veterinary medicine.

The Indians had a good knowledge of herbal preparations and were not averse to using them as poisons and weapons. Candragupta (ruled 321-297 BC), who founded the Mauryan Empire, and was the first emperor to unify most of India, had a strategist, Kautila, who sounds like an early version of Machiavelli. Kautila was instrumental in helping Candragupta to overthrow the Nanda Dynasty, and wrote a book on statecraft, the *"Arthasastra"*, in which he gave details of numerous poisonous weapons emphasising their propaganda value. Perhaps his most frightening suggestion was to tip arrows with the blood of animals suffering from rabies. Kautila also suggested remedies for these weapons, probably the first recognition that biological weapons are two-edged swords that might cut the user. Not surprisingly, Kautila was alternately praised for his statecraft and condemned for his ruthlessness.

Greek Medicine

It is impossible to determine how much of their medical knowledge the Greeks obtained from other sources such as Egypt, but they were the first people to develop rational medicine free of magic, shamanism, witchcraft and religion. This was an extension of the ideas of the philosophers of the sixth century BC, who attempted to explain the environment in non-supernatural terms. The Roman physician Celsus, credits Hippocrates as being the first to separate the practice of medicine from philosophy and religion, although it is probable that this started several generations earlier and was a gradual process. Only a small amount of pre-Hippocratic material survives, some of it attributed to Alcmaeon of Croton whose work is dated to the early fifth century BC. This suggests that medicine was being separated from religion before Hippocrates, although there is considerable disagreement whether Alcmaeon was in fact a doctor. Certainly by the time of Hippocrates, Greek doctors considered disease to be a natural phenomenon rather than a supernatural one, and were looking for both the cause and a rational cure.

The Greeks had a long history of medicine, starting with Asklepios (Aesculepius). Legend states he was one of the warriors who fought in the Trojan War around 1000 BC and his two sons were described by Homer as also being skilled physicians. One of them, Machaon, healed Menalaus after he was struck by a Trojan arrow, and also treated Philoctetes, who had been injured by a poisoned arrow and abandoned by his fellow Greeks on the way to Troy, as the wound smelt so badly. Some legends claimed that Askelepios was the son of Apollo, the God of Medicine, other legends claim that Apollo passed the secrets of medicine to the centaur, Chiron, who taught Asklepios.

Castor and Pollux, the twin sons of Zeus were also considered to be healers, and later became associated in Christianity with the saints Cosmas and Damian, the patron saints of physicians.

The Greeks had an excellent knowledge of plants and their pharmaceutical properties[20]. One of the earliest documented examples of biological warfare was the poisoning of drinking water during the First Sacred War in the sixth century BC. The city of Kirrha had been attacking pilgrims visiting the sacred shrine of Apollo at Delphi, and the other Greek City States banded together to deal with the problem. Apollo, the father of medicine, cursed Kirrha and the rest of the Greeks probably

---

20   The words pharmacy and pharmacist are both derived from the Greek word *pharmakon,* which means drug or poison.

considered they were carrying out his instructions. The water into the city was cut off and then reinstated several days later after it had been poisoned with extracts of aconite, also known as monkshood or wolf's bane. This extremely poisonous plant was dedicated to Hecate, the Queen of Hell, and was the plant traditionally used in Greek mythology by the witch, Medea, in an attempt to poison the hero Theseus. It still causes fatal poisoning today usually being mistaking for horse-radish.

In the case of Kirrha, the inhabitants drank the poisoned water, and those who survived were slaughtered whilst helpless with diarrhoea. Very small doses of aconite were used by physicians, such as Hippocrates, as a purgative to treat problems caused by intestinal worms, larger doses paralyse the nervous system and cause death. Several versions of this story are known, and the suggestion has been made that the proceedings were regarded with such abhorrence that attempts were made to spread the blame. Two of the people implicated were Solon, the sage of Athens, and Nebros, an Asklepiad, who was claimed to be an ancestor of Hippocrates. It is probably the first suggestion of a doctor being involved in waging biological warfare, and it has been suggested that it was possibly the origin of the Hippocratic oath, as Hippocrates was attempting to undo the damage caused by one of his ancestors, and ensure it never happened again.

In the aftermath of the Sacred War, the Greek City States reached an agreement that poisoning drinking water was an unacceptable form of warfare. Presumably this only applied to fellow Greeks, as the Athenians did it in 478 BC as part of their scorched earth policy against the Persian invaders.

Whilst the Greeks may have regarded using chemical warfare against fellow Greeks as abhorrent, they had no qualms about using the Scythians as mercenaries. They were notorious for poisoning barbed arrows by dipping them in either hemlock, or a combination of snake venom and rotting flesh. If the poison did not kill their enemies, then there was an excellent chance of them dying of tetanus or gangrene. The psychological effect of such weapons was (and still is) immense, and the Scythians defeated the Romans and Persians, who were both terrified of them.

The chemical and herbal knowledge of many of these ancient cultures is frequently underestimated today, to give just one example, by 424 BC the Boeotian allies of the Spartans had created a primitive flame-thrower based on pitch and sulphur, which was used as a siege weapon.

By the eighth century BC, Asklepios was being invested with supernatural powers, and his emblem of the serpent was frequently depicted as the symbol of healing. The symbol of twin serpents wrapped around a staff was known as a caduceus, and was carried traditionally by Hermes and Mercury, the Messengers of the Gods. It was also carried by Greek and Roman heralds, and a version with a single serpent is still used to denote medicine today, and may be seen in the badge of the Royal Army Medical Corps. Some authors have suggested that the serpent is the Guinea worm (Ch 4) being wound out of a lesion on a piece of stick. The Guinea worm is described in a number of early writings and is thought to be the fiery serpent of the Bible (Ch 1). This ancient medical practice is described by both the Greeks and Romans, and many traditional healers still treat infections of the Guinea worm in this manner.

Over three hundred temples were dedicated to the cult of Asklepios at its peak, the centre being at Epidauros. This contained a hospital, where the priests dispensed medicines, together with baths, a theatre, a stadium, hotels and a library. It was thought that Asklepios would visit patients in their dreams whilst they slept and give advice that would cure them. Many of these temples were based in areas possessing the hot springs that are common in volcanic areas such as Greece. Such springs have been, and still are, used widely in the treatment of problems such as rheumatism, arthritis and skin complaints. Evidence suggests that much of the priestly treatment was based on sensible advice regarding diet, rest and the use of herbal treatments of various types, reinforced by magic.

A number of medical schools appeared throughout Greece, one of the earliest being the medical school of Croton, derived from the philosophy school founded in the late sixth century BC by Pythagoras of Samos[21]. The most famous member was Empedocles, who taught that there were four elements, earth, air, fire and water, and four qualities, hot, cold, moist and dry. His philosophy was that health depended on the harmony of the elements of the body, and disease was caused by an imbalance. This ultimately produced the theory of the four humours of the body that so bedevilled medicine for the next two millennia[22]. Empedocles also realised that swamps produce disease, and stopped an outbreak of fever (apparently malaria) in Selinos in Sicily, by draining the adjacent marshes. A series of coins was struck to commemorate this and show a sacrifice being made to Asklepios.

Fifth century BC vases showing doctors holding clinics have been found by archaeologists. These show that by this time doctors were secular, independent of the temples and priests, and were obviously highly regarded, two generations before Hippocrates.

The best known centre of Greek medicine however, was on the island of Cos. Hippocrates (*ca* 460-377BC), sometimes known as "*the father of medicine*" was assumed to be a member of the "medical school" of Cos, indeed Plato refers to him as the "*Asklepiad of Cos*". Numerous documents known as the *Corpus Hippocraticum* have been attributed to him. Whether any of them were actually written by Hippocrates is uncertain, but

---

21   Pythagoras is better known today for his influence in mathematics, especially geometry.

22   Geoffrey Chaucer (*ca* 1340-1400) describes the Doctor of Physik in *Canterbury Tales* (written in the 1390s) as follows.

> *"He knew the cause of every malady*
> *Whether of hot or cold or moist or dry*
> *And where engendered and of what humour*
> *He was a very perfect practitioner".*

they appear to be the collective teachings of the Cos "medical school", of which Hippocrates seems to be the most senior member[23]. Until this time, Greek medical tradition is mainly oral.

Evidence suggests that there were originally approximately seventy documents of which about sixty survive. The collection is obviously written by a number of different physicians with very different styles, and the style of writing in the documents suggests that at least a century separates the earliest and latest. Part of the *Corpus Hippocraticum* includes a treatise on epidemics consisting of seven books, written by at least two authors. These documents describe both malaria and tuberculosis, they make it obvious that malaria was a very serious problem[24], and that TB was recognised as contagious. Smallpox, syphilis and bubonic plague are not mentioned, suggesting that these diseases were not known in the Greek world because the symptoms of all three are fairly obvious, even to the untrained observer. Some authors think that Hippocrates does mention buboes that might suggest plague, but the context is ambiguous, and could refer to the swollen glands that are found in numerous diseases. Rather curiously, Hippocrates does not mention the Plague of Athens, which would have occurred during his lifetime, leading one to suspect that it may be described in the missing portion of the *Corpus Hippocraticum.*

Other epidemic diseases described by Hippocrates include an outbreak of (possibly) mumps on the Island of Thassos in the northern Aegean, and an epidemic in what is now modern day Turkey, that may have been either whooping cough or diphtheria. Diarrhoea, dysentery and pneumonia are described, and it appears that dysentery was a serious problem

---

23   Two other physicians frequently mentioned with Hippocrates are Praxagoras and Chrysippus. Praxagoras was the mentor of Herophilus, who was mentioned earlier.

24   The Greeks had recognized by this time that malaria was associated with marshes.

in the army, suggesting overcrowded barracks with inadequate sanitation. Another part of the *Corpus Hippocraticum* is *De aere, aquis et locis* (Concerning air, water and places) which is a study of human ecology. This lays a lot of importance on diet, and comments that, *"our nature is the physician of our diseases"* and suggests that the role of the doctor is to encourage self-healing. The importance of the *Corpus Hippocraticum* is that it emphasises the observation of the individual patient, stresses the importance of putting the symptoms into the correct sequence and then using these to deduce the nature of the disease. This is obviously the method still used by physicians today.

Many of the documents from the Cos medical school were copied, and subsequently appeared in the Great Library of Alexandria in Egypt around 200 BC, where a medical school had started around 300 BC. From there they were later incorporated into Islamic medicine.

The Greeks also practiced surgery as well as medicine, around 400 BC the surgeon, Diokles of Karystos, invented instruments for removing barbed arrow heads from wounds without causing further damage to the victim.

ROMAN MEDICINE

In early Roman medicine, the head of the household treated families by making sacrifices to the gods and using herbal remedies. There were a large number of gods, and if the cure did not work, the wrong god had been invoked or the sacrifice had been inadequate. Pliny the Elder suggested that Romans had done without doctors for centuries and did not need them. At a later date, rich families had their own physician who was usually a Greek slave skilled in medicine. Public doctors were of low social status, there was no regulation of medical practitioners and they were frequently little better than quacks.

Physicians and surgeons in the Roman Army had their own corps and uniform, and were well trained and respected and

Roman military doctors in distinctive uniforms are depicted on Trajan's column, the record of Roman campaigns against the Dacians.

The most important Roman doctor was Claudius Galen of Pergamon (129-216 AD), a Greek living in Rome, who regarded Hippocrates as the most influential figure in medicine (after himself). Galen is alleged to have stated that, "*I have done for medicine what Trajan did for Rome when he built roads and bridges. It is I alone who have showed the true path of medicine, Hippocrates mapped the path, but I have trodden it*". Galen had an excellent knowledge of physiology and anatomy from time spent working as a physician to gladiators, and he wrote a great deal, providing us with a large amount of information on ancient medicine. Much of his work was translated into Arabic around 850 AD. He is thought to have written over five hundred texts, the main one being "*Ars Magna*" which effectively became the bible of medicine for the next fifteen hundred years. Although some of Galen's observations were important, for example, he also made the connection between the expansion of cities into marshland and fever (malaria), his influence was such that some of his incorrect ideas influenced and impeded the study of medicine until well into the Renaissance period. Galen did realise however, that water passing through lead pipes could be a problem, and a number of his prescriptions stipulate that water supplied through lead pipes should be avoided. Perhaps one of the most important aspects of Galen's writings today, is that he makes us aware of some of the earlier information and manuscripts that have been lost. Unfortunately, a considerable amount of Galen's work was also lost following a serious fire in his drug store.

Galen considered that four humours, blood, phlegm, melancholy (black bile) and choler (yellow bile) were found throughout the body, and that sickness was caused by an imbalance of these humours. Each humour was characterised by a pair of qualities, of which there were four, wet, dry, hot and cold. Blood was hot and wet, choler was hot and dry, melancholy was dry and cold whilst phlegm was wet and cold. These produced the four temperaments, sanguine, choleric, melancholic and phlegmatic, with each individual being placed in one of these categories. Treatment of an imbalance was by application of the opposite, thus as blood was hot and wet, an excess of blood could be cured by blood-letting, the application of leeches or by dosing the patient with a cooling or drying medicine. Fevers were thought to be caused by excess blood putrefying and could be cured by bloodletting, whilst excess bile could be cured by inducing vomiting or diarrhoea.

Many of Galen's teachings were followed for nearly fifteen hundred years, and although the Arabs did question some of them, it was not until the time of Renaissance physicians and alchemists, such as Paracelsus (1493-1541), that many of Galen's ideas started to be challenged and eventually overthrown.

Galen was not the only Greek physician living in Rome whose influence was important in later centuries. The Greek physician Dioscorides, who served in the Roman army, wrote a collection of medicinal and pharmaceutical texts in the first century AD. His book *"De Materia Medica"* written between 41-68 AD, that details about one thousand drugs and herbal remedies, was first translated into English in 1665, and used widely in English medicine until the eighteenth and nineteenth centuries. One of the herbal preparations mentioned is *Aloe vera*, which he claimed stopped the spitting of blood and cured genital ulcers. Modern research has shown that extracts kill the bacterium *Mycobacterium tuberculosis*, the causative organism of tuberculosis (Ch 11), and heal sores caused by the *Herpes* virus.

Another doctor of note was Aulus Cornelius Celsus, who wrote an encyclopaedia of which only the medical portion, *De Medicina*, survived. This disappeared for centuries, was rediscovered by Pope Nicholas V in the fifteenth century, and was one of the first medical texts to be printed. This work is the source of much of our knowledge of Greek medicine. Celsus also had some very modern ideas about the treatment of wounds, recommending that they should be kept clean and washed with mild antibacterial agents such as spirits and vinegar.

The Romans did not introduce many new ideas in medicine, they mainly recycled Greek ones. On the other hand, they were very good at practical aspects of medicine, such as the organisation of hospitals, especially military ones, and also the organisation of many aspects of public health, such as the piping of clean water into towns via aqueducts, an idea that may have been copied from the Etruscans. There was however a huge gulf between rich and poor in Rome; although the rich could afford to have water piped into their homes, the poor had to collect it from public fountains.

Whilst the basic idea of hospitals in Europe goes back to the Greeks, who probably got the idea from Egypt, the organisation required to run an effective hospital on a large scale is definitely Roman, and was honed by the Roman military machine. The military base at Novaesium in Germany had a hospital with forty wards, a pharmacy, its own kitchens, refectory and administration buildings. In Britain, large amounts of the herb centaury, a member of the gentian family, have been found in military bases. This was used widely to dry septic wounds, and was named after the centaur, Chiron, who in mythology taught man the secrets of medicine. By 325 AD, the emperor, Constantine the Great, had decreed that every cathedral city in the empire should have a hospital.

By the end of the fourth century, Christianity had become the official religion of the Roman Empire. Rome had been seriously weakened by numerous epidemics, and if something unseen and not understood, is killing a large percentage of the population, any religion promising an after-life has a considerable advantage. There is also a Christian tradition of helping the sick that would have reinforced the message.

Many of the miracles of the New Testament are medical, raising the dead, healing the sick (e.g. lepers) and casting out devils. The image is therefore of Christ the Healer who transfers his healing powers to his disciples, *"He called his twelve disciples together, and gave them power and authority over all devils and to cure disease"* (Luke 9.1). The Christian church therefore assumed that Christ's divine healing powers had devolved to them, and medical practice passed into the hands of the Church, a situation that more or less continued until the middle of the second millennium AD.

The church line was that disease was a punishment for sin, and if God decided to cure the patient (sinner), this would be done by divine intervention. Saints were invoked to intercede with God on behalf of the sick person and some of these saints became identified with some of the earlier Roman gods. Saint Sebastian, the patron saint of epidemics, is usually depicted as a beautiful young man being shot with arrows. In mythology, the arrows of Apollo (who is also a beautiful young man), rained diseases on humans and as St Sebastian survived the arrows it enabled him to protect people who had been attacked in a similar manner.

Pre-Columbian Medicine in the Americas

Very little evidence exists regarding pre-Columbian medicine in the Americas as the Spanish destroyed most of it, frequently on religious grounds. The small amount that can be found mentioned in Spanish documents, indicate that the Aztec and Inca cultures had a large pharmacopoeia based on plants, which was used for a wide variety of treatments. The most important of the herbal products to come out of the Americas was the bark of the *Cinchona* tree that contained the alkaloid quinine, used for treating fevers and malaria (Ch 16).

Islamic Medicine

Islamic mathematics, science, cartography and medicine were far in advance of Western European knowledge of these subjects from the eighth to the twelfth centuries. The numerals 1-9, which we use today, all came to the West from Arabic sources although their origins were Hindu. They also developed the concept of zero and the use of the decimal point. These ideas replaced the cumbersome Roman numerals that had been used for centuries, and were transmitted to the West by trade, travelling scholars, the Arab conquests that started in the seventh century and the crusades that started in the late eleventh century. The importance of the Arabs to mathematics is seen by the use of words such as zero, zenith and algebra, all of which are derived from Arabic words. A similar situation is found in chemistry, words such as alchemy, alcohol, alkali and elixir are all Arabic in origin although the meanings have changed somewhat.

The main problem in early Islamic medicine was the clash between the priests and mystics, who believed that illness was the Will of God, and thus could only be cured by prayer, and the doctors or hakims who believed in secular medical practices. The theologians and priests finally gained the upper hand and Islamic medicine and science went into a steep decline by the twelfth century. This decline was exacerbated to a considerable extent by the destruction of many Islamic cities by the Mongols in 1219, and again in 1258. In addition to destroying Baghdad and other cities, they also destroyed the qanats (the covered irrigation channels), thus destroying the infrastructure of the irrigation system. Although Baghdad was rebuilt, it was destroyed again in 1384 by the army of Tamerlane who boasted that he found a city and left a mountain of skulls.

Much of early Islamic medicine was a collection of rules emphasising both physical and spiritual (mental) health. Islamic medicine is to some extent a descendant of classical Greek ideas and practices. Many of the Greek ideas were carried eastwards by the Nestorians (after they were expelled from Byzantium for heresy in 431 AD), and adopted initially by the Persians, and then by Islam. Islam was an extremely open society at that time, prepared to accept ideas in science and medicine from a wide range of sources, including Christian, Jewish, Persian, Hindu and pagan ones. The importation from Greek sources did cause problems later as the Nestorians translated Greek into Syriac (the language of ancient Syria, a relative of Aramaic), and Syriac into Arabic. When these Arabic documents were translated into Latin, so that Islamic ideas of medicine could reach Western Europe after the Crusades, the Greek originals had frequently become badly distorted following three or four translations. By this time, very few people in Western Europe could read the original documents in classical Greek as the study of this had virtually vanished after the collapse of the Western Roman Empire in the fifth century.

Islamic doctors were highly regarded from the ninth century onwards, with much of their teaching being used in medieval Europe. Islamic science and medicine reached their height during the reign of the Abbasid caliph al-Mamun, (the son of Harun al-Raschid [of the Thousand and One Nights]), who reigned in Baghdad from 813-833 AD, a period known as the Golden Age[25]. Al-Mamun created the House of Wisdom in Baghdad. This was a combination of royal library, academy of scholars (university) and state translation bureau containing thousands of books, at a time when western monasteries were considered rich if their library contained a few dozen manuscripts.

The caliphs continued to support the medical school in Gondeshapur (Jundashapur) that had been established by the Persians, and a medical library was founded in Baghdad in the ninth century, during the reigns of Harun al-Raschid and

---

25   The Abbasid caliphs defeated the Umayyad caliphs in 750 AD, and in 762 they abandoned Damascus as the capital of the caliphate and relocated to Baghdad. After the death of Harun al-Raschid, there was a civil war between his sons, Amin and al- Mamun, in which al-Mamun was successful. In 861 AD, the ruling caliph was assassinated by his bodyguards initiating a civil war that lasted for nine years. The Abbasid caliphate was the last time that the Muslim world was politically united.

al-Mamun. This was under the control of a doctor known in Europe as Mesue the Elder (Yuhanna ibn Masawaih), who was personal physician to the caliphs, and whose writings included work on leprosy and various fevers. Islam encouraged public medicine and care, and the rich frequently paid for charitable works such as the care of the poor and the provision and staffing of hospitals.

Other major centres of Arab learning sprang up, including Cordova and Toledo in Spain, which was under Muslim rule at this time. After the fall of the Umayyid Caliphate, the sole surviving Umayyid prince, Abd al-Rahman, fled to Spain and eventually became ruler of Cordova. This city became a centre of learning to rival Baghdad with huge libraries, one of which was reputed to contain four hundred thousand volumes.

Important Arab/Persian doctors of the period included Rhazes (Abu al-Rhazi, *ca* 865-930), a polymath best known as a doctor, who wrote a medical encyclopaedia of over twenty volumes that was a compendium of Greek, Syrian, Indian and Arabic medicine. He was also a chemist who contributed to the knowledge of a wide variety of pharmacological drugs and herbs. He is best known in Western Europe however, as the doctor who first distinguished between smallpox and measles, writing a treatise that was translated into both Latin and Greek, and hence into many modern European languages. Unusually for the age, he also wrote a book querying numerous aspects of Galen's work.

Another important Arab polymath, widely regarded as a doctor, was Avicenna (980-1037), known as the Prince of Physicians, whose tomb is still a place of pilgrimage. His book, *"Canon of Medicine"*, was used and quoted in European medical schools until the seventeenth century. Avicenna (Abu ibn Sina) gave a very accurate account of leprosy, and although there are earlier descriptions in the Bible, and by Hippocrates and Galen, they are very general and could apply to a number of skin complaints. He also wrote an epidemiological account of various rash-producing diseases. Although the postulated cause of these diseases was totally incorrect (an extension of Galen's four humours theory), he was aware that the later in life a person encountered such diseases, the more serious the outcome would probably be. One book he wrote refuted astrology as the cause of disease, at a time when astrology was a major influence on many aspects of life. Avicenna was also reputed to have invented the process of distilling volatile oils from plants[26], and fifteenth century Hebrew translations of his *"Canon of Medicine"*, contain illustrated pages showing him teaching his pupils in the corner of a well stocked pharmacy, an indication of the importance of drugs in Arabic medicine.

Although surgery was considered inferior to medicine, the first illustrated surgery text written by Abu al-Qasim al-Zahrawi of Andalusia (936-1013, known in the West as Albucasis), was used to teach surgical procedures in European medical schools for about five hundred years. He also invented numerous surgical instruments that were the prototypes of many still in use today, and in addition, provided the first known description of the genetic disease, haemophilia (bleeding disease).

The surgical work of Albucasis was translated by Gerard of Cremona, one of the most important twelfth century translators, who also translated the work of Avicenna. Another important translator was Hunayn ibn Ishaq (Johannitius) who translated the work of Galen into Arabic, and also corrected it where he perceived mistakes and limitations. One of the major problems for the translators, especially when translating from Greek into Arabic, was to find the appropriate scientific or medical term, as in the initial stages Arabic did not have an extensive scientific vocabulary. The Romans had the same problem when translating from Greek to Latin, and Lucretius, writing in the first century BC, uses an extremely convoluted style.

---

26   The word alcohol was originally derived from an Arab word meaning anything that could be distilled.

Stephen of Pisa (Stephen the Philosopher) translated the *"Royal Book"*, a medical encyclopaedia written in the tenth century by al-Abbas al-Mujisi (known in the West as Haly Abbas) from Arabic to Latin. The importance of this particular piece of scholarship was that Stephen prepared a glossary of Arabic and Greek medical terms with Latin translations and commentaries that was used in Western Europe for centuries.

Part of the reason for the success story of translation and the rapid spread of knowledge, is probably due to the introduction of paper from China into the Arab Caliphate in the mid-eighth century. Paper was much cheaper than vellum or parchment and is simpler to use, making it easier to both copy and store books leading to the development of extensive libraries. By the end of the eighth century, there was a paper-making factory in Baghdad.

Hospitals were also established under Islam. One founded by Ibn Barmar, Vizier to Harun al-Raschid, in the early ninth century, contained both doctors and pharmacists, and also provided training for medical students. Students who had completed their training in medicine and pharmacy, were required to pass exams before being issued with licences allowing them to practice. At this time there was very little organised medicine in Europe, and the Holy Roman Emperor, Charlemagne, sent to Harun al-Raschid requesting a doctor for his court, and was sent a Jewish doctor, Rabbi Mahir.

Islamic medicine was significantly more advanced than European medicine by the end of the Crusades. Numerous influential books had been translated from Arabic into Latin and still influenced some thinking in western medicine as late as the seventeenth century. However, by the end of the sixteenth century, the flow of ideas had started to be reversed, and Islamic doctors were beginning to follow European practices in the treatment of certain diseases such as syphilis.

By the mid-seventeenth century, ibn Sallum, physician to the Ottoman sultans, was referring to the practices of Paracelsus.

JEWISH MEDICINE

Jewish medicine was an important source of material to the medicine of many other cultures, as the Diaspora of 70 AD, which expelled the Jews from the Holy Land, meant that many of their theories relating to medicine were spread throughout the Old World. Jewish medicine was based to a large extent on the Old Testament (especially Leviticus), probably written about 1,000 BC and the Talmud, a set of rules written between *ca* 700 BC-200 AD. The central thrust of Jewish medicine was hygiene and public health measures associated with the prevention of disease, and relatively low priority was given to therapy or surgery.

Much of their medicine related to the fact that personal cleanliness was considered necessary for religious purity and medicine was therefore a by-product of religious ritual. Many of the early physicians were rabbis and unusually for early cultures, there was very little reliance on magic. Their ideas on public health were very advanced for the period, and they formulated rules for controlling diseases. These were based on the belief that many diseases were spread by personal contact and contaminated food and water; for example, no wells for drinking water were allowed near cemeteries. They suggested the best ways of dealing with epidemics were isolation of the sick person, avoidance of flies and fumigation.

Perhaps one of the most important comments on Jewish medicine of the period was that the Sultan, Salah ah Din (Saladin), who died in 1193, appointed the Jewish Rabbi, Moses ben Maimon (Moses Maimonides), from Cordova in Andalusia, as his personal physician. Maimonides wrote widely on medical matters including a list of public health rules that would be considered acceptable today.

POST ROMAN MEDICINE IN WESTERN EUROPEAN

The early Christians frequently regarded disease as a divine punishment for sin, and as such, the only cures were prayer and penance. As a result, medicine was based to a large extent on prayer, blessings, exorcism, and the laying on of hands. Whilst this may have been of some use for problems of mental health, it was of no use at all in dealing with practical matters such as the epidemics that swept Western Europe during the Dark Ages[27]. A small number of monasteries, in countries such as Ireland, would have had monks skilled in herbal medicine, but their medicine would still have involved large amounts of prayer.

The Saxon remedies in Dark Age Europe were based on a mixture of herbal medicine reinforced with large doses of magic, sorcery, and astrology. Many of the illuminated Anglo-Saxon manuscripts of the period depicting recipes for cures, show a worm (serpent or dragon) being driven out of the afflicted person by the treatment. Worms were blamed for many ills, heart-worms in the case of sudden death and tooth worms were thought to cause tooth decay. By around 1100 AD, much of the medical knowledge available in England was being prescribed by monks, with many abbeys and monasteries having an infirmarer, or herbalist, skilled in the use of medicinal herbs, who was also responsible for the infirmary or hospice. The intercession of saints was also important, and one of the main shrines in England was that of Thomas Beckett at Canterbury, which was famous for curing disease (making Canterbury rich in the process). Many of the Saxon ideas about medicine persisted in England until the thirteenth century.

27   The term Dark Ages is usually taken to refer to the period between the end of the Western Roman Empire (late fifth century AD) and the formation of the Holy Roman Empire (800 AD), a time about which there is relatively little contemporary information. Many historians now refer to this period as the Early Middle Ages, to avoid the connotations of barbarism and ignorance usually associated with the term Dark Ages. Much of this association is due to the influence of Edward Gibbon (1737-94) who wrote, *"Decline and Fall of the Roman Empire"*.

In medieval times, the causes of disease were frequently thought to be celestial. A single cause could lead to a number of different diseases, depending on the humours of the person infected. It was also thought that a single disease could arise from a number of causes, and that diseases could change into each other, under the influence of astrological phenomena, such as the alignment of the planets and stars. Chaucer in the *Canterbury Tales,* describes the "Doctor of Physik" as *"skilled in astrology"*[28] and the University of Bologna had a professor teaching medical students about the influence of astrology on the body.

The most notorious of these astrologer physicians, albeit at a somewhat later date, was Michel de Notredame or Nostradamus (1503-1566). He gained great notoriety for his book of poems entitled *"Centuries"* published in 1555, which claimed to predict the future, and in 1560, he was appointed physician to the French king, Charles IX. Belief in his predictions still has a wide following today, with many people believing he prophesied World War II and numerous other major events of the twentieth century.

One of the features of the twelfth century was the development of numerous organisations of warrior monks, who founded hospitals to tend sick pilgrims in the Holy Land. These included the Knights of St John, the Templars and the various Teutonic Orders of Knights. A further development of the late twelfth and thirteenth centuries was the foundation of large numbers of lazarettes, hospitals dedicated to the treatment of lepers (Ch 11). It is estimated there were nearly 20,000 lazarettes or lazar houses in Europe in the thirteenth century. In the fourteenth century as the incidence of leprosy fell, many of them became plague hospitals (pest houses)[29].

---

28 Chaucer obviously had a low opinion of doctors, whom he claimed, *"loved gold"*. He was not alone in this opinion, as the Monkey Window in York Minister, made around 1325, depicts monkeys as doctors, one of them examining a patient and another examining a flask of urine.

29 The concept of isolation, or quarantine of infectious people, first

The first recognisable, non-Islamic, medical school in Europe after the Dark Ages appeared in Salerno in Sicily in the ninth century, which by the eleventh and twelfth centuries was known as the Civitas Hippocratica (City of Hippocrates) due to its fame. Tradition has it that the medical school was founded by four doctors, one Jewish, one Muslim, one Latin and one Greek. Major features of this medical school were that it was secular, and did not require students to be priests, and also accepted women and Jews as students. Salerno is thought to be the oldest European university having a curriculum prescribed by the state; in 1140, Roger II, King of Sicily passed an act requiring students wishing to practice medicine to pass exams, the penalty for failure being imprisonment and confiscation of all of their goods[30]. The following century, his grandson, Frederick II, King of Sicily and Holy Roman Emperor (who was known to his contemporaries as Stupor Mundi [the Wonder of the World]), decreed a curriculum requiring medical students to study logic for three years, and medicine, including surgery, for a further five. No one was allowed to practice medicine until he had been examined and approved by the Faculty at Salerno. He also recognised pharmacy as a subject distinct from medicine, and laid down a code of ethics for both.

European medical schools such as Bologna, Paris, Padua, Oxford and Cambridge sprang up in the thirteenth and fourteenth centuries. Montpellier University was teaching medicine in the early twelfth century, and a Faculty of Medicine was formed in 1221, although the Papal Bull establishing the university only dates from 1289. The medical school at Paris however, still only contained a handful of books at the end of the fourteenth century, reflecting the fact that medicine was not regarded as a major subject, compared with subjects such as theology, canon law and logic. Medical schools at this time

---

appeared as a response to leprosy, and is mentioned in the Bible.

30   That no doubt concentrated a few minds, one wonders what the effect of such an edict would be on the student population today.

still had their syllabus constrained by the Church; they were mainly recycling the theories of the ancients, such as Galen, and most academic disputes were over the precise translation or meaning of some ancient, frequently obscure and incorrect text.

A number of important European teachers are found during this period, one of the most eminent being the Franciscan monk, Roger Bacon (1220-1292), who taught at Oxford. He is reputed to be the European discoverer of gunpowder, although the Chinese had been using it since about the ninth century, and is also alleged to have used a simple microscope to study cells. However, his greatest contribution to science and medicine was that he did not accept the teachings of the ancients, but considered that theories should be proved by experiment, an idea that is now universally accepted, but which at that time was totally revolutionary and heretical. Whilst Bacon is alleged to have used a microscope first, there are suspicions that he obtained the idea from his mentor, Robert Grosseteste (Bighead) (1175-1253), Bishop of Lincoln and Chancellor of Oxford University, who wrote various treatises on the sciences. The few original thinkers, such as Bacon, took their lives in their hands, and stood a considerable risk of being accused of heresy. Bacon himself was imprisoned by his fellow Franciscans, for original thinking, during the last few years of his life.

By the fifteenth century, certain doctors such as Paracelsus (1493-1541) were starting to challenge some of the old ideas of medicine. Paracelsus was born Phillipus Theophrastus Aureolus Bombastus von Hohenheim, but by the age of twenty-six had changed his name to Paracelsus. The implication is obvious, Para (beyond) the well-known Roman physician of the first century, Aulus Cornelius Celsus. His attitude was probably not helped by his name, an aureola being the corona around the sun, or the radiant halo shown around the heads of Christ and the saints in paintings. Paracelsus originally trained as a metallurgist, then as a doctor, and became an army surgeon before travelling widely around Europe and the Near East.

Amongst the more important ideas of Paracelsus was the suggestion that specific diseases require specific medicines, such as laudanum and sulphur, not cure-all panaceas. He also realised that the dose of medicine is important, that more does not always equal better, and a large dose of something that kills, may be a cure in a small dose. Finally, he considered that theory should be derived from practice, that is, if something works it should be accepted, if it does not, it should be rejected. Paracelsus upset his colleagues in many towns so successfully, that he had to move at frequent intervals to stay in front of the avenging mob. He publicly demonstrated his disapproval of the work of earlier physicians when he burned the books of Galen and Avicenna in the market place of Basle, surrounded by a crowd of cheering students. Whilst many medical colleagues would no doubt have been appalled by his burning the books of the ancients, it is probable that they regarded the fact that he taught in the vernacular rather than Latin as his most heinous crime, as this put knowledge within reach of the common man. A number of them claimed that he only taught in the vernacular because his Latin was so poor, and it is obvious that he was a seriously abrasive character. Many people think that we get the word "bombastic" from one his middle names, "Bombastus", but the Oxford Dictionary claims that it is derived from a sixteenth century word meaning the cotton or wool used to pad out clothing.

Some of the ideas of Paracelsus were decades, if not centuries, before their time. He claimed that if the physician prevented infection, Nature would heal a wound herself, and he also attempted to immunise people against plague by giving them pills of bread containing minute portions of excreta from plague victims. It is not known whether this treatment worked, but he did not catch plague himself.

Paracelsus was not right all the time, some of his ideas were seriously flawed, but he was like a breath of fresh air blowing through the musty corridors of medieval medicine. Perhaps the contribution of this unusual scholar can be summed up in the following sentence. It is alleged that a number of his books and publications were placed on the *Index Expurgatorius* (the list of condemned books) by the Catholic Church, but in spite of this, many doctors and scientists today would regard him as being the architect of the modern day union between chemistry and medicine.

In much of Europe, the early physicians did not carry out surgery, and regarded surgeons as their inferiors, and for hundreds of years surgery was performed by barbers. Barbers were originally found in monasteries as the monks were required to be clean-shaven and wear tonsures. In many orders, they were also required to undergo blood-letting at regular intervals, but in 1163, the Pope passed a decree that forbade the clergy to shed blood with an edged weapon. This was aimed at warrior priests, such as the Prince-Bishops of Durham, who regularly led armies into Scotland[31]. The result was that the blood-letting role was turned over to the barbers.

The Master Surgeons Guild was formed in 1348, whilst the Guild of Barbers received their charter in 1462 from Edward IV. The two guilds were amalgamated in 1540 by Henry VIII, with the members being given the title "Master". In a classic piece of inverse British snobbery, doctors who have progressed to the level of surgeon drop the title "Doctor", and are still addressed as "Mister".

The union lasted until 1745, when the surgeons and barbers parted company. The barbers lost their medical role, and now there is only a striped pole outside the premises, reminiscent of blood and bandages, to remind the public that they once carried out blood letting and other minor operations. The

31   They got around this minor inconvenience by using a mace that inflicted crushing injuries, instead of a sword or battle-axe that inflicted cutting ones.

Royal College of Surgeons, however, did not receive its charter until 1800.

The organization of the Barber Surgeons in London in 1540, marked the beginning of some control over the qualifications of those who performed operations. In England, Henry VIII had passed an Act early in the sixteenth century regulating medicine, and forbidding unlicensed people to practice. Anyone practicing medicine in the area around London had to be examined by the Bishop of London or the Dean of St Pauls, plus four doctors of physic. In 1518, Thomas Linacre, the physician to Henry VIII, received a Royal Charter to found the Royal College of Physicians, and became its first president. This charter gave the College the power to regulate medicine, and fine anyone practising without a licence. Following the founding of the Royal College of Physicians, Henry passed further acts incorporating the Apothecaries and Barber-Surgeons into the college. Although the Royal College of Physicians was a very small guild containing no more than twenty to thirty members, it was extremely powerful as it had direct access to the king.

One of the successors of Linacre was Dr John Caius, (see the sweating sickness [Ch 1]) who produced a set of rules and procedures for the Royal College in 1555. Cauis made medicine a core part of the syllabus whilst master at Gonville and Cauis College, and also obtained a royal charter allowing students to dissect executed criminals, even although the Church opposed it[32, 33].

The problem of the availability of bodies for dissection was not regularised in Great Britain until the early 1830s. Whilst

32   Dissection was considered part of the punishment, as it was widely believed that on Judgment Day, the dead would arise from their graves to be judged. No burial and no grave equated with no resurrection.
33   In 1300, Pope Boniface VIII published a Bill forbidding the dissection of bodies, the intention was to curtail the trade in body parts as holy relics, but it also stopped the study of anatomy. At Montpellier, one of the premier medical schools of the fourteenth century, there was one dissection every other year.

the bodies of executed criminals were occasionally used, there were never sufficient to supply all the doctors and medical students wishing to acquire them. The earliest account of body snatchers and resurrectionists appears in 1738; these dug up newly buried corpses and sold them to medical students who asked no questions. The situation became so bad that many families would pay for grave watchers, to sit over the graves of recently deceased relatives, until the body had decomposed sufficiently to be of no use for dissection purposes.

Matters came to a head in Edinburgh in the 1820s with the murders committed by William Hare and William Burke. Hare owned a boarding house and in 1827 an elderly man with no friends or relatives died there, so Hare and Burke sold his body to Dr Knox's School of Anatomy for £7-10s. This was obviously easy money, so over the next year, the pair murdered at least sixteen people and sold their bodies to the same establishment. They were eventually caught and the scandal ruined Dr Knox; Hare turned King's evidence and Burke was hanged in January 1829 and his body publicly dissected (but not at Dr Knox's establishment). Burke's skeleton is still on display at the Anatomy Museum in Edinburgh.

In 1832, the law was changed allowing corpses to be used for dissection purposes as long as all the relatives of the deceased person agreed and the remains received a Christian burial.

Whilst major advances in medicine were continuing, the role of the apothecary was also increasing; the apothecaries were descended from the Guild of Pepperers founded in 1180. In 1316, these were joined by the Guild of Spicers, and in 1428 they became the Worshipful Company of Grocers. Apothecaries as members of the Grocers Company sold spices, perfumes, herbs, spiced wine and drugs[34]. The apothecaries petitioned James I in 1617, and The Worshipful Society of Apothecaries was formed by Royal Charter. Initially they prepared medicines

---

34   The Latin word, apotheca means a storehouse for herbs, spices and wine.

for the physicians, but in 1815, they were granted the right to practice medicine and the Society was allowed to examine and licence candidates to provide a minimum qualification for doctors. By the middle of the nineteenth century, five out of six medical students were enrolled by the Society of Apothecaries, who provided a route into medical practice that was a great deal cheaper than the traditional route through university. It was a route taken by many important doctors of the nineteenth century such as John Snow (Ch 12).

One of the most important apothecaries, Nicholas Culpepper, was born in 1616, and fought in the English Civil War when he was seriously wounded, but luckily recovered. He translated the Pharmacopoeia used by apothecaries from Latin into English in 1649; this was a massive task, as many of the Latin measurements and terms had no obvious equivalent in English. The English names of many of the plants used were also difficult to translate (this was a century before Linnaeus), as many of them had numerous colloquial names depending on the part of England in which they were located. Culpepper corrected many of the mistakes found in earlier Latin editions and added numerous detailed instructions on how various medications should be prepared and used.

In addition, Culpepper attacked (in 1650) medical astrology that was still regarded as an important part of medicine. In the mid-seventeenth century, accusations of witchcraft against apothecaries were common, and indeed the last execution for witchcraft in Britain did not take place until 1722.

His most important work was published in 1652, the "*English Physition* (*sic*)" which became better known as "*Culpepper's Complete Herbal*". This book listed all the medicinal plants and herbs growing in England, and described their appearance, use and preparation. It was unique at the time as it only described plants growing in England, and emphasised the use of cheap, easily available material, and eliminated all references to exotic or non-existent materials such as unicorn horns.

One doctor, Thomas Sydenham (1624-1689), who fought in the Commonwealth Army during the English Civil War has been called the English Hippocrates. He emphasised the importance of careful examination of the patient, insisting that his students must attend the bedside as this was the only place they would learn medicine. He made a close study of epidemics and is regarded as one of the founders of the science of epidemiology. He also introduced the use of laudanum (an alcoholic preparation of opium) to England, and popularised the use of Jesuits bark (quinine) to treat malaria.

One of the greatest physicians of the day was William Harvey (1578-1657) who studied at Gonville and Cauis College, Cambridge, and also Padua. Whilst at Padua, Harvey studied under the successors of Andreas Vesalius, the great sixteenth century Belgian anatomist. Vesalius who was a professor at the University of Padua had published "*De fabrica corporis humani*" (Concerning the composition of the human body) in 1543. Many of the illustrations in his book, made directly from observations, challenged Galen's theories, although in common with many of the doctors of the day, he hesitated to challenge Galen directly.

When Harvey was examined by the College of Physicians for the right to practice medicine, the ability to memorise large portions of Galen's work (in Latin) was still essential. Indeed, one reformer was complaining about the influence of Galen as late as 1665, giving rise to the saying, *"ubi tres medici, duo athei"* (where there are three doctors, two are atheists) because of the classical (pagan) knowledge required to qualify as a physician. The Church still greatly influenced medicine and it was not until the Printing Act of 1643, that the power to licence the publication of medical texts was taken from the Bishop of London, and given to the Royal College of Physicians.

Harvey was an extremely political individual and as part of his career progression he became an enforcer for the Royal

College of Physicians. This involved raiding the premises of apothecaries who were accused of practising medicine illegally. He was one of only four physicians who remained in London during a major epidemic of plague in 1625. It was during this period that the apothecaries took over the role of providing medicine for much of the population of London especially the poor.

Harvey became a doctor at St Bartholomew's Hospital and physician to King Charles I, enjoying considerable royal patronage, and also acting as tutor to his young sons, the future kings Charles II[35] and James II. In 1628, he published (in Latin) his most famous work, *"De moto cardis"* (On the motion of the heart), which described the circulation of blood, and refuted the *"earlier ebb and flow"* theory of the movement of blood around the body. This was not translated into English for another quarter of a century, and Harvey was forced to tread carefully to avoid offending the politically powerful disciples of Galen and Avicenna whilst presenting modern knowledge. He also carried out a considerable amount of work on fertilisation, anatomy and embryology, and was so far in advance of his time that some of his theories were not confirmed until the early nineteenth century[36].

By the time of Harvey's death it may be said that medicine in England had slowly but surely started to enter the modern age, although the ability to study Greek and Latin texts in the original was still a requirement for a medical degree as late as the nineteenth century, and a grammar school qualification in Latin was essential for entry into some medical schools in Britain until well into the twentieth century.

---

35   After the restoration of the monarchy in 1660, following the Commonwealth, Charles II was responsible for the foundation of The Royal Society.

36   The importance of Harvey can be seen by the fact that he is one of the supporters of the heraldic device of the British Medical Association.

CHAPTER 3

A History of Microbiology

Micro-organisms may be defined as those biological organisms that cannot be seen without the use of a microscope. Microscopes are generally thought to have been invented at the beginning of the seventeenth century, although there are suggestions that they may have been used before this date (Ch 2). Two types are found, the first being simple microscopes made of a single lens, these have a high magnification and are based on the same principle as a magnifying glass. Magnifying glasses are able to increase the size of an image by several times, and had been known for hundreds of years before microscopes, being described by Archimedes (*ca* 287-212 BC).

The second type of microscope is the compound microscope made up of two lens, an eyepiece and an objective lens, held in a straight line by a body tube. All modern microscopes are of this type, and typically are used at magnifications up to a maximum of approximately 1000x, which approaches the theoretical upper limit of an optical system using white light. The first known compound microscopes were made in the Netherlands around 1600, by the lens makers, Hans and Zacharias Jannsen, a father and son team.

By the middle of the seventeenth century, the existence of organisms too small to be seen with the naked eye had been suspected for many years, but although the French philosopher Rene Descartes (1596-1650) described a crude microscope, the magnification was not sufficient to detect micro-organisms. In 1665, Robert Hooke (1635-1703), who was a founder member of the Royal Society (founded in 1662 by Charles II), published

"*Micrographia*" in which he described using a microscope to study thin slices of cork, and gave the first description of cells. He also described a number of microbiological phenomena including moulds (filamentous fungi) growing on the surface of leather, and bacteria which he concluded were alive.

The first major discoveries in microbiology were made by Anton van Leeuwenhoek, a Dutch merchant (1632-1723), who wrote frequently to the Royal Society in England, which elected him as a Fellow in 1680. Although he spoke only Dutch, his letters were translated into English and published widely. Many of his letters to the Royal Society coincided with a Dutch king, William III (William of Orange) on the throne of England from 1689-1702. Van Leeuwenhoek worked with simple microscopes, whose magnifying powers are an intrinsic property of the curvature of the lens used and cannot be changed. By using of a variety of different lenses and lighting methods, he was able to obtain magnifications ranging from about 50x to approximately 300x. He constructed hundreds of these simple microscopes, a small number of which survive in various museums. He was extremely secretive regarding their manufacture, and the methods he used to prepare the glass lenses by grinding have been lost, but we do know that making them required considerable technical competence. No one was allowed to handle his microscopes, not even the Russian Tsar, Peter the Great. Van Leeuwenhoek prepared the samples himself and would only allow observations.

Van Leeuwenhoek made numerous discoveries with his simple microscopes including demonstrating the existence of spermatozoa and red blood cells. However, he is mainly remembered for his discovery of micro-organisms, as he described all the main groups of unicellular micro-organisms (which he called animalicules), including bacteria, yeasts (a unicellular form of fungus), algae and protozoa. The first known representation of bacteria is shown in one of his drawings published by the Royal Society in 1683, and he described many types of cells so accurately that we can still recognise his descriptions today. In many of his letters, he also emphasised the vast numbers of micro-organisms found in many natural habitats.

Van Leeuwenhoek was strongly opposed to the theory of spontaneous generation (see later), and was able to show that it did not occur in a number of species, such as weevils in flour, which had previously been thought to multiply in this manner.

Nearly a century after van Leeuwenhoek, Muller, a Danish zoologist studied bacteria (from Greek, *backterium,* meaning little stick), and was able to distinguish different types on the basis of their shape. Later still in 1838, Ehrenberg published his work in which he divided different types of micro-organisms into various groups using names, some of which are still used, although their context has changed to a greater or lesser extent.

Much of van Leeuwenhoek's work could not be repeated by his contemporaries. The reason for this was that most of his contemporaries, including Robert Hooke, used compound microscopes. Intrinsically these are greatly superior to simple microscopes, but the early ones had severe optical defects known as spherical and chromatic aberration due to the poor quality of the lens. Spherical aberration is caused by the fact that light rays passing through the centre of a lens are bent less than those passing through the edges, and therefore focus at a slightly different distance producing a blurred image. Chromatic aberration is caused when white light passes through a lens and is broken up into the colours of the spectrum. These different colours are bent at slightly different angles as they pass through the lens and do not refocus together, thus producing an image that is fringed with a spectrum of colours. These problems greatly reduced the efficiency of the earlier compound microscopes, and prevented them being focused on very small objects such as bacteria. The problems of chromatic and spherical aberration were not solved until 1824 and 1830 respectively, and after this period the compound microscope started to produce significantly better results than the simple microscope. The solution to chromatic aberration was the achromatic lens discovered by the father of Lord Lister (see later).

Further developments, in the early twentieth century, involved the introduction of microscopes using ultraviolet light; this enabled a higher magnification to be used, and allowed some of the larger viruses to be seen for the first time. The first electron microscope appeared in the early 1930s, and the first commercial model was built in England in 1935. These machines ultimately produced magnifications in excess of 250,000x, enabling viruses to be seen in great detail.

MIASMAS AND SPONTANEOUS GENERATION

During the two centuries after van Leeuwenhoek, considerable energy was expended in attempting to prove or disprove two theories. The first of these was the miasma (from a Greek word meaning to defile or pollute) theory, which suggested that all diseases are caused by "bad air". One aspect of the miasma theory that still lingers today is the belief in the benefits of "fresh air". The second theory was that of spontaneous generation but more of this later.

The idea that bad air causes diseases goes back to Greek and Roman times, and numerous references to it can be found. One of the earliest is in the *"Anabasis"*, written by the Greek general Xenophon, who led his army across hundreds of miles of hostile territory in Asia Minor (March of the Ten Thousand), after their defeat at the battle of Cunaxa in 401 BC. Xenophon advised his men to always camp in healthy places and avoid swamps.

This knowledge was put to practical use by the Sicilians when defending Syracuse against the Athenians in 415-413 BC, and the Carthaginians in 397 BC. Sicilian generals manoeuvred them into camping in the swamps and both armies were destroyed by fever, probably malaria. A similar fate appears to have overcome the Gauls attacking Rome in 390 BC, who also camped in the marshes around the city.

The Romans were also aware of the problems. Marcus Terrentius Varro (116-27 BC) stated that, *"Precautions should be taken near swamps…they breed certain minute creatures which cannot be seen, but which float in the air and enter the body through the mouth and nose and cause serious diseases"*. In the first century BC, Titus Lucretius Carus (*ca* 100-55 BC) wrote in *De rerum natura* (on the Nature of Things), *"In the earth there are atoms of every kind. There must be countless atoms flying around that are pestiferous and poisonous"*. He considered that when these harmful atoms accumulated in the mist the *"air causes disease"*. He also thought that variations in the air from country to country caused different diseases[37]. It is obvious from these statements that both Varro and Lucretius had considered the possibility of unseen micro-organisms capable of causing disease, and the comments of Varro were endorsed by Pliny the Elder.

By the fourth century AD, these possibilities had been extended to include water, the Roman strategist, Vegetius, writing that, *"Dirty water is like poison and causes plagues"*. He also claimed that the water *"becomes corrupt"* and *"diseases arise if an army stays too long in one place"*.

In the Middle Ages, many diseases were thought to be spread by miasmas that could be kept at bay by the use of pomanders containing sweet smelling flowers or herbs. This belief would have been fostered by the foul smelling streets full

---

37   Lucretius was a follower of the teachings of the Greek philosopher Epicurus. Some of his ideas on science were two thousand years in advance of their time, and what is even more unusual is that Lucretius wrote them in hexameter verse. This was greatly complicated by the fact that at this time, Latin did not have equivalent words to describe many of the Greek scientific ideas, and he was forced to express many of his thoughts in an extremely convoluted form. The early Christian Church considered the ideas of Lucretius so dangerous and revolutionary, that they spread the rumour that he was mad in an attempt to discredit his work.

of rubbish and sewage. The miasma theory persisted until well into the nineteenth century, and was one of the main obstacles faced by pioneers such as Dr John Snow (see Ch 12). A few eminent people, including some doctors, believed miasmas caused disease until the early twentieth century.

The theory of spontaneous generation has also had a long history, and in ancient times it was accepted without challenge that some animals and plants could generate spontaneously under certain conditions. However, experiments carried out in 1665 by an Italian physician, Francesco Redi, showed that maggots in meat developed into flies, and that if the meat was protected from flies with muslin, maggots did not appear as the flies had been unable to lay their eggs.

It is considerably more difficult to disprove the theory of spontaneous generation in micro-organisms for a number of technical reasons, and it was not until the end of the nineteenth century that this theory was finally abandoned by most scientists.

An Italian monk, Lazarro Spallanzani (1729-99), a professor at the University of Pavia, carried out numerous experiments in the eighteenth century disproving spontaneous generation, by showing that microbes did not appear in heated and sealed flasks, but did appear in unsealed ones. His work was continuously challenged by people carrying out flawed and poorly designed experiments, their main claim being that the air in the sealed flasks had been changed by heating it.

One of these was John Needham, a Catholic priest, who claimed to have proved spontaneous generation in 1748, by boiling broth and then observing *"animalcules"* in it. Spallanzani claimed that he had not protected the broth from the air, and this was supported by Schwann, in 1837, who showed that if meat broth was boiled, it remained unspoilt as long as any air coming into contact with it had also been heated. Again however, claims were made that the air had been changed by heating it.

Another Italian, Bartolomeo Bizio, also carried out experiments in the early nineteenth century in attempts to disprove the *"Blood of Christ"* miracle. This occurs when red spots are formed on the consecrated bread and wafers used in the Christian mass. Bizio examined this phenomenon microscopically, described the spots as a fungus, and was able to show that they could be passed to fresh damp bread after handling the contaminated bread. We are now aware that this phenomenon is caused by the red-pigmented bacterium, known as *Serratia marcescens* that grows rapidly on damp bread.

In spite of these demonstrations, in the middle of the nineteenth century, the French chemist Pouchet carried out numerous technically flawed experiments that appeared to support the theory of spontaneous generation. Pouchet's work caused the French Academy of Science to offer a prize to any scientist who could finally settle the problem. Louis Pasteur (1822-95) was awarded the prize after a series of experiments, the most famous of which demonstrated that if broth sterilised by heat was kept in a swan-necked flask open to the air, it remained sterile. The main feature of these flasks was that the neck was sufficiently tortuous to cause any bacteria contained in air entering the flasks to impinge on the sides, and not reach the broth. The important fact was that the air had not been altered in any way. This was one of the main objections to earlier experiments where sealed systems had been used or the air had been heated. With these experiments of Pasteur the *"Germ Theory"* had arrived, but it would be some years before it was accepted by the majority of people including a number of doctors.

The early microbiological work of Pasteur, who had trained as a chemist, was on the fermentation of wine, which he showed was due to yeast. He also worked on the spoilage of wine, which he referred to as a disease of wine, and was able to prove that this was caused by bacterial contamination. This was of considerable industrial and economic importance, as many breweries did not brew beer during the summer months because the possibility of spoilage was so high. Pasteur was able to show that the spoilage was due to the presence of bacteria in the beer, and he developed the technique of gentle heating of materials, such as wine, to prevent spoilage. This procedure became known as pasteurisation, and was later applied widely to milk to control bovine tuberculosis (Ch 11), and also became a major factor in the successful development of the food canning industry.

Further work was carried out on diseases in silk worms, which were damaging the French silk industry, and this led to several interesting theories, one being that specific human diseases might be caused by specific micro-organisms.

An English physicist, John Tyndall, a contemporary of Pasteur, carried out a series of experiments in support of him. Tyndall's work showed that some types of micro-organism were able to exist in two forms, a vegetative form which was easily destroyed by boiling for five minutes, and a spore form which is extremely resistant to heat. Some of these spores are able to withstand heating in boiling water for periods of up to six hours at the end of which they were still capable of germination and growth. These experiments of Tyndall, and further experiments by Ferdinand Cohn, showed that the failure of many of the early experiments carried out to disprove spontaneous generation, was due to inadequate sterilisation. These ideas, and the work of Pasteur led to the development of sterilisation procedures, including autoclaving, in which material is treated under pressure, at an elevated temperature above the boiling point of water.

MEDICAL MICROBIOLOGY

The Roman philosopher, Lucretius had suggested *"the seeds of disease"* in the first century BC, and this germ theory of disease was expanded by Giralamo Fracastoro (1485-1553) of Verona, in 1546, in his book *"De contagione et contagiosis morbis"* (On Contagion and contagious diseases). This was the first attempt at a scientific explanation of infection, diseases, "germs", their transmission and the cause of epidemics. Fracastoro (Fracastorius) was considerably in advance of his time, but his work vanished into obscurity until his theories were resurrected by Pasteur and Koch in the nineteenth century.

He described three methods of infection, direct contact between individuals, infection by fomites (derived from *fomes*, a Latin word meaning kindling or tinder), and infection at a distance (droplet infection) (Ch 6). The only one he missed was infection transmitted by vectors, a phenomenon not recognised by medical science until the last decade of the nineteenth century. Fracastoro considered the causes of disease to be invisible seeds of contagion that he called *"seminaria"*, and thought that smallpox had its own specific seminaria. He also realised that seminaria were capable of being transmitted through the air, and must have the power to reproduce themselves. In addition, he described the disease typhus (Ch 13), which appeared at the end of the fifteenth century, and recognised the contagiousness of pulmonary TB or consumption. In an earlier publication in 1530, he had described syphilis (in poetry), a disease that appeared at the end of the fifteenth century, and suggested mercury and guaiacum wood as cures (Ch 14).

In 1762, Marko Plenčič (or von Plencig) (1705-86) published a book based on the ideas of Fracastoro. He was convinced that infectious diseases were caused by living *"contagia"*, and suggested that certain specific diseases had a specific microbial aetiology. Plenčič described scarlet fever and suggested that it entered the body either through the skin or respiratory system. These ideas were extended to crops, and by 1813 it had been shown that some fungi could cause diseases in cereal crops, and in 1845 it was realised that a fungus was causing the potato blight in Ireland.

In spite of these demonstrations, and the work described earlier by people such as van Leeuwenhoek, many doctors in the first half of the nineteenth century refused to believe that organisms as small as bacteria could cause diseases in humans. They still believed in the *"miasma"* theory, and considered that diseases were caused by foul smells from rotting corpses causing sickness when they encountered a person with a weakened constitution. Many also still believed in the spontaneous generation theory, a later and more sophisticated version of which held that bacteria and parasites were the products of a diseased system, not the cause of it.

One of the major problems of medical microbiology was the lack of understanding of the transmission of infectious diseases from person to person, even though Fracastoro had described three of the four methods of transmission three centuries earlier.

The German epidemiologist, August Hirsch, published a *"Handbook of Historical and Geographical Pathology"* between 1860-4 in German, with a revised edition in English twenty years later. In this, he described various nineteenth century epidemics ranging from ergotism, erysipelas (a streptococcal infection of the skin), scrofula (a form of TB) to typhus. He suggested that the Plague of Justinian (540 AD) was the first definite manifestation of bubonic plague in Europe, although he considered the epidemic described by Rufus of Ephesus in North Africa in the third century AD, may also have been bubonic plague. Hirsch also recognised that some diseases are contagious (passed from person to person), whilst others are not.

The indirect transmission of puerperal fever (childbirth fever) was recognised as early as the late eighteenth century in publications by British doctors, such as Charles White and Alexander Gordon. An American doctor, Oliver Wendell Holmes, published an article in 1843 in the Boston Medical Society, detailing precautions to be taken by doctors attending childbirths. All of them stressed the importance of cleanliness. Holmes is probably better known in the USA as a poet, and as one of the people responsible for saving the warship "USS Constitution" from the breaker's yard.

Another doctor, Thomas Kirkland, suggested cross contamination from one patient to another, and this theory was supported by a series of doctors at the beginning of the nineteenth century. In 1847, Ignaz Semmelweis (1818-1865) of Vienna, published an article that was essentially a modern statistical survey of the epidemiology of this disease. Semmelweiss recognised that puerperal fever was spread by doctors using corpses to practice obstetric techniques, and then moving from morgue to patient, without washing their hands. He realised that thoroughly washing the hands between patients greatly reduced the risk of infection, and insisted that doctors under his control should wash their hands in chlorine water, before examining pregnant patients. Within a year, the mortality rate from puerperal fever in his ward fell from 11% to 3%. Ironically, Semmelweis died at the age of forty-seven from a generalised infection of the bacterium *Streptococcus*, the same organism as that causing puerperal fever.

By this time, Jacob Henle (the mentor of Robert Koch, [see later]) had postulated that smallpox pustules contained *"the contagion for pus"*, that this contagion must be alive, and could be transmitted from patient to patient. He also published an essay in 1840, suggesting that specific *"contagia"* or living organisms caused specific diseases but could not produce sufficiently rigorous proofs.

A further example of indirect transmission or transmission by fomites was demonstrated in 1854 by John Snow, in another early epidemiological survey, when he showed that contaminated drinking water was responsible for the transmission of cholera (Ch 12). Snow further proposed that the organism responsible for causing cholera had *"the property of reproducing its own kind"* in the gut of the victim. Prior to this, a group of English doctors had described the *"comma shaped"* bacterium of cholera in the faeces of cholera victims, and shown that it was also present in the drinking water of infected areas, but not in the drinking water of non-infected areas. A government/medical sub-committee however, considered that *"whilst a "virus" (sic) could cause cholera, the main cause was a miasma"*.

The introduction of anaesthetics such as ether in the 1840s meant that operations could become more complicated, and take considerably longer as the problem of shock was greatly reduced. However, another problem, that of wound infection or sepsis became much more serious. Florence Nightingale (1820-1910), of Crimean War fame (1853-6), was one of the first people to publicise the mortality rates found in hospitals from nosocomial infections (infections acquired in hospital, [from *nosocomium*, the Latin word for hospital]), based on her experiences in the military hospital of Scutari. Her attention to cleanliness led to the death rate from hospital acquired infections falling from over 40% to 2% in one year. Although she was able to reduce infection rates by cleanliness, her reasoning was incorrect. She thought that the filth generated a miasma, which caused diseases, and that if filth was eliminated, the miasma would also be eliminated.

The surgeon Joseph Lister, later Lord Lister (1827-1912), who was aware of Pasteur's work on fermentation and putrefaction, considered that sepsis might arise from wound infection by micro-organisms. Lister greatly reduced the rate of sepsis in the 1860s where he worked in Glasgow Royal Infirmary, by the sterilisation of instruments and the widespread use of disinfectants such as carbolic acid (phenol or German creosote) during and after surgery. In 1865, Lister treated a boy with a compound fracture of the leg; until this time it had been standard practice to amputate in these circumstances. Lister treated the wound with carbolic acid, it remained free of infection and healed completely. Prior to Lister's work which was published in 1867, the mortality rate from bacterial sepsis following amputation was typically of the order of 45%, mostly caused by bacteria of the genus *Streptococcus,* which also caused puerperal fever, erysipelas, scarlet fever and tonsillitis. Following the introduction of Lister's antiseptic techniques, the percentage mortality rate fell to single figures. Antiseptic surgery was rapidly replaced by aseptic surgery (the elimination of bacteria from the surgical environment). In view of the fact that this knowledge has been available for nearly 150 years, it is ironic that the rate of nosocomial infections caused by organisms, such as methicillin resistant *Staphylococcus aureus* (MRSA) and *Clostridium difficile*, has been rising rapidly in many developed countries over recent years.

Lister's theories were also tested on the battlefield during the Franco-Prussian war of 1870-1, the Prussian army which adopted them had far better results for treating wounds than the French, who ignored them in spite of the work of Pasteur. Lister's work was also rejected by the American Surgical Association in 1882.

The implication of bacteria as specific disease agents was first shown by a study of anthrax, a disease of animals occasionally transmitted to humans. Studies by Davaine in the 1860s showed that bacteria are always present in the blood of diseased animals, but never present in the blood of healthy ones, and that inoculating the blood of a diseased animal into a healthy one caused anthrax. Further work by Pasteur on anthrax, produced an attenuated (weakened) strain of bacteria that could be used in the preparation of a vaccine against the disease (the history of vaccines is considered in Ch 7).

A number of experiments on anthrax were carried out in the 1870s by Robert Koch (1843-1910), who passed the organism causing the disease through a series of mice, and then through a series of tubes of sterile culture medium. The contents of the final tube of culture medium were injected into an animal, when it again caused the characteristic symptoms of anthrax. At all stages of his experiments, in both mice and the test tube, Koch was able to demonstrate the characteristic *Bacillus anthracis* by microscopy and photography. In an extension of this work, Koch demonstrated the specificity of the disease organism, when he was able to show that other species of the bacterial genus *Bacillus* were not able to cause anthrax.

These experiments led to publication of a paper on the "*Aetiology of Infectious Diseases*" published in English in 1880, which became known as Koch's postulates (Ch 12), although much of the groundwork for these rules had been laid by Henle (Koch's mentor), in the 1840s. Although it was possible by the beginning of the twentieth century to apply Koch's postulates to many bacterial diseases, there was still considerable controversy, as numerous diseases could not be shown to obey these rules. It is now known that many of these diseases are caused by viruses. These could not be demonstrated using the technology of the late nineteenth and early twentieth centuries.

Koch's forerunners were aware that specimens taken from medical samples were mixed, and contained a number of different types of bacteria. Lister had isolated pure cultures of pathogenic bacteria from mixtures by working at very high dilutions. The rationale behind this method is to dilute a sample repeatedly, until only one bacterium is present in a container. Obviously when this is grown in culture, it will produce a pure strain as it is derived from a single cell. However, the process is extremely lengthy and tedious and requires considerable technical expertise.

Koch made major advances in the development of microbiological media, including the development of solid media using agar, a chemical derived from seaweed. This greatly simplified the separation of bacterial specimens into pure cultures. The idea of using agar came from Frau Hesse, the wife of a doctor, Walter Hesse, who worked with Koch for several months in 1881. Fanny Hesse had heard about agar from friends who lived in the East Indies, where it is used for cooking. The use of agar (which melts at 100°C and solidifies at 50°C) to solidify media allowed the isolation of pure cultures, and the identification of a number of medically and industrially important bacteria. Prior to this, attempts to grow bacteria on a solid medium had been limited to using slices of potato and moist bread. Although gelatin had been used to solidify media, it has the major disadvantage of liquefying at around 28°C, which is below the temperature of the human body (37°C), and the temperature required for the growth of many pathogenic bacteria. An additional problem with gelatin is that it is degraded by many bacteria, agar on the other hand is only broken down by a very small number of marine micro-organisms.

Koch also perfected many of the practical techniques of working under conditions of sterility. He was an extremely careful experimental worker, who demonstrated proofs of his theories at each stage, which played a major role in establishing many of the experimental techniques of bacteriology.

Other important practical applications included the development of Petri dishes, small saucer-like dishes with a cover. Prior to the development of these, all work had been carried out under belljars that are large, cumbersome and extremely inconvenient. There is controversy over whether Petri, who was an associate of Koch, should have been given credit for the invention of these dishes; there is published evidence that at least one other bacteriologist, Frankland, had been using them for some time before Petri.

Koch's greatest triumph however, was his work on tuberculosis (Ch 11). By the latter half of the nineteenth century, tuberculosis, also known as consumption or the white death, was causing an estimated 20% of all deaths in Europe. In the seventeenth century, it was estimated to have caused 25% of all deaths in London in non-plague years. Technically, work on the tuberculosis causing bacterium, *Mycobacterium tuberculosis,* is difficult. The organism is very slow growing, requires complex media for growth and is extremely difficult to stain with dyes, making microscopy very tedious. Koch was able to demonstrate his postulates again, this time using guinea pigs as laboratory animals, and this work culminated in him receiving the Nobel Prize for medicine in 1905. However, even Koch could not get it right all the time. He considered that the bovine strain of TB was not transmitted to humans by drinking contaminated cows milk, and his opinion probably impeded the fight against the disease for a number of years. There were also severe criticisms over his claims for tuberculin (a protein extract of the tuberculosis organism) and its therapeutic powers, after the deaths from tuberculosis of several individuals who had been treated with tuberculin.

Koch was also able to demonstrate the causative organism of cholera, and develop the concept of disease *"carriers"* (Ch 1). In addition, his group worked on the isolation of the causative organism of bubonic plague (Ch 9), but was beaten to its discovery by the Swiss microbiologist, Alexandre Yersin, after whom this organism is now named.

Despite all the honours heaped on him, Koch's private life in later years was a mess following an acrimonious divorce from his first wife, and marriage to a second wife, a teenage actress about one third his age.

Two major schools of bacteriology developed, one under Koch in Berlin and one under Pasteur in Paris. Considerable rivalry existed between them, exacerbated to a considerable extent by the Franco-Prussian war of 1870-1. Koch, whose patron was the Kaiser, was openly scornful of Pasteur and the French school, and criticised Pasteur's use of liquid media as careless. Although solid media were crucial for the early work on the isolation of various bacterial species, we now know that some of the typical behaviour of bacteria is lost when they are grown on solid media in pure culture.

The German school concentrated on the isolation of the causative organisms of a number of major infectious bacterial diseases such as tuberculosis, cholera, typhoid and plague. The French school concentrated on the inter-relationships of the disease-causing organism and its host, an approach leading to the development of a number of vaccines. Following the work of Koch and Pasteur, public immunisation of children for a number of diseases was made available free of charge in 1871, and was made compulsory in a number of countries during World War I.

Other major advances in microbiology were also made by a number of people. Patrick Manson (1844-1922) was a British Medical Officer in China in the 1870s, who saw many cases of elephantiasis. The autopsies of victims showed filarial worms (Ch 4) in their lymph tissues, and Manson reasoned that they must somehow be transported to the outside world, and then find their way to another human host. Manson fed mosquitoes on people infected with filarial worms and was able to demonstrate worms in the mosquito. He made one serious mistake however, he did not realise that the infected mosquito would bite a second person and thought that somehow they contaminated drinking water, which was then consumed by the victim. At this time, it was a common misconception that mosquitoes only had one blood meal during their lifetime.

This was followed by a realisation that insects were a major factor in the transmission of numerous diseases. In 1885, Sir David Bruce showed that the protozoan *Trypanosomas,* the causative organism of African sleeping sickness, was transmitted from one victim to another by the bite of the tsetse fly.

In 1880, Charles Laveran (1845-1922), a French Army doctor discovered the malarial parasite in the blood of infected people, and the British Army doctor Sir Ronald Ross (1857-1932), discovered the role of the mosquito in the transmission of malaria about twenty years later in India (Ch 16). Ross had corresponded at some length with Manson who made the suggestion that he should examine mosquitoes. Both Laveran and Ross received the Nobel Prize for their research. This was followed by the work of Walter Reed (1851-1902), an American Army doctor, whose team discovered the role of mosquitoes in the transmission of yellow fever (Ch 17), a few years after Ross's discoveries.

In 1864, Pasteur demonstrated that rabies, which is now known to be a viral disease can be passed from one animal to another, whilst Mayer made a similar discovery relating to plants and their viruses in 1886. By the late nineteenth century, it had become obvious that infectious agents fell into two categories. Most infectious agents, such as bacteria, could be removed from a liquid by passing it through a filter with a sufficiently fine mesh, and these were visible with a light microscope. Others however, could not be removed, these were referred to as viruses and could not be seen with an optical microscope. For many years, their existence could only be inferred, although Martinus Beijerinck studying Tobacco Mosaic Virus (TMV) in 1898, showed that they were able to reproduce in living plant tissue.

In 1935 Wendell Stanley was able to crystallise TMV and demonstrate that it was largely protein, he received the Nobel Prize for this work in 1946. Later, it was shown to also contain a small quantity of the nucleic acid, ribonucleic acid (RNA). All viruses have now been shown to contain either RNA or deoxyribonucleic acid (DNA), but never both, unlike all other biological systems that always contain both types of nucleic acid. The first photographs of viruses were obtained in the 1940s using primitive electron microscopes. As more sophisticated machines and photographs became available, it became obvious that viruses occurred in a wide variety of shapes and sizes, the pox viruses being amongst the largest and most complicated.

CHEMOTHERAPY

The work of Pasteur had led to a great deal of information about host immunity to diseases and the use of vaccines. Vaccines are preventative measures, that is, they prime the immune system of an individual to react quickly when exposed to a disease, and thus stop people getting the disease, or at least reduce its severity. As such, they have had a major impact on the control of a number of dangerous infectious diseases such as smallpox, yellow fever, polio, measles and diphtheria. They have also greatly reduced the number of battlefield casualties from diseases such as gangrene and tetanus. Vaccines however, have very little effect on a disease whose symptoms have already appeared in an individual.

Paul Ehrlich (1854-1915), a German doctor who had worked with Koch, proposed a theory of immunity based on the body's recognition of dangerous molecules, and the specific neutralisation of these molecules. He received the Nobel Prize for medicine in 1908 for this work. Ehrlich is, however, better remembered today for his research on chemotherapy, the treatment of disease using drugs. He initiated a systematic search for chemicals showing selective toxicity, that is, they would destroy the disease-causing organism, but not damage the host organism. This approach was called chemotherapy, and was initially based on what was known as *"vital staining"*, the fact that some dyes will specifically stain certain disease-causing micro-organisms, but not the host cell. One example was the dye Methylene Blue, which stains malarial parasites in human blood. When used in an attempt to treat human malaria, the dye showed a small effect, but insufficient to make it clinically useful. This small success however, caused Ehrlich to reason that if the dye did not stain the host cell, it should be possible to produce a selectively staining dye, to which had been attached a toxic agent capable of killing the malarial parasite or other microbial cells. Two later derivatives of the dyes Ehrlich worked with are Suramin (derived from the dye Trypan Red), which is effective against African sleeping sickness, and Mepacrine (a similar structure to Methylene Blue) that was used widely against malaria. Suramin, introduced in 1920, is interesting as it was the first effective antimicrobial agent that did not contain a toxic metal atom such as arsenic or mercury.

A related aspect of *"vital staining"* was the empirical discovery by the Danish microbiologist, Christian Gram, in 1884, that some bacteria would stain with a combination of certain dyes whilst others would not. Gram was unable to ascertain the reason for this, but was able to show that it was reproducible. We now know that this difference is related to fundamental differences in the cell wall chemistry of different groups of bacteria, and results in bacteria being divided into two major groups for medical purposes, Gram positive and Gram negative. This is of major importance medically, as certain antibiotics, such as the penicillins, will preferentially attack the cell wall of one group rather than the other.

The use of chemicals to control specific diseases and medicinal problems had been known in some cases for a long time. The Romans used honey to treat wounds and numerous plant and herbal remedies were used by early Chinese, Greek, Roman, Arabic and medieval doctors to name but a few. One of the earliest chemicals to be used in medicine is probably opium (derived from the poppy [*Papave somniferum*]), whose use is thought to date back at least 6,000 years. It was certainly used in classical Greece, where it was sacred to three gods, Hypnos, the god of sleep, his twin brother Thanatos, the god of death, and Morpheus, the god of dreams (hence the name of the drug, morphine).

Many of these cultures were well aware of the use of herbal preparations, poisons and their antidotes, indeed in Homer's Odyssey (written in approximately the eighth century BC), Odysseus (Ulysses) is advised to take *"Moly"* to protect himself against the poison used by the witch Circe. *"Moly"* was probably a preparation of the snowdrop (*Galanthus nivalis*), which is an antidote to poisonous plants such as the thorn apple (*Datura stramonium*). This remedy however, was unusual for the time, in that it is a specific antidote to a certain type of poison. In most cases in antiquity, the antidote to poisons was merely an emetic to make the victim vomit, and hopefully get rid of the poison before it did too much damage.

Herbal remedies were widely used during the Dark Ages and Middle Ages by religious foundations, and monasteries generally maintained herbal gardens containing a wide range of medicinal plants. One well-known example of herbal remedies still in use today is the bark of the cinchona tree, also known as Jesuit's bark, which contains quinine and has been used to treat malaria and fevers for hundreds of years. The use of extracts of bark from the willow (*Salix alba*) was mentioned by Hippocrates, who was aware of the analgesic (pain relieving), and anti-pyretic (fever reducing) properties of willow. Another example, meadowsweet (*Spiraea ulmaria*), was used as an analgesic and anti-inflammatory agent, and research in the nineteenth century showed that the active ingredient of both willow bark and meadow sweet was salicylic acid. The bitter taste of this and its side effects causing stomach irritation, led to the compound being modified in 1897 to form acetyl salicylate. This was patented in 1899 as aspirin (A for acetyl and spirin from *Spiria*), and is probably the most widely used drug ever developed.

Very few of the worlds plants have been fully screened for their medicinal properties, even although approximately half of the twenty-five or so best selling drugs in today's world are based on natural products of plants and fungi. Recent examples of important chemicals isolated from plants are the very valuable anti-cancer drugs, vincristine and vinblastine from *Catharanthus roseus* (Madagascar periwinkle) and taxol from the bark of the Pacific yew, *Taxus brevifolia*. This can cause serious environmental problems as the Pacific yew is a rare species and collection from wild plants is unsustainable. Luckily in this case, taxol can also be obtained from the clippings of *T. baccata* (English yew).

Attempts to alleviate this problem have been made in a number of cases using tissue culture. This technique consists in taking some of the tissue from a plant and growing it under sterile conditions in the laboratory. The principle is relatively simple but the practicalities are considerable, one of the main ones being keeping the cultures from becoming contaminated with bacteria or fungi. Whilst tissue culture is effective sometimes, in many cases the tissue cultured does not produce the desired chemicals.

Many pharmaceuticals are prepared from plants grown in plantations, typical examples are morphine obtained from opium poppies, the heart drug digitoxin from *Digitalis lanata,* a member of the foxglove family, the steroid contraceptives are derived from the yam, and the ergot alkaloids are produced from rye seeded with the fungus *Claviceps purpurea.* The drug may just be isolated and purified from the plant tissue, or it may be modified chemically before use. One problem is that as the pharmaceutical compound is derived from a natural source, there may be variations from batch to batch, and it is essential that purified material is carefully standardised.

A further problem is that in herbal medicine, whole plants are frequently used and over-exploitation of these can cause shortages, creating price fluctuations and leading to plant substitution and adulteration. Unfortunately in many cultures practicing herbal medicine, plants taken from the wild are seen as more efficacious than the same plant grown or cultivated commercially, which raises the emotive question of sustainable yields.

A major objection of many people is that drugs are synthetic, and not natural. Many drugs are however, identical to those found in nature, aspirin for example is now made synthetically as it is a lot cheaper than isolating it from *Spiraea,* and there are numerous other examples such as the antibiotic chloramphenicol. Many other drugs, for example, the antibiotics of the penicillin group, are made using what are known as semi-synthetic processes. This consists of growing cultures of the fungus, *Penicillium,* purifying a parent compound made by the fungus, and then altering this chemically, to produce a wide range of penicillins, each one having a slightly different activity against various groups of bacteria.

Other chemicals, in addition to plants and their extracts, were used medicinally, including certain elements. Mercury containing ointments had been used to treat syphilis since the sixteenth century, although in this particular case the treatment was probably as dangerous as the problem. Similarly, another element, the poison antimony was alleged to have been used by the alchemist, Basil Valentine on his fellow monks, in order to test its *"healing"* properties. A number of authors have queried whether Valentine actually existed, or whether he was a figment of the imagination of Paracelsus (Ch 2).

Paracelsus is usually credited with introduction of laudanum (an alcoholic extract of poppy) to Europe, and in the nineteenth century, opium and its active constituent, morphine were used to treat a wide range of real and imagined ailments including pain relief, pacifying babies and controlling diarrhoea. Hypodermic needles were invented in the mid-nineteenth century and were used by society ladies to hold morphine parties. By the end of the nineteenth century, irresponsible use of opium had led to widespread addiction. The authorities initially tolerated the situation to a considerable extent. However, the situation eventually became so bad that the government was forced to take notice, and in Britain, addiction to opium became to a large extent the driving force behind the introduction of the "Dangerous Drugs Acts", leading to the control of this and similar chemicals.

Other examples of the early use of specific chemicals for medicinal purposes are also known. In the 1860s, Chesshire had realised that blindness, caused by bacterial eye infections in newly born children, could be cured by the application of silver nitrate solution to the eyes, a treatment continued in the USA until replaced by antibiotics in the 1940s.

The use of arsenic containing compounds was also widespread throughout various parts of the world. Chinese medical books written around 200 BC describe the use of realgar (arsenic sulphide) to treat scrofula (Ch 11), and arsenic oxide was used widely in China as an anti-malarial agent, whilst the use of arsenic sulphide is described by Hippocrates. In Styria, a region of Austria, white arsenic (arsenic trioxide) was used in the seventeenth century as a prophylactic against plague.

Ehrlich however, modified a large number of compounds (over 600), and eventually in 1910 produced an arsenic-containing compound known as salvarsan, number 606. This was effective at treating syphilis and related diseases and was only supplanted by penicillin in 1945. The two important features of Ehrlich's work were the screening of large numbers of compounds for antimicrobial activity, and the deliberate synthesis of chemically modified compounds related to a parent compound known to have antimicrobial activity. Essentially, these are still the techniques used today in the search for antimicrobial drugs.

A small number of other compounds were developed using the principles of Ehrlich. The next major breakthrough in chemotherapy was made in the 1930s by Gerhard Domagk (who received the Nobel Prize in 1939[38]), for the discovery of the compound prontosil, which is active against many groups of bacteria. Domagk worked for Bayer and was researching azo dyes when he discovered prontosil. This compound displays a property known as *"lethal synthesis"* which is found in many molecules. It is inactive in the test tube, but in animals, prontosil breaks down in the liver into sulphanilamide, the

---

38   He was not allowed to accept it until 1947, because of the policies of Nazi Germany.

active form of the drug. A wide range of *"sulpha"* drugs were developed, and although their use has to a large extent been superseded by the antibiotics which are more effective in most cases, they are still widely used in veterinary medicine, and also in the treatment of a few specific human diseases.

The discovery of sulphanilamide was also responsible in an indirect way for the development of much of the legislation attached to the sale of drugs in the modern day. In 1937, patients in Oklahoma, USA, who had taken a sulphanilamide preparation began to die in agony, further cases followed in other states. Post mortem examination showed catastrophic failure of internal organs, especially the liver and kidneys. All the victims appeared to have taken a preparation known as Elixir Sulphanilamide, supplied by one company, S. E. Masengill, based in Tennessee. The company chemist, Harold Watkins, had no formal qualifications and had been dissolving sulphanilamide in di-ethylene glycol (DEG) to sweeten it, and make it more palatable, especially to children. DEG is one of the main ingredients of antifreeze and the company had not bothered to test its effect on animals before using it. When challenged by officials from the Food and Drug Administration (FDA), Watkins swallowed a large dose of the preparation in an act of bravado, to prove there was nothing wrong with it. He was fighting for his life within twenty-four hours.

The FDA took emergency action and managed to recall approximately 97% of the lethal mixture, but the remainder caused over one hundred deaths, and nearly three hundred people were left with long-term illnesses.

The company claimed it had not broken the law; in this it was technically correct, as the existing Food and Drug Acts at that time only prohibited the mislabelling of medicines, it did not prohibit the sale of medicine containing useless or even poisonous ingredients. The company was eventually fined the equivalent of about £7,000, the maximum possible for selling a preparation labelled an elixir, a term implying that it contained ethyl alcohol.

The case caused public outrage, and the result was that in 1938, the Federal Food, Drug and Cosmetic Act came into law, which forced companies to prove that their products were safe before selling them. In a final act of the tragedy Watkins, who was one of the people to survive the poisoning with DEG, was unable to live with the situation; he shot himself several months later.

The great chemotherapeutic advance in the treatment of disease was the discovery of the antibiotics. Technically, these are compounds made and excreted by certain micro-organisms that are toxic to the growth of other micro-organisms, although the term is now generally used to describe any anti-microbial compound. The first of these compounds to be discovered was penicillin by the English bacteriologist, Sir Alexander Fleming (1881-1955), in 1929. He discovered that certain fungi of the genus *Penicillium* excrete a chemical (penicillin). This was able to inhibit the growth of the bacterium, *Staphylococcus aureus,* that is responsible for causing boils and septicaemia. Although Fleming was unable to completely purify penicillin, he did use partially purified preparations to treat localised skin infections. In recognition of his work, Fleming received both a knighthood and the Nobel Prize in 1945.

Mycotherapy (the use of moulds to treat diseases) was used widely during the 1930s and early 1940s. This consisted of growing antibiotic producing moulds on bandages that were then applied to wounds. Whilst the work of Fleming had obviously given this type of approach scientific respectability, there was an extensive folk medicine based on the use of moulds. Mould therapy was used by the ancient Egyptians, is mentioned in early Jewish texts, and the application of mouldy bread as a poultice was used widely in many societies. One seventeenth century English work specifically praises the use and effectiveness of moulds growing on human skulls.

Further work on penicillin was continued by a British group led by Howard Florey and Ernst Chain at Oxford in 1939/40. They were able to produce, purify and stabilise it and by 1941, it was being given to patients with advanced septicaemia[39]. Both Florey and Chain received the Nobel Prize at the same time as Fleming.

The work was continued in the USA during World War II, and by 1944 several technical advances had led to huge amounts being produced. Ultimately a large range of commercial penicillins were synthesised. One of the major difficulties in production is that the strain of *Penicillium* that produces most penicillin, when grown on a solid agar surface, is not necessarily the strain that produces most when grown in a fermenter containing liquid cultures (the method of commercial production). Germany did not start active research on penicillin production until 1942 and German scientists were never able to produce it in sufficient quantities to have any military value.

There was considerable controversy when A. J. Moyer, a US employee, claimed patents on penicillin and was granted them. The Oxford group had not patented penicillin on the grounds that public money was used to develop them, and the public should benefit. Millions of pounds in royalties were diverted to the USA and were the source of great acrimony for many years.

Although they were the first group of antibiotics to be discovered, the penicillins still remain one of the most effective and widely used groups of antibiotics, as they show high levels of selective toxicity (the ability to kill a disease-causing organism without damaging the host). Their selective toxicity is based on the fact that they destroy the cell wall structure of many bacteria, which contains a number of chemicals not found in the human body.

---

39   At this time, the antibiotic was so valuable and in such short supply that excreted material was re-isolated from the urine of the patient and reused.

This work was followed by the discovery of a second group of antibiotics, the streptomycins by Selman Waksman, who also won the Nobel Prize in 1952. These compounds first became available in 1947, and are derived from the bacterial genus *Streptomyces,* commonly found in soil; it is this bacterium that gives soil its distinctive smell. The award of the Nobel prize in this particular case was marred by accusations that Waksman had not given sufficient credit to one of his co-workers. Although the co-worker was not awarded a share in the Nobel prize, he was able to mount a successful legal challenge to the assignment of patents. The importance of the streptomycins was that they could destroy some bacteria not attacked by the penicillins, and were also able to kill *Mycobacterium tuberculosis,* the causative organism of tuberculosis.

A large number of antibiotics are now known, but only a relatively small number of these are used chemotherapeutically, the rest all have major problems of side effects on the host, or some technical problem obviating their use. The rate of discovery of new and effective antibiotics has declined considerably in recent years, and it is probable that a majority of the useful ones have already been discovered and exploited. In the last thirty years or so, most new antibiotics have just been a chemical modification of an already existing class[40], and during this period very few new classes of antibiotics have been discovered and introduced into general medicine.

A major and potentially very serious problem in the use of antibiotics is the increase in bacterial resistance to this type of treatment. Much of this problem is due to the widespread inappropriate use of antibiotics to treat relatively trivial infections, such as sore throats. A further aspect is the use of antibiotics in the farming industry to speed up the rate at which livestock gains weight, which has obvious commercial implications.

The use of *"broad spectrum"* antibiotics is also causing problems. These are antibiotics that kill all bacteria including

---

40   Frequently referred to as me-too antibiotics.

the beneficial ones. The use of broad spectrum antibiotics has been described as *"carpet bombing the microbial population"* and is an important factor in the development of microbial resistance. A bacterium frequently causing problems in hospitals is *Clostridium difficile.* This organism occurs naturally in the gastro-intestinal tract of about 3-5% of the population but the other beneficial bacteria that colonize the gut compete with it, preventing it becoming a problem. When someone is given a broad-spectrum antibiotic the beneficial bacteria are killed leaving *C. difficile* to proliferate without competition. The result is that it colonises the whole gut causing severe diarrhoea that frequently kills the patient.

Tuberculosis is probably the most serious long-term example of resistance and this is discussed later (Ch 11). The best known example is probably the antibiotic resistance demonstrated by *Staphylococcus aureus.* This bacterium, commonly found on the skin, causes boils, abscesses and blood poisoning and is a common cause of post-operative infections. The first recorded case of penicillin resistance was in 1947 only four years after penicillin G, the first penicillin, became commercially available. In 1952, almost all hospital infections caused by *Staphylococcus* could still be treated with this compound. By 1982, penicillin G was effective in less than 10% of cases, and by 1992, one of the most effective penicillins, methicillin, was also ineffective in a large number of cases, giving rise to the term MRSA (methicillin resistant *Staphylococcus aureus*[41]). The misuse of antibiotics causes the susceptible bacteria to be killed, leaving the more resistant ones to flourish. By the early 1990s, many staphylococcal infections could only be treated with the antibiotic vancomycin, occasionally referred to as the *"antibiotic of last resort"*. Reports of resistance to this were

---

41   This bacterium, frequently referred to as a "superbug" by journalists, was first recorded in the 1960s, only a couple of years after methicillin became available. The appearance of MRSA is a classic example of Darwinian evolution (Ch 5) with humans providing the selective pressure in the form of penicillin-based antibiotics.

also starting to appear, especially amongst a group of bacteria known as the enterococci. A further problem of resistance relates to cost, methicillin is about ten times more expensive than penicillin G, and vancomycin is even more expensive.

Resistance to a wide range of other antibiotics is also becoming more common, as also is the transfer of antibiotic resistance from one group of bacteria to another[42]. Frequently, this involves the transfer of antibiotic resistance from a relatively innocuous group of bacteria to an extremely dangerous group. What is even more worrying is the fact that in many cases, resistance to as many as five or six totally unrelated antibiotics is transferred from bacterium to bacterium as a single step. The agent carrying out this transfer is a piece of deoxyribonucleic acid (Ch 4) known as a plasmid. The general consensus of opinion amongst microbiologists is that these plasmids are degenerate bacteriophage (bacterial viruses), that retain the ability to infect new bacterial hosts but have lost the ability to kill them.

As a result, many doctors fear that we will soon have reverted to the pre-antibiotic era in terms of the treatments available for bacterial diseases. A recent development in this direction has been the use of maggots to treat wounds containing necrotic (dead) tissue, a treatment used widely during the Napoleonic wars, the American Civil War and World War I for the treatment of gangrenous wounds. The application of maggots grown under aseptic conditions is now being used in many countries to treat recalcitrant wounds and antibiotic resistant infections. The use of medicinal leeches to remove blood clots is another move in a similar direction, whilst the use of bacterial viruses (bacteriophage) to treat a variety of diseases was used widely throughout Russia and its satellite countries for much of the twentieth century.

---

42   The speed at which resistant bacteria are appearing is outstripping the rate at which new antibiotics are discovered, and drug companies are running desperately in an attempt to keep up.

Although there is a considerable range of chemicals available for the treatment of bacterial diseases, there are relatively few compounds effective against diseases caused by viruses. Viruses cause a large number of infectious diseases including some of the most dangerous ones known, such as smallpox, yellow fever, measles, HIV/AIDS and Ebola. The few drugs that are available are frequently very expensive, for example, treatment of a patient suffering from HIV/AIDS in the UK and USA, using the latest drugs available, has been estimated at approximately £1,400 (US$2,300) per month. Whilst a doctor may well prescribe an antibiotic for an elderly person suffering from influenza, which is a viral infection, this is done solely to stop the development of a secondary infection of pneumonia caused by bacteria. The antibiotic has no effect on the course of the viral flu infection.

The reason for this paucity of chemotherapeutic agents effective against viruses is due to the mode of reproduction of the virus. Viruses are only capable of growth inside a host cell, and effectively subvert the host cell's metabolic systems for their own purposes. The result is that it is generally extremely difficult to destroy a virus without causing serious side effects in the host organism.

Some diseases are caused by organisms other than bacteria or viruses. Malaria (Ch 16) is one example, being caused by members of the protozoan genus, *Plasmodium*. Chemotherapy of diseases of this type is also extremely problematical as the basic cell pattern of *Plasmodium* is of the same type as that found in humans. This means it is technically very difficult to synthesize chemotherapeutic agents that do not produce serious side effects upon the human host. Some of these diseases are not major killers in their own right, but produce a seriously debilitated population who become highly susceptible to other diseases caused by bacteria and viruses. In the case of diseases caused by members of the metazoa, such as Schistosomes (Ch 19), treatment becomes even more difficult.

Finally, it is worth pointing out that although antibiotic research is generally considered to be the glamorous side of microbiology, the lives of far more people have been saved by non-glamorous aspects of microbiology, such as vaccination, the provision of clean drinking water and the efficient disposal of sewage.

BIOLOGICAL WARFARE

Perhaps one of the most worrying aspects of microbiology in the twentieth century was the development of biological weapons that contravene all civilized values. Fighting disease is seen as virtuous, and to cause disease is regarded as totally unacceptable. Many people regard bioweapons as totally repugnant, but this attitude completely ignores the realities of politics. The brutal fact is that if these weapons are available they will be used, and indeed have been used already. Some scientists are of the opinion that man cannot improve on the lethal nature of diseases honed by thousands of years of epidemics and evolution, although this is debatable given recent advances in genetic engineering. However, what man has done with great efficiency is to improve on the delivery systems of such weapons, and the speed with which the disease can be spread.

Biological weapons are extremely dangerous for a number of reasons. Studies by the USA suggest that they are very much more effective than conventional, chemical or nuclear weapons. They are also much cheaper to produce than nuclear weapons, putting them within reach of many more countries and their manufacture is much easier to keep hidden. Detection of biowarfare capability is difficult as a fully operational biowarfare laboratory could be set up in a small, apparently innocuous warehouse.

Further problems are caused by the fact that micro-organisms suitable for biowarfare are frequently difficult to separate from those of the normal environment, indeed they may be identical to those of the normal environment, and it can therefore be difficult to recognise a biological attack even after it has occurred. Once an attack becomes imminent, knowing what to immunise against, and having enough vaccine to do so, also become major problems. Finally, once biological weapons have been used, they are impossible to control, and are at the mercy of prevailing weather conditions, such as wind direction, temperature and rain.

Biological weapons have been used prior to the twentieth century, for example, the French, Americans and British are all reputed to have given North American Indians trade blankets impregnated with smallpox in the eighteenth century. There are also numerous medieval accounts of dead bodies of both humans and horses being hurled into besieged cities using giant catapults. The development of biological weapons on a grand scale however, was a twentieth century phenomenon.

One of the main problems in the international control of these weapons is that the technology required for their development is dual-purpose technology, this means that the techniques used for legitimate biotechnology and weapons production are the same. Any country having the technology to ferment beer or wine, or produce antibiotics or vaccines on a large scale, also has the capability to produce biological weapons. For example, many vaccines against viral diseases are inactivated viruses, so that to develop the vaccine it is necessary to grow the virus. The result is that the technology to produce micro-organisms on a large scale is widespread, with well over one hundred countries having biological warfare capability of some form or another.

What differs from country to country is the capability to deliver a payload in the form required to make it highly effective. Even the capability of delivering a warhead hundreds or thousands of miles is not necessary, a slurry or powder (milled to the correct particle size) of bacteria, such as anthrax, placed in an underground railway system, could be spread very effectively by the slipstream of passing trains. As such, micro-organisms make a very effective terrorist weapon and were used in this manner in the Tokyo underground system by the Aum Shinrikyo religious sect in 1995. This was done on at least four occasions, but was ineffective, probably due to problems with the particle size, so they then used the nerve gas sarin, and caused about a dozen deaths. This was not the first use of micro-organisms by terrorists. In 1984, the Rajneeshee cult in Oregon contaminated salads with the bacterium *Salmonella,* and caused over a thousand cases of food poisoning in attempts to influence voting patterns in local elections.

Whether the attack is effective or not is immaterial, the public knowledge that there are individuals or groups *"out there"*, who are prepared to make use of such weapons is frequently sufficient to cause mass panic and chaos.

Terrorist attacks involving the addition of botulin toxin to the water system (the only realistic way to use it), a scenario much beloved by thriller writers, would not work, as water treatment systems in developed countries would rapidly degrade the toxin. In addition, although the toxin (which works by blocking nerve impulses and paralysing muscles) is one of the most deadly biological toxins known when injected, the lethal dose by ingestion is about one thousand times greater. The toxin does have a legitimate medical use for treating uncontrollable twitching of muscles. The use of botox for beauty treatment is however, an accident waiting to happen, sooner or later someone will get the dosage disastrously wrong. There has already been at least one accident with botox treatment involving a number of victims, although in this case it appears that the problem was a contaminated batch of botox, supplied from an unregistered laboratory.

Following the terrorist attacks on the World Trade Centre on 11th September 2001, anthrax was used as a biological weapon to attack various government departments in the

USA, causing the first cases of pulmonary anthrax in the USA for twenty-five years, and ultimately five deaths. No terrorist group appears to have been involved in the attacks and the FBI identified a single individual as being responsible, an individual however with specialist knowledge and access to the military (Ames) strain of anthrax. This is resistant to many of the antibiotics normally used to treat the disease. He also had access to specialist milling equipment to produce the optimum sized particles for biowarfare. The suggestion has been made that the organism may have come from Fort Detrick itself, the American germ warfare centre. If these suppositions are correct, it demonstrates the ease with which biological weapons can be deployed.

The biological community has been notoriously lax over the security of micro-organisms in the past. Many deadly organisms were available from various culture collections as long as the request came from an apparently reputable source. Cultures and information on growing them are freely available between laboratories and on the internet.

In 1925, the Geneva conference banned the use of biological warfare, however, a number of countries assumed that if it was worth banning, then it must have potential value. Japan developed an extensive programme between 1931-45 run by General Ishii, and carried out in Manchuria (Pingfan Institute) by the infamous Unit 731. It was even alleged that the Japanese laced fruit with cholera organisms in 1931, to disrupt the League of Nations Commission studying the Japanese seizure of Manchuria. The programme run by Unit 731 used local people and Japanese dissidents as test subjects infecting them with numerous diseases including anthrax, bubonic plague, typhoid and yellow fever. After World War II, the Stockholm International Peace Research Institute estimated that the Japanese had killed over ten thousand people in laboratory experiments, and several hundred thousand in field operations.

There were serious epidemics in Manchuria between 1946-8, and the Chinese were convinced that these had been caused by retreating Japanese troops releasing infected animals in 1945. It is extremely difficult to establish the extent of the experiments. The Americans gave a blanket immunity from prosecution for war crimes to Ishii and his team, in order to obtain their results, after discovering that they had used human guinea pigs. The main concern of the USA over this matter appears to have been that the knowledge of the deal would become public and cause the USA severe political embarrassment.

In World War II there was significant preparation for biological warfare, by all the major belligerents, based on inaccurate intelligence reports suggesting that the other side was preparing for biological warfare. The Japanese claimed after World War II that the Russians had also used biological weapons, especially cholera and bubonic plague. German intelligence sources indicated that the Russians had started biological warfare research in the 1930s. It was alleged that the USSR had carried out trials in Mongolia, and that in 1941, a prisoner had escaped causing an epidemic of plague that killed up to 5,000 people.

In 1956, at the height of the Cold War, Marshal Zhukov stated that all future wars would be fought using a variety of weapons including biological ones. The USSR agreed at a biological warfare convention in 1972 to ban the development, testing, production, stockpiling and deployment of such weapons. However, in 1979 an outbreak of anthrax killed hundreds of people near Ekaterinburg. The Russians claimed tainted meat was to blame, but the USA claimed that an accidental release had occurred at a local military facility after the failure of a biological filter. In 1992, President Yeltsin admitted that the American version was correct. In 1997, Ken Alibeck, the second in command of the Russian biological warfare programme, defected to the West, and reported that the Russians had developed genetically engineered anthrax resistant to all antibiotics and were stockpiling approximately twenty tonnes of smallpox virus that could be converted into weapons at short notice.

Sir Frederick Banting (the discoverer of insulin), who received the Nobel Prize for Medicine in 1923, applied for a grant for biological warfare research from the Canadian government in 1940. The work involved mixing bacteria with sawdust and spraying it from a plane. A group was set up at Porton Down in the UK to study the feasibility of biological warfare. By the end of 1940 it had determined that the most effective method of spreading diseases was aerosol production to form particles, which would be inhaled. Tests were carried out, mainly on anthrax, and one test site, Gruinard Island off the west coast of Scotland, was contaminated so badly that it was not pronounced fit for human habitation until 1990. The targets used were sheep, but at least one experiment was alleged to have gone wrong when a corpse floated to the mainland, infected mainland sheep and possibly killed several people. The affair was censored under wartime regulations.

The USA began their biological warfare programme in 1943 at Fort Deytrick, and had developed a large offensive programme by 1969, which had involved tests (some of which were fatal) on both military and civilian personnel. In many cases, the personnel involved had no knowledge of the fact that tests were being carried out and that they were being used as targets. Nixon renounced US use of these weapons in 1969. It is thought however, that this renunciation was due to the realisation that there is no really effective defence against biological warfare, and the US had realised that their own research programme was a threat to their own security.

Other countries have developed biological weapons, the most notorious case recently being Iraq. Iraq had used chemical weapons against both the Kurds and Iran in the

1980s, but although Iraq admitted to having missiles armed with biological warheads, these were not used in the Gulf War in 1991. The most probable reason for their non-use was threatened retaliation with nuclear weapons. The question of whether Iraq had destroyed their biological and chemical weapons was a major reason for the second Gulf War.

Human Genome Project

One of the major biological initiatives of recent years has been the human genome project that aims to identify, and relate the genes found in humans to their function. Whilst the intention is to identify genes causing diseases such as cancer, with the ultimate intention of providing gene therapy, this knowledge, in common with many scientific discoveries, could also be put to alternative uses. It has become obvious from the progress of this project that various ethnic groups have small, although significant differences in their DNA frequencies. These differences lead to differing susceptibilities to certain diseases, such as diabetes and various types of cancer. This raises the possibility of producing ethnic weapons, that is weapons aimed at certain ethnic groups as specified by their gene frequencies.

The weapon would be made by using genetic engineering to attach a disease-causing virus to a chemical (probably a nucleic acid sequence), able to recognise specific sequences of the human genome, in the ethnic group targeted. One genetic marker would not discriminate sufficiently, but if several genetic markers occur at a high rate of frequency in the target population, then the possibility of producing a highly specific weapon becomes feasible. The possibility of this type of weapon being developed has been raised significantly by the total synthesis of the polio virus. Whilst polio is only a relatively simple virus, it is obvious that if polio can be synthesised, more complex and modified viruses will follow sooner or later. This would appear to be the ultimate weapon as it would destroy a substantial percentage of the target population, but leave buildings, infrastructure and one's own troops untouched. Whilst this might seem to be the nightmare scenario of science fiction, given recent advances in gene recognition and genetic engineering, the possibility of such weapons is probably less than a few decades away.

It is not necessary for biowarfare to be aimed at a human target, biological weapons aimed at crops could cause economic devastation to a country. Those countries most at risk are countries such as the USA, Canada or countries of the former USSR, where vast areas of monoculture crops such as wheat, barley, maize and rice are grown.

The use of fungal diseases such as rusts, smuts and wilts against cereal crops could cause massive economic damage, famine and political destabilisation. It may not even be necessary to destroy large areas of crops, even small outbreaks could result in a crop being blacklisted by the World Trade Organisation, and most countries operate a quarantine system for diseased crops, especially unprocessed ones. Food riots are already a normal feature of many countries when price rises of staple foods occur, and the blacklisting of a staple food could easily destabilise the economy of a small or poor country.

The production of such a weapon would be simple. Plant pathogens are spread naturally by wind and insects, and there is no need for genetically modified plant parasites. Naturally occurring plant pathogens, which have been locked in an evolutionary arms race with plants for thousands of years, are probably already as effective as anything that could be produced in the laboratory. A further advantage is that plant pathogens are so widespread naturally, that it would be extremely difficult to determine whether the disease was a natural occurrence, or as a result of an enemy attack. The problem might not even be an enemy attack; it could be a company attempting to gain a commercial advantage. For example, a company exporting an exotic crop from country A, might decide to introduce the disease into country B where a different company was operating, in order to eliminate the competition.

CONCLUSION

As a final note to this chapter, it should be mentioned that there was a considerable over-optimism towards the defeat of infectious diseases during the 1960s. In 1967, the US Surgeon-General stated, *"It was time to close the book on infectious disease"*. When we look at the numbers of people today infected by various diseases, this has to be considered one of the most unfortunate remarks ever made by a doctor. There are an estimated world-wide total of thirty to forty million cases of AIDS; an estimated three to five hundred million cases of malaria, of whom about three million die each year, mainly children and pregnant women; a minimum of five million deaths each year of children under the age of five from gastro-enteritis in one form or another; three million deaths per year from tuberculosis, and about two hundred thousand children die each year from measles. These figures are almost certainly a considerable underestimate, and no doctor or microbiologist today would have the temerity to suggest that infectious diseases are a spent force. They represent one of the most serious challenges that the human species faces in the immediate future.

CHAPTER 4

Pathogenic Micro-organisms; Know the Enemy.

BIOLOGICAL CLASSIFICATION

The classification and understanding of biological systems underwent a massive reorganisation during the last quarter of the twentieth century. Prior to this period, living organisms had been classified to a large extent on their appearance, and in the case of bacteria on their chemical properties and reactions. As a result, during the first part of the twentieth century, five Kingdoms were recognised in the biological world, Bacteria, Protozoa, Fungi, Plants and Animals.

Major advances in the understanding of nucleic acid chemistry has meant that the classification of organisms is now arranged on the structural similarities of certain types of Ribonucleic Acid (see later) found in all organisms. The result has been a major realignment of the inter-relationships between organisms over the last three decades or so, with a recognition that the greatest biological diversity is found in the microbiological world.

Three domains of organisms are now recognised, the first and second being the Bacteria and the Archaea (the Ancient Ones), both of which have a simple type of cell structure known as prokaryotic[43]. The third group are the Eukarya, a group of organisms having a more complex cell structure, of a type

---

43   The terms prokaryotic and eukaryotic are both derived from a Greek word, *karyos* meaning a seed or kernel. Thus eukaryotic means true seed, that is, a nucleus in the cell, and prokaryotic means before seed, that is, no nucleus present in the cell.

known as eukaryotic. The domain Eukarya includes Protists, Algae, Fungi, Plants and Animals. Protists are regarded as those members of the Eukarya existing as single cells, but this includes a wide variety of different cell lineages or phyla (a phylum can be defined as a major cell lineage).

The Archaea are thought to be the earliest forms of cellular life and evolved in ecosystems such as hot springs and geysers. They are of great interest in geochemistry and of increasing interest in industrial microbiology and chemistry, but so far, none have been shown to have any role in causing disease and are therefore of no further interest in this book.

Seventeen (at least) major groups (phyla) of the domain Bacteria are known, and have been grown in the laboratory. Numerous others have been identified from circumstantial evidence but have so far defied attempts to culture them.

DISEASE CAUSING ORGANISMS

Infectious diseases can be caused by a number of different types of entities. These include viruses, bacteria, fungi, protists and metazoa (metazoa means many cells). Diseases may also be caused by prions and algae, although prions fall into a somewhat different category.

VIRUSES

Viruses are the simplest disease causing entities, their name is derived from a Latin word meaning poison (hence the word virulent). It was not until the late nineteenth century that the word virus came to mean an infectious agent.

The simplest viruses consist of a core of a chemical, known as a nucleic acid, surrounded by a protein coat. The core may be either Ribonucleic Acid (RNA) or Deoxyribonucleic Acid (DNA), but never both. This core is organised into a sequence of genes carrying the genetic information of the virus. Although the nucleic acids contain the genetic information of the virus, they lack certain parts of the information needed to reproduce the virus, and therefore use the host enzymes (biological catalysts[44]) for the synthesis of some of their components.

The coat of the virus varies in complexity, at its simplest it is comprised of protein[45] only, although some viruses do have more complex coats. No matter how complex the coat is, it has similar functions in all viruses. It protects the nucleic acid and it also enables the virus to recognise receptor molecules on the cell surface and thus gain entry into susceptible host cells. The coat is however, the weak link of viruses causing disease in animals as it is the proteins in the virus coat that are recognised by the defensive system of the host, and which initiate the immune response of the host.

Viruses are incapable of multiplying unless they enter a susceptible cell[46], and in the absence of an appropriate host cell, they are effectively inert. The virus multiplies by entering the host cell, taking it over, and then subverting its biochemical mechanisms to make more viruses. Once it has entered the host cell, the virus enters an eclipse phase, where it apparently disappears for a period of time. The length of the eclipse phase varies widely depending on the disease. At the end of the eclipse phase, a large number of new virus particles (hundreds or thousands) are formed, these are released from the infected cell, and each one is able to infect a new susceptible cell. There are a number of different variations found on this basic theme depending on the virus involved.

The central theory of nucleic acid replication and function was originally proposed by Crick, who suggested that DNA had two roles. The first of these was to replicate itself accurately from generation to generation, and the second was to dictate

---

44   A catalyst is a molecule that speeds up a reaction without being changed itself. The rate at which the reaction is speeded up varies widely, but in some cases the catalysed reaction may be more than a million times faster then the uncatalysed reaction.

45   Protein molecules consist of long chains of compounds known as amino acids.

46   This may be any type of cell including animals, plants or even bacterial cells.

the structure of RNA (a process known as transcription). The role of RNA was to dictate the structure of protein (a process known as translation). This is summarised in Figure 4.1.

Figure 4.1

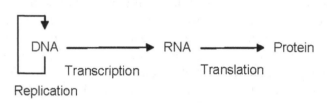

This theory was modified slightly by the discovery of the RNA viruses when it was realised that RNA viruses must also be able to replicate themselves without the involvement of DNA. The modification of the theory showing the replication of RNA viruses is shown in Figure 4.2.

Figure 4.2

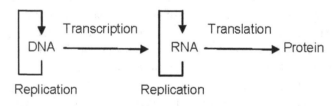

The greatest challenge to the theory came with the discovery that some RNA viruses are able to dictate the structure of DNA, a process known as reverse transcription. These viruses are now known to consist of an extremely important group referred to as the RNA *retro*-viruses. A diagram incorporating this further modification is shown in Figure 4.3.

Figure 4.3

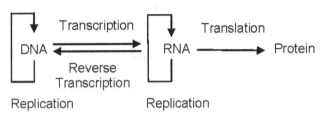

Three groups of viruses are therefore recognised, the DNA viruses, the RNA viruses and the RNA *retro*-viruses. Each of these groups is then further subdivided with a variety of features being used to achieve this.

Viruses are considerably smaller than bacteria, the polio virus which is amongst the smallest is only 28ηm, whilst one of the largest are the pox viruses at approximately 200ηm (the abbreviation ηm stands for nanometre, one billionth [10^{-9}] of a metre).

There has been considerable discussion over a long period of time concerning the origins of viruses. Did they evolve from more complex parasites that lost various bits and pieces until they were forced into a dependence mode of existence? Alternatively, are they pieces of nucleic acid that were excreted from organisms and developed into a quasi-species of their own? Are they alive or not? They have frequently been described as being, *"edge of life"*.

Research into disease-causing viruses and the chemicals attacking them is difficult, as it is necessary to grow a culture of susceptible cells first, and then culture the virus on these host cells. Whilst the theory of this is not particularly difficult, there are some major practical problems, such as contamination, to be overcome.

PRIONS

Transmissible Spongiform Encephalopathies (TSEs) (also known as prion diseases), include a number of diseases such as CJD (Creutzfeld-Jacob Disease) and BSE (Bovine Spongiform Encephalopathy). They have been receiving considerable publicity over recent years, but have been known for a long time. The first documented disease of this type, scrapie, was recorded over 200 years ago in sheep and goats. Kuru in humans in New Guinea has also been known for many years and was transmitted by ritual cannibalism. When someone important died or was killed, their brain was eaten to gain their wisdom, and transmission of the disease was only stopped when a ban on this practice was enforced.

Some of these diseases appear to have a genetic origin, whilst others are acquired from some food source. TSEs are fatal once clinical symptoms appear, and in the case of the acquired ones, there is frequently a very long (usually years) incubation period between first exposure and the appearance of the disease, making it extremely difficult to pinpoint the source. There is no conventional immune response.

A common feature of all these diseases is degeneration of the brain and spinal cord tissue leading to impaired transmission of nerve impulses, and part of this process involves a host protein known as the prion protein. During a TSE infection, an abnormal form of this protein is deposited in excessive amounts in the spinal cord, brain and nervous tissue. The infectious agents causing these diseases are unlike any conventional pathogens, and their nature was controversial for a long time. One theory, now discredited, suggested that they were small conventional viruses.

The theory now accepted is that it is an altered physical state of the normal host prion protein. This abnormal shape propagates itself by initiating a chain reaction causing other normal prion protein molecules to adopt the abnormal state. Any given sequence of amino acids making up a protein will twist and fold itself into a 3-D structure dictated by the amino acid sequence. This 3-D structure is usually unique, but in some proteins there are two alternative possibilities. The normal brain contains only one of these alternatives, but in the abnormal brain the protein flips to the alternate shape leading to chemical changes in the brain. It has not been possible as yet to produce infectious prions from normal prions in the laboratory.

Perhaps the simplest analogy of prion behaviour is to imagine a large number of square boxes piled up on top of each other to make a stack. If one of the boxes at the bottom of the heap is forced into a diagonal shape, then it will be necessary for all the boxes to take up a diagonal shape before the stack fits neatly together again.

BACTERIA

Many people consider all bacteria to be dangerous because of their association with certain diseases. A large number are however beneficial, they decompose rubbish and are an integral part of the water purification and sewage disposal systems. They are also found in ecosystems such as the human gut where they play a major role in stopping harmful bacteria gaining access to the body. They have an important industrial role in the making of products as diverse as cheese, yoghurts and some antibiotics.

Bacteria belong to one of the two groups of organisms known as procaryotic cells. They are very small, typically one to two microns in length (a micron is one millionth of a metre 10^{-6}), usually unicellular, are normally surrounded by a very strong cell wall and are relatively simple in organisational terms. They contain both DNA and RNA (the genetic information being carried by the DNA molecule), and a wide range of different proteins, producing a complicated immune response from any host organism they infect.

As mentioned earlier, at least seventeen major groups are found, a number of which contain disease-causing bacteria.

However, medically it is usual to divide pathogenic bacteria into four main groups depending on their shape and their reaction to the Gram stain. The two most common shapes are the cocci (singular coccus), which are round cells approximately one micron in diameter, and rods which are cylindrical, about one micron in diameter and two to three microns long. They are usually found singly, but in a few cases may occur in short chains. A few bacteria exist as tightly coiled spirals, these include organisms such as *Treponema*, the causative organism of syphilis. They tend to be much longer than other bacteria and considerably thinner.

Bacteria are then subdivided into Gram-positive and Gram-negative groups based on the stain developed by Christian Gram (Ch 3). All the Gram-positive bacteria occur in one phylum of the seventeen mentioned above, but the Gram-negative bacteria that are medically important fall into several different phyla. The result is that for practical purposes, the vast majority of medically important bacteria are split into four groups, Gram-positive cocci, Gram-positive rods, Gram-negative cocci and Gram-negative rods. Pathogenic bacteria are found in all four of these groups, with further subdivision to generic and specific level usually being carried out by several means, including a number of biochemical tests.

One important test is whether the bacteria are motile. Motility is conferred by the possession of flagella and the presence of flagella is an important factor in both the identification and determination of the antigenic makeup of the bacterium. A second important feature is the ability of the organism to use oxygen. Bacteria that are able to do so are known as aerobic, those that cannot use oxygen are anaerobic.

One group of organisms that used to be considered separately were the *Rickettsia*, but these have now been shown to be bacteria. In the older literature, they are frequently considered to be a halfway stage between bacteria and viruses.

The *Rickettsia* are a group of micro-organisms transmitted by arthropod parasites, such as fleas, ticks, lice and sand-flies. They are bacterial in appearance and have many of the typical chemical features of bacteria, but they have a reduced set of genes and are dependent on a host organism for much of their energy supply and the synthesis of some of their structural components. It has been impossible to culture many of them outside a host cell which has hindered research into antimicrobial compounds effective against them. They are all pathogens, and can be divided into several main groups based on the clinical diseases they cause. The most important of these organisms causes typhus (Ch 13).

An important feature of the RNA phylogeny that has developed over the last few years is that it has enabled us to realise relationships within the bacterial domain that were not always obvious previously. This has proved useful in attempting to understand the ability of pathogenic bacterial genera, such as *Escherichia, Salmonella, Shigella* and *Yersinia* to exchange genetic material with each other. Bacteria are able to exchange DNA in an extremely promiscuous manner using a number of different mechanisms, the donor bacterium does not even need to be alive. In 1928, Griffith carried out experiments on bacteria of the genus *Streptococcus;* some of these can exist in two forms depending on whether they possess a capsule around the cell. This is a polysaccharide found in smooth (S) cells but which is absent in rough (R) cells. This might seem to be a mere technical difference, but if S cells are injected into a mouse, the mouse dies within a couple of days from septicaemia. However if R cells are injected into a mouse, it survives. The capsule of the S cells protects the bacterium from phagocytosis (Ch 7) or engulfment by the defensive white cells of the mouse. Griffith found that if live R cells are mixed with dead S cells and injected into a mouse, the mouse dies and live S cells can be isolated from it's blood. Later research showed that the R cells were scavenging DNA from the dead S cells and using it to transform themselves into S cells. This type of behaviour has been shown to be responsible for the acquisition of antibiotic resistance by a number of bacteria.

Further experiments showed that many bacteria contain organelles known as plasmids. These plasmids are circular pieces of DNA capable of passing from cell to cell and transmitting a number of biochemical properties from the donor bacterium to the recipient. This includes the ability to transfer resistance to about half a dozen antibiotics in one step. The worrying fact is that the antibiotics do not need to be in the same family, they could be in six widely dispersed chemical groups.

From a practical point, bacteria in the laboratory are frequently divided into four groups depending on the inherent danger of the organism under consideration. These groups are defined as follows

- Group 1. An organism unlikely to cause human disease.
- Group 2. An organism that may cause disease, and which might be a hazard to laboratory workers, but is unlikely to spread throughout the community. Effective treatment is usually available.
- Group 3. An organism that may cause serious human disease, and is a serious hazard to laboratory workers. It might spread through the community, but effective treatment is usually available.
- Group 4. An organism causing severe human disease, and which is a serious hazard to laboratory workers. There is a high risk of spread through the community and there is no effective treatment.

Laboratories for handling micro-organisms are designed to cope with various levels of containment, depending on which of the above groups is involved.

Most bacteria are able to grow independently of a host cell and it is possible to culture them on special growth media. They reproduce by binary fission, that is each bacterium divides to become two identical daughter cells. The speed of replication is frequently extremely rapid, many bacteria are able to divide every 20-30 minutes. To put this into perspective, if there is one bacterium at time zero, dividing every 30 minutes, then there are over one million after ten hours, and approaching seventeen million at twelve hours.

The numbers of bacteria found in natural habitats are immense, for example, sour milk could easily contain one hundred million bacteria (10^8) per millilitre. Van Leewenhoek commented on this aspect of microbiology as long ago as the seventeenth century in a number of his letters to The Royal Society.

FUNGI

Fungi belong to a group of organisms of the eucaryotic cell type. Cells of this type have a far more complicated level of organisation than the procaryotic bacterial cell. Relatively few fungi are pathogenic for animals, although a considerable number (e.g. rusts, smuts and wilts), are extremely important plant pathogens in economic terms. Fungi have two basic shapes, the yeasts, which are single celled fungi shaped somewhat similarly to a rugby ball, and mycelial fungi that grow as threads (hyphae). Medically important fungi frequently show dimorphism, that is they appear as yeasts in infected humans but take up a mycelial shape when grown on solid media in the laboratory. The vast majority of fungi are non-motile with the exception of a few of the more primitive aquatic groups.

Mycologists divide fungi into four main groups on the basis of the appearance of their sex organs. In medical terms, fungi infecting humans can be divided into two broad groups, those causing superficial skin infections and those causing systemic diseases. Two of the most well known of those causing skin infections are athlete's foot and ringworm. Although these are highly infectious, and can cause cosmetic problems, they are not life threatening and are generally just an itchy nuisance. Fungi causing systemic diseases are generally extremely dangerous even in previously healthy individuals. The general incidence of this type of disease has risen significantly in recent years, due to the rise in patients compromised immunologically and those suffering from conditions such as cancer, diabetes and AIDS.

Fungi that are important animal pathogens include the yeast, *Candida albicans,* causing vaginal thrush which may be sexually transmitted. This organism can also cause life-threatening infections in AIDS patients (Ch 1). Another fungus seen more frequently in recent years and causing severe lung infections in immune compromised patients is *Histoplasma.* This has an interesting history as it is found in high levels in the dust of old tombs inhabited by bats. When these are entered for the first time, the archaeologist stirs up the dust, breathes in large numbers of the organism, develops a serious lung infection and the Pharoah's curse strikes again.

One major problem with fungal infections is that due to the similarity of fungal cells to human cells, there are relatively few antibiotics available to treat fungal diseases that do not also cause serious side effects in the human host.

Further problems are caused by certain fungi that produce toxins and alkaloids that may cause different types of food poisoning and cancer. One well known example from history (described as early as the ninth century), was the ingestion of ergot alkaloids causing the disease known as St Anthony's Fire (Ch 1). The cause was the fungus *Claviceps* growing on rye used to make bread.

ALGAE

The Algae are a large group of eucaryotic organisms, which are very diverse structurally, and are found in considerable numbers in both fresh and seawater. They range from microscopic species to the giant kelps that may be over 50 metres long. Algae are not generally a major problem and do not cause infectious diseases, but a few of the microscopic species are able to form blooms (red tides), in which vast numbers grow and cause serious ecological problems.

Two types of bloom are found, the first type is caused by algae that do not produce toxins. However, the huge numbers of algae produced remove all the oxygen from the water, suffocating other species present. The problem continues after the death of the algae as their decay causes massive bacterial growth leading to further oxygen depletion of the water. Recently, large amounts of algae (seaweed) washed up on the French coast have generated toxic quantities of hydrogen sulphide as they decayed. This has caused the deaths of several animals and at least one suspected human death. One of the ten plagues of Egypt may have been an algal bloom of this type.

The second group of bloom forming algae produce some extremely powerful toxins, such as saxitoxin, which is approximately one thousand times more deadly than strychnine. Some of these toxins will kill fish and other species but are harmless to filter feeding shellfish, such as mussels and clams. Shellfish concentrate these toxins, they get into the food chain and ultimately finish up in humans, where they cause gastro-intestinal and neurological problems, and in a small number of cases, death. One of the earliest recorded cases of this happening was during the expeditions of Captain George Vancouver to survey the west coast of Canada in 1793. A landing party ate contaminated shellfish at an area now known as Poison Cove, and after showing *"sickness, giddiness and numbness",* one of them died. Vancouver noted in his log that the local Indians had a taboo prohibiting the eating of shellfish when the sea was phosphorescent, a common indication of the presence of toxin-producing algae.

PROTOZOA

Disease-causing protozoa, and the next group discussed, the metazoa, are frequently referred to as parasites. Protozoa and metazoa are eucaryotic cells, and although most protozoa are unicellular, they are considerably larger than bacteria, being up to fifty microns across. They can be distinguished from algae by a lack of the photosynthetic pigment chlorophyll, and from fungi by the fact that most of them are motile. They are a very large and extremely diverse group of protists occurring in several phyla of the Eukarya. Only a relatively small number cause human disease, but the disease causing ones are spread across different phyla and cause a number of extremely important diseases.

The protozoa can be conveniently subdivided into several groups depending on the way they move. The first group are the flagellates, the defining feature of these being the possession of one or more flagella. These are long filaments at one end of the cell that beat in a whip-like manner and propel the organism through the surrounding medium. Many flagellates (the euglenoids) contain pigments enabling them to carry out photosynthesis (utilisation of the light energy of the sun), but if the pigments are lost they become saprophytic (feeding on dead organic matter) or predatory on bacteria. Some photosynthetic flagellates are able to grow in vast numbers, and produce neurotoxins that poison and contaminate other forms of life, such as shellfish, and as such can get into the human food chain with serious results.

The flagellate group contains a number of dangerous pathogens. These include *Trichomonas vaginalis,* an organism causing a common sexually transmitted disease that is usually asymptomatic in men, but produces a vaginal discharge in women. Undetected infections may cause infertility, but frequently the presence of this organism is an indication that a more serious sexually transmitted disease may be present.

The most dangerous flagellate is *Trypanosoma brucei*, the causative organism of African sleeping sickness (Ch 16). This is spread by the bite of the tsetse fly (*Glossina*), and renders large areas of sub-Saharan Africa very dangerous to humans and domesticated animals. Many species of wild animals act as reservoirs for this particular protozoan making any prospect of its control highly unlikely. A second member of this genus, *Trypanosoma cruzi*, causes Chagas disease, a disease of tropical America, sometimes known as American sleeping sickness. This is transmitted by bedbugs.

A number of these disease-causing organisms pass through different forms whilst inside the human host, making it very difficult to control them using drugs; drugs effective against one form of the disease are frequently ineffective against other forms.

The second group of protozoa are the ciliates that possess a large number of cilia (short filaments around the circumference of the cell). These beat in unison, and when seen under the microscope look like the oars of an ancient galley. The only important parasite in this group is *Balantidium coli*, which lives in the large intestine, and frequently causes a serious form of dysentery that may be fatal.

The third group are the amoeboid protozoa. These have no fixed form, and move across surfaces by flowing over them. They feed by forming pseudopodia (false feet), which flow around food particles and engulf them. By far the most serious pathogen in this group is the organism *Entamoeba histolytica*, which causes amoebic dysentery. This feeds on the wall of the large intestine causing abscesses and bleeding ulcers. It is spread by means of cysts passing out in the faeces that contaminate food crops and when these are eaten uncooked, a new host is infected.

The final group of protozoans are the sporozoans, all of which are parasites. These are non-motile and many are transported from host to host by a vector. One member of the group is the genus *Plasmodium,* the causative organism of malaria (Ch 16) which is spread by certain species of mosquito. Approximately half the world's population are at risk from this disease, it infects an estimated three to five hundred million people, causes an estimated three million deaths a year, and is one of the major diseases of the tropical and sub-tropical world.

A number of protozoan diseases have been increasing in frequency in recent years. These include diseases caused by *Pneumocystis* and *Cryptosporidium,* both of which are found widely in immune compromised patients (e.g. AIDS victims). *P. carinii* causes an unusual form of pneumonia, which is frequently fatal in AIDS victims. The organism is usually considered to be a protozoan, but its relationship to other protozoa is debatable and recent work using RNA phylogeny suggests it may be more closely related to the fungi. *Cryptosporidium* is a member of the Sporozoa and causes intestinal problems; it is transmitted by the oral/faecal route and has been recognised as a serious problem in water supplies in recent years, causing at least one major epidemic in the USA involving hundreds of thousands of people (Ch 12).

Pathogenic protozoa have been very difficult to grow in the laboratory until recently, and this has hindered research into their disease relationships and control. A major problem in the development of vaccines to control these diseases is that many protozoan parasites are antigenically very complex. Many of them are able to alter their antigenic profile at regular intervals, apparently in a random manner, thus presenting a difficult moving target for the defensive immune system of the host organism. In addition to this problem, many protozoa have life cycles that involve them passing from one organ of the body to another, and drugs effective against the parasite in one organ frequently have no effect when a different organ becomes infected.

METAZOA

The metazoa are organisms composed of many cells. Some of these multi-celled organisms are important parasites and include various parasitic worms such as round worms, tapeworms and flukes, all going under the general heading of Helminths. Humans may be the final host or intermediate host depending on the parasite involved. The final host is the one in which the sexually mature form of the parasite is found, the intermediate host(s) is the one containing an immature form of the parasite. The level of infection caused by these organisms is high, especially in the tropics and sub-tropics. Although some of them can kill very heavily infected hosts, (the World Health Organisation quotes the annual death toll due to schistosomiasis as 200,000), the major problem is that they usually produce a debilitated population, whose resistance to other infectious diseases caused by organisms such as bacteria, is greatly reduced.

Helminths tend to cause non-life threatening diseases and chronic long lasting infections that the host is frequently unable to eliminate. They differ from bacteria and viruses in that the immune system frequently does not recognise them as foreign. If these infections are eliminated either with drugs or naturally, the host is liable to re-infection very rapidly.

Probably the most significant of these diseases are the gastro-intestinal nematodes, which are thought to infect in excess of one billion people world wide, and schistosomiasis (also known as bilharzia), caused by the schistosome (blood fluke), which is thought to infect up to 250 million people in the tropics (Ch 19). With the exception of schistosomiasis, these parasites are not dealt with elsewhere in this book, so they are considered in some detail here.

ROUND WORMS

Round worms are cylindrical white worms whose name Nematoda is derived from *"nema"*, the Greek word for thread. About fifty species of nematode are parasitic in humans but of these only about a dozen occur commonly. The most important one is *Ascaris lumbricoides,* which inhabits the human intestine, and may be as much as a foot (30cm) long. The female is considerably larger than the male, and lays up to two hundred thousand eggs daily, which pass out with the host's faeces. These develop into immature worms inside the eggs, and if the eggs are swallowed by a suitable new host, they are released into the gut. Once released, the immature worms burrow through the intestine wall, and move around the host's body through the blood vessels, eventually finishing up in the host's lungs. They bore into the bronchi, ascend to the mouth of the host and are swallowed, eventually finishing back in the intestine, where they grow into adults. The damage to the host generally occurs during the migration of the young worms, the adults in the intestine are relatively harmless, unless they cause an intestinal blockage.

The major problems of parasitism caused by *Ascaris* are found in areas where human faeces are used for fertiliser on food crops that are not going to be cooked. Whilst this practice may sound unpalatable, it has allowed land in areas such as China and Japan, to be used for intensive farming for many generations. The problem can be alleviated to a considerable extent by allowing the faeces to dry out for several weeks before using them, a process which kills the eggs.

Another roundworm causing serious levels of parasitism is the American hookworm (*Necator americanus)* that occurs in the South Eastern states of the USA. The name translates as the American killer, but it is more usually translated as the American murderer which is rather more emotive. This parasitic worm attaches itself to the lining of the intestine and sucks the blood of the host. The eggs again pass out with the faeces and hatch into larvae that are capable of boring through human skin and infecting a new host. The host, who is frequently a young child, may be infected very heavily leading to severe anaemia and lack of physical energy. To a large extent, the disease can be controlled by disposing of faeces in a sanitary manner and avoiding contact between skin and infected soil by wearing shoes.

A further roundworm parasitising humans to produce the disease trichinosis, is *Trichinella spiralis,* which is usually caught by eating contaminated pork that has not been cooked sufficiently. In this species, the adult worms are found in the human gut, and the female produces eggs that hatch inside her body forming live larval worms. These bore through the intestine wall into blood vessels and are carried around the body, eventually boring into muscles. Once in the muscles they grow to about one millimetre in length, and then form cysts. There is no further development unless the host dies and is eaten by a new host when the worm enters a new cycle. The damage is caused when large numbers of the larval worms migrate through the body causing serious muscle damage, and in severe cases death. The disease is controlled in Western Europe by the examination of meat by trained government inspectors who have the power to impound and destroy contaminated produce.

Other roundworms infecting humans include the Guinea worm, also known as the Medina worm and dragon worm, that is found widely in Central Africa, India, Egypt, Arabia and throughout the Middle East. It has the distinction of being the first parasite to be shown to require an intermediate arthropod host by the Russian, Alexei Fedchenko, in 1870.

Humans are infected when they drink unfiltered water, containing an infected crustacean known as *Cyclops.* The stomach acids digest the *Cyclops,* the larvae are released and migrate from the intestine to connective tissue, where they mate and the male dies. The female worm matures to produce millions of live larvae that are kept in her uterus and then migrates to the skin of the human host and releases a toxic compound causing a painful blister to form. This breaks when the skin is plunged into cold water releasing the larvae that infect a new *Cyclops,* and the cycle starts again.

When the adult worm (which may be up to one metre long) reaches the surface of the skin, it can frequently be seen, appearing as a coiled varicose vein. At this point, local healers may remove it by winding it out on a piece of stick. Whilst this is effective, if carried out by a doctor using precautions against infection, when carried out by an untrained person gangrene may develop resulting in the loss of a limb. The human host has no acquired immunity and re-infection is common.

There are no drugs effective against the disease and there is also no vaccine. However, humans and *Cyclops* are the only two hosts and the disease can be controlled relatively easily by passing all drinking water through a fine filter to remove the infected *Cyclops* (these are about one millimetre long), and persuading infected people to stay out of the water, until the mature worm has been removed. In 1986, the WHO started a programme for the elimination of the guinea worm, and the number of cases has fallen from around four million in 1986 to a few thousand by 2009. About eighty to ninety per cases of the remaining cases occur in the south of Sudan, a war zone, and eliminating these will be a serious problem. However, dracunculiasis is probably going to be the second disease to be eliminated after smallpox.

The final group of roundworms acting as serious parasites in humans are the filarial worms. Several important types are found in the tropics and sub-tropics, the common feature is that they are all spread by biting insects. Adult worms of the species *Wuchereria bancrofti* are about 10cms long, and live in the lymph glands of humans, who are the final hosts. The female produces larvae known as microfilaria that migrate to the surface blood vessels and undergo no further development unless the infected human is bitten by mosquitoes of the correct species. Once in the mosquito, the larvae mature and eventually migrate to the proboscis of the mosquito. When the mosquito bites a new victim, the larvae are deposited onto the skin and then penetrate the bite wound to enter the new host. The adult worms cause a slow inflammation of the lymphatic system, eventually causing it to become blocked. The connective tissues, usually in the legs, become swollen causing the condition known as elephantiasis. In many people, an infection does not progress to elephantiasis, in those that do, there appears to be an over-reaction of the immune system of the host.

Another vector borne filarial worm, *Onchocerca volvulus*, causes a serious disease in much of West Africa known as river blindness. This is carried by small blood sucking insects known as blackflies. When a human is bitten by one of these insects carrying the infective larvae, the larvae migrate through the skin causing inflammation and the host forms fibrous tissue around the worms known as nodules. These worms may also cause elephantiasis, but the most serious problem is that if they enter the eyes, they cause severe damage resulting in blindness. The disease can be controlled relatively easily using a drug known as invermectin.

Tape Worms

The second major group of worms parasitising humans are the Cestodes or tapeworms. The adult forms of most tapeworms are long, flat and ribbon-like organisms living in the intestine of vertebrates. Tapeworms have no mouth or digestive systems, they feed by soaking up food that has already been digested by the host organism.

The most common tapeworm in humans is probably the "beef tapeworm", *Taenia saginata"*, which may be thirty feet long. This consists of a small head, which holds onto the intestine by means of four suckers and a series of body sections, the most immature being immediately behind the head, and the most mature furthest away. The worms are hermaphrodite and eggs develop in each individual body section. As the eggs mature, the section containing them detaches from the worm and passes out with the faeces. These are deposited on pastures and the eggs are eaten by cattle. Once inside a cow, the shell is digested, the embryo bores its way through the wall of the intestine, and is carried by the blood stream to muscle tissue. On entering the muscle tissue, the embryo forms a bladder with the inverted head of the new tapeworm on its inner wall. When rare or uncooked beef is eaten by a human, the bladder is digested, the head of the tapeworm is everted, attaches to the intestine of the new host and the process is then repeated.

The pork tapeworm *Taenia solium* behaves in a similar manner but obviously the bladders are found in pigs. Occasionally, an infected human infects him/herself with the embryo, and the bladder then develops in the human host. If this occurs in muscle then the damage is not usually serious, but if it occurs in the brain or other organs, it may be fatal.

Both beef and pork tapeworms can be controlled by rigorous examination of meat in slaughterhouses and thoroughly cooking meat.

Some species of tapeworms spend their adult life in other mammalian species, and only spend the immature stage in humans. One example is *Echinococcus granulosus,* in which the adult lives in the intestines of dogs. If a human swallows the eggs, these develop into very large bladders known as hydatid cysts that may grow to the size of a tennis ball. Obviously, if this occurs in the brain, the results are likely to be fatal. From the point of view of the tapeworm, the infection of humans is a dead-end as they are unlikely to be eaten by dogs; the normal host for the immature worm are sheep and cattle. It can be controlled by worming dogs at regular intervals and thorough personal hygiene after handling a dog.

Flukes (Flat Worms)

The third group are the flukes or Trematodes, a group of parasitic flatworms. As already mentioned, the most important of these is the schistosome, (Ch 19); unlike some of the following trematodes, schistosomes have only one intermediate host.

The large liver fluke, *Fasciola hepatica*, is the most widespread geographically, and occurs in large numbers of sheep and cattle, causing severe stock losses. The number of humans infected worldwide has been estimated at two million. This fluke only has one intermediate host, a species of snail, and when the cercaria (the immature form of the fluke) leave the snail, they form cycts on grass and other vegetation which is eaten by the final host. Humans are infected by eating unwashed salad vegetables. The symptoms include liver disease, inflammation of the bile ducts and in serious cases, severe anaemia.

The Chinese liver fluke, *Clonorchis sinensis*, is typical of liver flukes involving two intermediate hosts. This is found in China and Korea, although it has been eliminated to a large extent in Japan. In this case, the adult fluke in the human host produces eggs that pass out in the faeces and are eaten by fresh water snails. The immature fluke passes through an asexual reproductive cycle to produce cercaria, which are released into the water and bore into fish, especially members of the carp family. Once in the muscles of the fish, they encapsulate and remain there until the fish is eaten by the final human host, when the fluke is released into the gut, and makes its way to the liver and bile duct. The disease can be controlled by thoroughly cooking the fish.

Although the number of people attacked by metazoa is of the order of millions world-wide, they generally receive very little publicity and the public is largely unaware of the problems they cause.

CHAPTER 5

The Evolution of Urban Man

INTRODUCTION

Two commands may be regarded as hard-wired into all living species, these are *"Survive and Reproduce"*, and for a species to be successful, the obvious requirement is to survive long enough to reproduce[47].

Evolution in all species can be regarded as the result of two forces; the first is mutation whilst the second is selection. A mutation is a random change in the nucleic acid sequence of a species and mutations may be beneficial, neutral or deleterious to the species. A beneficial mutation is one that gives an organism a survival or reproductive advantage and such a mutation will, no matter how small, over time, spread throughout the gene pool of the species. A neutral mutation is one that confers neither an advantage nor disadvantage. The spread of these throughout the gene pool of a species will be determined by chance. Some will be diluted out of the gene pool relatively quickly, whilst others will spread throughout the species. Those that survive may be subjected to one or more further mutations, which again may be advantageous, neutral or deleterious. A deleterious mutation is one that places the organism at a disadvantage in the survival or reproductive race[48].

---

47   It is worth making the point that we all are the descendants of ancestors who were survivors; if our ancestors had not survived to breeding age, we would not be here today. This may seem like stating the blindingly obvious, but it is amazing the number of people who have never considered this thought.

48   What is advantageous and what is deleterious depends

The second force involved in evolution is *"natural selection"*, and if left to nature, deleterious mutations are usually culled ruthlessly, normally within a generation or two (a very short space of time in evolutionary terms). Many people have no problem in understanding that evolution involves change or mutation, but they have considerable difficulty coming to terms with the selection part of the process and the elimination of unfit organisms. The blunt fact is that producing offspring for any species (including humans) is a gamble on genetic recombination. Reproduction might produce healthy offspring who are intelligent and athletic, or it might produce offspring that are mentally and physically disabled. In the case of animal species, the disabled are rapidly eliminated by predation[49]. All species must keep evolving just to maintain, let alone improve, their position in the survival stakes; as the Red Queen said in, *"Through the Looking Glass"*, *"It takes all the running you can do to keep in the same place"*.

The evolution of human epidemic diseases is closely linked to both our genetic evolution, and the social and cultural development of our society and it is impossible to separate them. The major problem facing the human species is that since the end of the last Ice Age (about 13,000 BC), our genetic evolution has not kept pace with the massive changes in our social behaviour during this period. As micro-organisms evolve much faster than we do, they have been able to take advantage of changes in our social development far more rapidly than the genetic evolution of the human species can take the appropriate counter-measures.

---

upon the perspective from which the mutation is viewed. If someone is suffering from a bacterial infection, from the human point of view, it is bad news if the bacterium mutates to antibiotic resistance. However, from the point of view of the bacterium, it has just made a beneficial mutation.

49   Modern humans living in developed countries are, to a considerable extent, shielded from the sharp edge of natural selection by our technology.

If we consider just one example of this problem, the super-volcano Mount Toba in Indonesia exploded approximately 73,500 years ago, producing one of the biggest volcanic eruptions in the last million years. On the basis of evidence from ice cores and seabed sediments, there was a *"nuclear winter"* thought to have lasted for about six years. At this time the human population was an estimated few thousand individuals. If we assume that a human generation for much of the time since then has been about fifteen years, then our species has passed through less than five thousand generations since the explosion. Bacteria multiplying once every twenty minutes, which is about the fastest they can multiply, would pass through five thousand generations in less than seventy days. When we consider figures such as these, the disparity in the evolution rate between humans and micro-organisms becomes obvious.

BASIC GENETICS

The basic rules of genetics were discovered by Gregor Mendel, a monk living in the Austro-Hungarian Empire, in the nineteenth century. Mendel first published his theories in an obscure German journal in 1865, and they languished there, generating only minimal interest, until their importance started to be realised in 1900. It is amazing that he was able to do such work at a time when the Catholic Church was dominated by the story of creation as described in the Book of Genesis. If the Church had been aware of the profound implications[50] these experiments would have over the next one and a half centuries, it is highly probable that the work would either have been severely censored or completely suppressed.

---

50   It is interesting to speculate on the influence that Mendel's work would have had on Darwin's theories, if Darwin had been aware of it. Darwin published the first edition of his *"Origin of Species"* in 1859, and died in 1882, which spans the period of Mendel's work. Although Darwin was not aware of Mendel's work, Mendel did have a German edition of the *"Origin of Species"*, but if he made the connection between his work and Darwin's, he did not publish his thoughts on it.

Mendel spent eight years carrying out research on peas, in particular the colour of their flowers and the colour and structure of the seed coat, using peas that bred true for the features in which he was interested. He was able to show that the inheritance of these features did not involve the blending of the parental characteristics, as Darwin had suggested, but that it could be predicted mathematically to give the probability of various discrete characters re-appearing in subsequent generations[51].

Scientists had attempted these types of studies on a number of different species previously, but had made the mistake of trying to explain the appearance of a whole organism based on the appearance of the parents. Many of them also made the mistake of choosing to study some feature that is not absolute, for example, height. A whole organism is so complex that any attempts at explanations at these levels were doomed to failure.

Mendel's stroke of genius was that he chose to study single characters, such as flower colour or seed colour, and was lucky in that he chose a plant in which the inheritance of these particular characters was simple, and which adhered closely to the basic principles. In the case of the pea, a single gene was responsible for the inheritance of flower colour and it exhibited either straightforward dominant (appearance) or recessive (disappearance) traits (we now call genes producing an either/or effect Mendelian genes). He explained his results by means of what he called factors (they were not called genes for another forty years). Each organism had two factors controlling a character, one factor inherited from the female parent, and one inherited from the male parent. Organisms containing two sets of factors are known as diploid. Diploid

---

51   A good analogy is shuffling a pack of playing cards. Although the order of the cards will change with each shuffle, the joker is always in there somewhere, and sooner or later it will appear at the top of the pack and the probability of it getting to the top can be determined mathematically.

organisms produce gametes[52] during sexual reproduction, the gametes only containing a single copy of the factor[53]. Gametes are egg cells and sperm in the case of animals, and ova and pollen in the case of plants.

Mendel was able to show that if two parent plants with different coloured flowers were cross-pollinated, then in the first generation (the F1), all the descendents produced the same coloured flowers (the dominant characteristic). However, when these F1 plants were self-pollinated, the recessive colour reappeared in the second generation (F2) in the ratio of dominant/recessive 3:1. This is now known as Mendel's First Law, or the Principle of Segregation.

If the two factors were the same, the F1 organism[54] was known as homozygous for that character, if they were different the F1 organism was heterozygous for the character. If the heterozygous state was present, then the dominant factor controlled the colour and masked the recessive factor, which apparently disappeared. However, the recessive factor could reappear in the F2 generation. The details are shown in Figure 5.1.

He was also able to show that if two different characters were considered, such as the colour of the flowers and the shape of the seed coat, they were inherited independently of each other, and neither influenced the inheritance of the other[55]. This became known as Mendel's Second Law, or the Principle of Independent Assortment, and can be used to explain the

---

52   It is surprising that the politically correct brigade have not got their teeth into the word "gamete"; it is derived from the Greek word "*gamos*" meaning marriage.

53   This is known as the haploid number.

54   F1 stands for First Filial Generation, F2 is Second Filial Generation.

55   This is not true in every case as it makes the assumption that the genes for the two characters are not very close to each other on the same chromosome. This assumption was correct for the examples Mendel studied.

Figure 5.1. Mendel's First Law

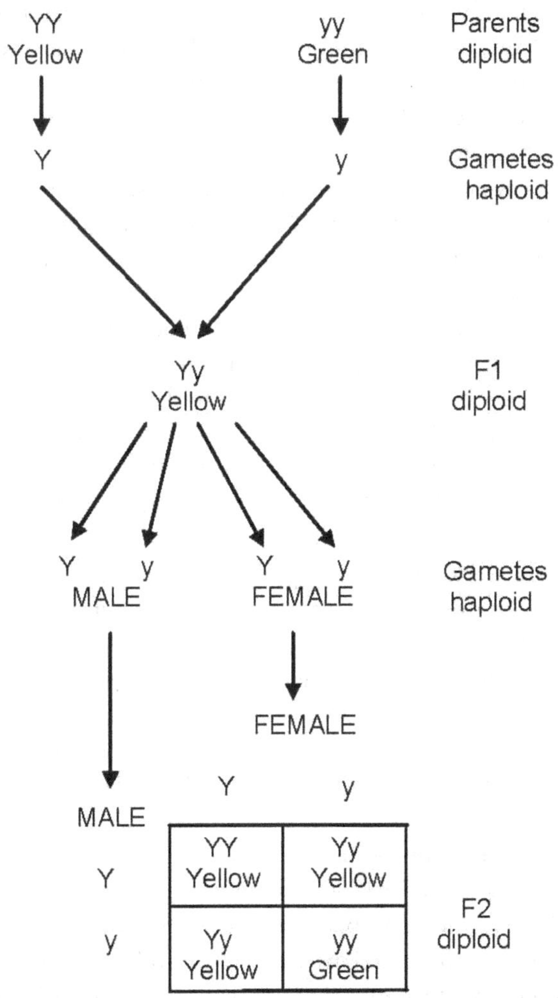

complicated ratios appearing when the inheritance of more than one character is considered. In Figure 5.2, which considers two characters, the combinations found in both grandparents reappear in the F2 generation, but two new combinations are found, each containing one dominant and one recessive character. The ratio found is 9:3:3:1, the nine being the number of descendants containing the two dominant characteristics, the threes each containing one dominant and one recessive characteristic, and one descendant containing the two recessive characteristics.

Alternative genes of this type are known as alleles or allelic genes. Occasionally more than two alleles are possible giving an allelic series, but each individual will only contain two of the possibilities, one inherited from each parent. One of the best known allelic series is the ABO blood group system.

Mendel was a long way ahead of his time, it was not until the 1930s that his work was linked to that of Darwin and the *"Theory of Evolution"*. It was not until the 1950s that the full implications started to be understood with the work of Watson and Crick, and their explanation of the chemical structure and function of Deoxyribo Nucleic Acid (DNA).

The work was based on probabilities, and Mendel reported the use of over 28,000 plants in his experiments. Statistically it would have been very difficult to obtain such good results, and the suggestion has been made that he either consciously or unconsciously manipulated the figures to fit in with his early observations. One important point about this work is that genetics relies on statistical probabilities, and, as in all statistical analyses, the larger the group studied, the more reliable the results become.

Mendel died in 1884 before his work was appreciated. He made no further contribution to science, but became abbot of the monastery in Brno, and spent the last years of his life embroiled in bureaucracy and arguments with the Austro-Hungarian Empire over the taxation of the monastery and church property.

Figure 5.2. Mendel's Second Law

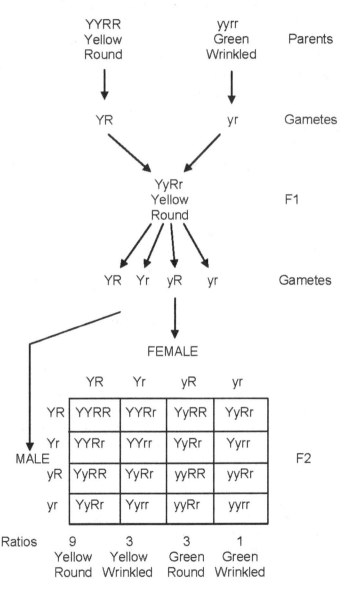

MUTATIONS

Several different types of mutation are found. The simplest of these are point or substitution mutations in which one base in the DNA sequence has been replaced by a different one. This usually, but not always, results in one amino acid in the protein chain being replaced by a different one. Whether or not this is an advantageous mutation depends upon the activity of the new protein compared with the old one.

A second type of mutation is an addition or deletion mutation. In this case, a base has either been added to, or deleted from, the DNA sequence. The result is a protein that has been altered significantly and usually bears little or no resemblance to the parent molecule. Mutations of this type are usually deleterious.

For many years it was thought that evolution was a slow and stately incremental progress that occurred by small mutations of the types mentioned above over thousands of generations. We now know however that there are a number of other types of mutation that may involve substantial changes to the cell, and produce bursts of evolution over relatively short periods. There is some evidence that *Homo sapiens* has undergone several rapid bursts of evolution including at least one in the last forty thousand years[56].

Many of these mutations involve sequences of DNA that can move around the genome of the cell and frequent consequences of these movements are alterations in the control systems of the cell. These sequences were first discovered in maize, but also occur in numerous other species. McClintock[57] who discovered them referred to them as jumping genes, but

56   In the case of *Homo sapiens* one of these major changes was in the gene controlling speech.

57   Barbara McClintock started working on jumping genes in the late 1940s and her work was initially subjected to ridicule by many other geneticists. She was awarded the Nobel Prize in 1983 at the age of eighty-one.

they are now known as transposons. In addition to jumping around the genome within a species, evidence shows that many of them can also jump from species to species by hitching a lift on a virus.

Transposons make up a significant portion of the human genome and appear to be distant relatives of *retro*-viruses such as HIV. The evidence suggests that they may be involved in certain human diseases such as haemophilia, some types of cancer and immunodeficiency diseases. They also play a major role in bacteria in the rapid evolution of antibiotic resistance and its transfer between different bacterial species. On the plus side, there is some evidence that they may have been involved in the evolution of antibody diversity in vertebrates.

HUMAN GENETIC EVOLUTION

It is now known that Mendel's factors or genes are arranged on chromosomes, which are thread-like organelles staining in the presence of certain dyes. The genes are not spread evenly along the chromosomes but occur as a mixture of gene rich and gene poor areas. Only about two to three per cent of human DNA codes for genes, the rest is frequently referred to as *"junk DNA"* and there is considerable controversy over its role.

Humans contain an estimated twenty thousand genes arranged on forty-six chromosomes (the human diploid number), the haploid number being twenty-three. This is roughly the same number and type of genes as are found in many other mammals, although the diploid number of chromosomes varies widely between species. Most of our genes are identical, or very similar to those found in chimpanzees (our nearest living relatives), the divergence between our DNA and chimpanzee DNA being only about 1.6%. There is some disagreement about when the human ancestor separated from the chimpanzee ancestor, but most biologists would consider six to seven million years ago to be a reasonable figure, based on both fossil and genetic evidence. A comparison of humans, chimpanzees, and various other species of apes and monkeys shows that the expression of genes in the blood and liver of all primates is very similar. The major differences are found in brain tissues, especially in the areas controlling speech, human brains differing considerably from those of other primates.

The main difference between mammalian species in general appears to be the way that genes are organised, controlled, and expressed. Although a wide variety of species use very similar genes, what differs is the order and timing of when they are switched on and off. It has been suggested that an estimated 16,000 human genes are subject to variation in regulation and expression.

The genetic variation between various members of the human species, *Homo sapiens,* is around 0.1%, and this small percentage difference accounts for much of the variation in appearance between individuals. J.B.S. Haldane was one of the first scientists to realise that different environments create different evolutionary pressures that cause the selection of varying genetic profiles. These evolutionary pressures would have ranged from environmental ones such as Ice Ages to a variety of diseases influencing the immune system. These pressures and our evolutionary adaptations to them would have produced what are perceived as "racial" differences today and include obvious differences such as the colour of the skin, shape of the nose, shape of the eyes and hair texture. What was a beneficial trait in one environment could be detrimental in another. The most obvious difference is skin colour, being dark skinned in the tropics gives better protection against UV light, whilst being light skinned in northern latitudes allows the synthesis of sufficient vitamin D in lower levels of UV light. The differences also include less obvious ones, for example, the varied responses of individuals to medical conditions such as asthma, allergies, and susceptibility to certain diseases, both epidemic ones such as smallpox and metabolic ones such as diabetes. Haldane was the first to suggest that the mutations in people with sickle cell anaemia and thalassaemias might have been selected in response to pressure from malaria (Ch.16).

The genetic variation is smaller than one would expect from a population as large and as geographically separated as *H. sapiens*, and this may be due to the evolutionary bottleneck our species passed through after the Mount Toba eruption.

There are two theories for the evolution of modern humans, the first is the *"multi-regional"* model, and the second is the *"out of Africa"* model. The *"multi-regional model"* suggests that an early form of human, *Homo erectus,* emigrated from Africa around 1.9 million years ago to various regions of the world and in each of these regions evolved independently into *H. sapiens.*

The *"out of Africa"* theory (which is the generally accepted one), considers that although *H. erectus* emigrated from Africa into other parts of the world, it only evolved into *H. sapiens* in Africa, about 150,000 years ago[58]. *H. sapiens* then migrated out of Africa about 60,000 years ago[59]. Assuming that the *"out of Africa"* theory is the correct one, *H. erectus* evolved into *H. neanderthalensis,* in Europe and into "Java" man and "Peking" man in Asia.

The migration of *H. sapiens* probably took place from the Horn of Africa into the Yemen, at a time when the sea levels were much lower than today. The number of migrations is controversial, most experts claim there was only one, a few claim there were several, but all agree that the total number of individuals involved was small. Considerable research has been carried out in recent years on the mitochondrial DNA[60],

---

58   This date is controversial, some experts consider it may have been earlier.

59   This date is also controversial; some authors think it may have been earlier, others consider a later date is more suitable. Africa was afflicted by severe droughts between 135,000 and 75,000 years ago; about 70,000 years ago the climate became wetter, creating conditions more favourable for human migration.

60   Mitochondria are small organelles found in the eucaryotic cell (Ch 4). There is a large amount of evidence showing mitochondria are descendants of bacteria that infected the ancestral eucaryotic cell. They are

which is only inherited through the female line, and the Y chromosome which is only inherited through the male line. All other chromosomal material has been shuffled through the genetic and mutational mechanisms that create diversity and individual variation. Although mitochondrial and Y chromosomal DNA are also able to undergo mutations, these mutations are limited and can be tracked more easily.

The evidence shows that all humans living today are descendants of a single female who lived about 200,000 years ago. A number of different mitochondrial subtypes are found amongst groups of modern day Africans, whilst only one subtype is found amongst non-Africans. It is generally considered that the evidence suggests that only one group of less than two hundred individuals, who were all closely related through the female line, left Africa and gave rise to all non-Africans living today.

Over a period of several thousand years, the descendents of some of these individuals would have made their way around the coasts of southern Arabia and Iran, around India and down through south-east Asia, making a living by beach-combing. About 40-50,000 years ago, a very small breakaway group would have made their way across to Australia. Genetic evidence shows that Australian aborigines separated from the Papuans of New Guinea about this time.

Other groups split off in the Middle East and made their way north into Eurasia, and a subsidiary group split off from these and moved back into North Africa. A further group migrated north-east reaching Siberia and the Arctic Ocean about 30,000 years ago. As these groups migrated, they would have displaced earlier populations of Neanderthal man. Whether humans replaced them by warfare, whether the Neanderthals were wiped out by some other factor such as disease or whether *H. sapiens* was better at acclimatising to environmental changes is unknown.

now indispensable, and their metabolic reactions provide our bodies with about ninety per cent of our energy requirements.

PARASITE PROBLEMS

Humans live in a three dimensional environment which exists in the vertical plane as well as the two horizontal ones. Our primate ancestors lived in the tropical rain forests but were forced to move onto the drier plains by major climate changes occurring in Africa around four million years ago. This would have brought them into contact with numerous new examples of the three Ps, prey, predators and parasites. Their diet would have altered over time from a vegetarian one, supplemented by insect grubs and the occasional bird's egg, to an omnivorous diet. Initially, carrion left from the kills of more powerful predators would have been scavenged, but over generations they would have learned to co-operate as groups for hunting large game, and this change in behaviour would have altered the spectrum of parasites infecting them. Zoonoses are parasites acquired from animal hosts and a wide range of zoonoses infecting primates and humans is found in Africa, suggesting that these relationships have had many generations to develop. Many zoonoses, such as *Plasmodium* (Ch 16) produce very little antibody response, and high levels of parasitism are found (Ch 6).

Some human parasites, especially those spending part of their life cycle in soil or water, would have been unable to survive frosts and ice at high latitudes in winter. Those parasites requiring vectors such as insects to transmit them would be influenced by the distribution and behaviour of the vectors, which would also need to survive.

When habitats change, the disease and parasitic profiles change, hot humid areas such as jungles and tropical swamps are high in parasites whilst cold or dry areas, for example, mountains and deserts, where there are wide temperature variations, are low in them. Therefore humans moving out of Africa into temperate regions were moving down a disease gradient[61], and were unlikely to encounter new parasites. On

---

61   This is not always true. Raw walrus meat may contain *Trichinella*, a parasitic worm infection (see Ch 4), normally found in infected,

the other hand a population from a temperate zone moving to the tropics encounters numerous dangerous parasites as they move up the disease gradient. During colonial times, the West Coast of Africa was known as *"The White Man's grave"* for very good reasons; indeed it was so notorious it gave rise to the following piece of nineteenth century doggerel.

> *"Beware, beware of the Bight of Benin*
> *One came out where twenty went in"*[62].

The mortality rate of European colonists and troops in India, Central America and the West Indies (known as the Fever Islands), was also extremely high.

The advantages and disadvantages of changing latitude and movement up or down a disease gradient can vary depending on local conditions such as the population density, contact between neighbouring populations and the supply of water, food, fuel and shelter. These local conditions can influence not only the human population but also any disease carrying vectors.

There were other differences in the disease profile between temperate and tropical regions. Non-tropical diseases are more likely to be bacterial or viral in origin, rather than metazoal or protozoal (Ch 4), and these usually provoke a strong immune reaction causing high level, long-lasting, host immunity. Bacterial and viral diseases therefore tended to be one-off, short-term infections, rather than long-term infections causing general debilitation. There are obvious exceptions such as tuberculosis (Ch 11) and HIV (Ch 18), but, generally, individuals falling ill with a bacterial or viral infection either recovered or died quickly, if they recovered, they usually had life-long or long-term immunity to that specific disease. Some of this immunity would have had a genetic basis and would been passed on to

---

undercooked pork. Arctic explorers have died from eating this type of meat raw, because of a shortage of fuel.

62   There are several different versions of this; the number going in varies between twenty and a hundred but they all agree on the same thing, only one came back out.

their offspring. Lactating females would produce antibodies in their milk, which would also pass to infants, providing considerable immunity to the specific disease during the first few months of life. The result was the resistance of individuals and the community to bacterial and viral infections increased slowly over generations. The population numbers would have risen as they moved out of the tropics into cooler or drier areas, with less exposure to parasites. In modern times, high levels of parasitism and disease are one of the major problems hindering the development of many tropical, under-developed countries, especially those of sub-Saharan Africa.

One factor in moving into a colder climate is that it involved the wearing of clothes, which create a new micro-environment. Clothes reduced the need for human adaptation to a colder environment, but created a new micro-niche for disease-carrying parasites such as lice[63], ticks and fleas. The scale of the problem caused by the presence of this type of parasite varies; they could range from being just an itchy nuisance to carrying life-threatening diseases (e.g. typhus, Ch 13).

One disadvantage of moving into a temperate zone is that the availability of food is more seasonal. In sub-tropical and tropical areas where there is plenty of rain, it is frequently possible to harvest several crops per annum, and food tends to be available for much of the year. In temperate zones, there are hot and cold seasons, and there is usually only one crop per year leading to a glut of food at harvest time and a shortage in late winter and early spring. Surplus food requires storage facilities leading to increased organisation. The ramifications of this are considered later in this chapter.

---

63   Genetic studies suggest the body louse (*Pediculus humanus corporis*) diverged from the head louse *(Pediculus humanus capitis)* about fifty thousand years ago. This time would have corresponded with humans moving into higher latitudes and the increased need for protection from the elements.

HUMAN MIGRATION

Migration in an East/West direction would not generally have caused serious problems with parasites, as it would have been along a disease gradient. There would have been some changes with movement between coastal and continental climates, desert and grassland, or alteration in altitude, but these would be relatively minor compared with migrations over large changes in latitude.

The early development of *H. sapiens* and other species of *Homo* in Africa did not seriously destabilise the continent ecologically, as numbers were only small[64] and they had spent considerable time co-evolving with other species, indeed it is probable that early hominids were prey rather than predators.

In many areas of the Northern temperate zones, the effect of human hunting on animal species was magnified by the changes in climate caused by the retreat of the last Ice Age (approximately 15,000 years ago). Temperate zones are much less diverse and complex biologically than the tropical rain forest and are more easily destabilised. In the Old World, the hunters had been moving out from their point of origin in Africa for tens of thousands of years, and game would have had time to adjust to their presence. The hunters were also generally moving away from the equator into colder and less favourable climates and took time to adjust to it, even though they had the advantage of moving down the *"disease gradient"*. The numbers of humans involved was still relatively small. It has been estimated that world-wide, the population of *H. sapiens* at the height of the last Ice Age (Last Glacial Maximum), about 22,000 BC, was less than one million.

In the Americas however, most of the big game disappeared at the end of the last Ice Age. These animals had no experience of organised hunting by humans and many large mammals became extinct in the Americas around the dates corresponding

---

64   Estimates of the number of *H. sapiens* about 130,000 years ago are of the order of 5-10,000.

to the Clovis culture[65], that is approximately 11,500 BC. Some authors consider that human hunting was not the reason for these mass extinctions and blame climatic changes and loss of habitat at the end of the last Ice Age. However, these animal species and their ancestors had experienced, and survived, ten ice ages during the previous million years, so it is reasonable to have expected them to survive the last one. They certainly continued to survive on Wrangel Island in the Arctic Ocean. A race of very small mammoths, only the size of a large pony, survived there until about 1,700 BC, suggesting that climatic changes were not responsible for extinctions; they only vanished when humans arrived. Computer simulations have shown that only a small amount of hunting is needed to destabilise an animal population, especially when the prey species is a large animal that reproduces slowly. A similar situation occurred in a number of other countries when humans arrived, these include New Zealand, Australia and Madagascar[66].

It is now thought that the Clovis Culture only lasted a relatively short time, possibly no more than a few hundred years and ended very abruptly. Excavation of numerous Clovis sites across North America suggest that this may have been due to some catastrophic event such as a comet exploding in the upper atmosphere or an asteroid strike somewhere on the

---

65   Named after the town of Clovis in New Mexico, where characteristic spear points were first found. Clovis points have been found from numerous widely separated sites, all dated closely to each other, suggesting an extensive trading network and a rapid spread of technological advances. Numerous skeletons of mammoths with Clovis spear points in their rib cages have been found across North America. A later series of spear points, known as Folsom points, developed between 11,000-9,000 BC. These however, are associated with the kills of Ice Age bison, suggesting that different groups of hunters concentrated on different types of prey, depending on what was available, presumably using a variety of hunting strategies.

66   In the case of Madagascar, one species that did not survive the arrival of man was the giant elephant bird. This however, is thought to have survived in legend and was the origin of the roc, the giant bird of the Arab stories of Sinbad the Sailor.

North American continent. A charred layer has been found, in all the Clovis sites examined, that contains numerous artefacts generally associated with such an event. Fossil remains of mega-fauna are found below this layer, above the layer there are very few. Although many experts agree with the theory of an extra-terrestrial event, there is considerable controversy over how widespread the effects were.

No crater consistent with an large asteroid strike dated to the correct period has been found, however, an air burst from some extra-terrestrial body would not have produced any large, recognisable impact crater. Alternatively, an asteroid strike might have been offshore producing a crater on the seabed that has not been recognised. The suggestion of such a catastrophe occurring is also consistent with the very narrow genetic base of the Amerindian population, the genetic diversity of this group being the lowest known of any racial group. This suggests that they went through a genetic bottleneck in which the population was reduced to a very small number of survivors.

The Ice Age finished around 13,000 BC, however, an extremely cold period known as the Younger Dryas[67] started approximately 10,700 BC and lasted about twelve hundred years. The effects were felt right across the Northern Hemisphere, the average temperature in Britain fell about 5°C and the forests of Scandinavia changed to tundra.

The evidence suggests that both the onset and the end of the Younger Dryas were extremely rapid, the onset taking about a decade[68] and the end only three years. The most probable cause of the rapid change back to cold weather is an alteration in the course of the Gulf Stream in the North Atlantic Ocean. This ocean conveyor belt carries warm water

---

67   So-named from the tundra wild-flower, *Dryas octopetala,* whose pollen appeared in vast quantities in core samples from about the time that the Younger Dryas period started.

68   Recent research on lake-bed sediments in western Ireland suggest that the onset may have been even more rapid, perhaps only a matter of months.

from the tropics to Britain and Northern Europe. As it cools in the north Atlantic it sinks and is carried back through the depths to the tropics where it warms up, rises to the surface and the cycle is repeated. Large volumes of fresh water coming off the Greenland icecap or out of the North American continent would displace it southwards. The cause of the Younger Dryas is thought to have been the release of vast volumes of cold fresh water from Lake Agassiz[69], on the North American continent, draining into what is now the St. Lawrence Seaway.

The rise in sea levels at the end of the last Ice Age was about one hundred and twenty metres (four hundred feet), and it is frequently assumed that this rise was gradual. Geological evidence however, suggests that there were at least six occasions involving catastrophic flooding when sea levels rose several metres within days. These were caused by huge lakes of melt water building up behind ice dams, and being released suddenly when the ice dam ultimately collapsed.

A number of authors have pointed out that the end of the Younger Dryas period corresponds with the beginning of the changes from a hunter-gatherer life style to agriculture, and have suggested that this event initiated these changes in the Fertile Crescent. The onset and collapse of the Younger Dryas event were both so rapid that a very swift cultural response would have been necessary on the part of any humans living in the Northern Hemisphere at this time.

The date for humans entering the Americas is controversial. For many years, most experts considered that there was one migration from Siberia occurring between 11-12,000 BC, which corresponds to the rise of the Clovis culture. This migration took place across an area known as Beringia. During the Ice Age, when sea levels were lower than they are today, Beringia was a land bridge, over a thousand miles wide, between Siberia and Alaska. There was also a corridor, free of

---

69   This lake, which was significantly larger than the modern day Great Lakes combined, was formed from melt water coming off the ice-cap at the end of the Ice Age.

ice, stretching from Alaska southwards into the Great Plains. This ice-free corridor passed between the Laurentide ice sheet to the east and the Cordilleran ice sheet to the west, and is unlikely to have been passable before approximately 12,700 BC. Not all experts agree with this scenario. Whilst there is considerable evidence for the presence of Ice-Age hunters in Beringia[70], it has been suggested that the actual migration routes from Asia to the Americas may have been by sea, along the southern coast of Beringia, with humans making a living from the kelp forests. Kelp beds are an extremely productive eco-system that would have provided hunters with shellfish, fish and marine mammals. These kelp beds appear to have stretched from Japan northwards, around the southern edge of Beringia and down the western side of North America as far as Lower California.

No coastal archaeological sites for these migrations have been found, but this is not surprising, as they would all have been inundated when the sea levels rose. Pollen analysis of sea-bed sediments that were dry land about 14,000 BC shows that there were a number of ice-free coastal areas between Alaska and the northern USA.

The existence of a pre-Clovis culture in the Americas has been an extremely controversial subject, and there has also been considerable disagreement as to whether one or several waves of immigration took place. Genetic evidence based on the evolution of mitochondrial DNA and the male Y chromosome, suggest that there may have been several (possibly three) immigration waves from Siberia, with the Inuit being the latest. Research on mitochondrial DNA suggests that the first of these migrations may have been as early as 20,000 years ago, and also suggests that these immigration waves were relatively small, each one consisting of no more than a few hundred individuals at most. Some experts claim that

---

70   Although it was so far north and extremely cold, Beringia remained ice-free because of the lack of precipitation.

this research is supported by analysis of Amerindian linguistic groups although this is controversial.

Numerous archaeological sites associated with human occupation have been found, but the dating of some of these has been very acrimonious, especially those claimed to have been pre-Clovis. Whilst the debate over the dating of many of these sites has still not been settled, a date of approximately 10,500 BC has been determined using radiocarbon dating for the upper layer of artefacts at the Monte Verde site in Southern Chile. However, a second distinct set of artefacts is also present at a lower level, these have been controversially dated considerably earlier. A further site at Cactus Hill, Virginia, has been tentatively dated to 18,000 years ago, and one at Meadowcroft, Pennsylvania, to approximately 17,000 years ago, whilst human coprolites, 14,300 years old, have been found in caves in Oregon.

The question of human migration from Siberia has been complicated by the discovery of Kennewick Man, whose skeleton, found on the banks of the Columbia River, is dated to approximately 7,300 BC. Initial examination of the more or less complete skeleton suggested that it was an early European, possibly an early nineteenth century fur-trader. The bones were then carbon-dated showing that they were over 9,000 years old. There was an immediate political furore with local Indian groups demanding the bones of an "ancestor", so that they could be buried at a secret, sacred site. A group of scientists sued to study the skeleton on the grounds that they were obviously not the bones of an Indian ancestor. The issue went to court, and the skeleton was finally examined in 2005, nine years after being discovered.

Skeletal remains of a small number of individuals (30-40), dated to pre 9,000 BC, have been found across the Americas. Most of these are represented by only a few bones, but they have very different dental patterns and facial appearance to Amerindian remains which are dated to post 9,000 BC. They show a greater similarity to Pacific peoples such as the Ainu of Japan[71]. Whether these people were wiped out by the Amerindians or assimilated into them is not known[72]. The skeleton of Kennewick Man however, bore signs of fighting with several fractured ribs, and a stone spearhead buried in the pelvis, the depth of the wound suggesting that the spear had been propelled by an atlatl. This had healed to the extent of bone starting to grow around the point. He was obviously part of a community and not a stray individual as he appears to have been given a formal burial.

The immigrants into North America would have taken no serious diseases with them for two reasons. Firstly, whenever these migrations took place, they were before the evolution of crowd diseases occurred in the Old World, and secondly, travelling thousands of miles through high latitudes, during an Ice Age, would have culled any sick individuals and acted as a cold filter destroying disease-carrying vectors.

The hunters were moving into a warmer climate as they moved southwards in the New World, and although this should have resulted in a serious increase in parasitism as they were moving up a disease gradient, the increase was nowhere near as great as moving into the tropics in the Old World would have been. The reason is that pre-Columbian America was free of many of the diseases that were widespread in the Old World. At least one account of travel in early seventeenth century South America details an expedition along the Amazon River without referring to fever, and says the inhabitants were numerous and healthy, a situation certainly not found in modern times. Whilst this statement cannot be substantiated with reference to the

71   The Ainu, who are still found on the island of Hokkaido in northern Japan, are probably the descendants of the Jomon whose culture is dated to 13,000 BC and possibly even as early as 14,500 BC.

72   The discovery of these remains has caused great political controversy in the USA. Many of the political demands of the Amerindians are based upon the fact that they regard themselves as the First Nations. Human remains of this type raise serious question marks over those claims.

health of the inhabitants, recent archaeological examination of the river banks of the Amazon certainly suggest that the pre-Columbian inhabitants were numerous and living in well-organised societies. It will be seen later that a major factor in the relatively disease-free state (i.e. contagious diseases) of the Amerindians immediately pre-Columbus was the lack of domesticated large animals.

THE SOCIAL DEVELOPMENT OF HUMANS

Diamond (1997) has discussed the development of human society in great detail in his book, *"Guns, Germs and Steel"*, which has had a considerable influence on subsequent authors. Human society started as small groups of hunter-gatherers, probably no more than a small number of related families numbering a few dozen individuals. The lower limit of size would have been determined by the number of adult males needed to form a hunting party capable of killing large prey. The upper limit would have been determined by the resources available within their territory. The various groups must have been in regular contact with each other, both for the purposes of trade and exchanging partners. A group containing only a few dozen individuals would not be viable over several generations, as interbreeding over a long period would have led to serious genetic defects appearing in the offspring as a result of *"cousin marriages"*[73].

73   *"Cousin marriages"* leading to genetic defects were a problem in rural areas of Britain before railways and canals encouraged the movement of people. Anyone carrying out family history research in isolated areas such as moorland or mountainous areas will be aware of how frequently the same family name occurs. There are several thousand of these genetic diseases, the vast majority of them only occurring rarely. These diseases occur in an individual when both parents are carrying a single copy of the defective gene, and the child inherits a copy from each parent. The double copy produces an individual with the disease in the clinical form. Two of the most common diseases occurring are cystic fibrosis (Ch 11) and sickle cell anaemia (Ch 16).

The problem is being seen in Britain today due to arranged *"cousin marriages"* within the ethnic community from the Indian sub-continent. Approximately fifty-five per cent of British Pakistanis are married to their

These bands would have been healthy as small groups cannot sustain crowd diseases, and they also moved frequently, leaving behind problems such as contaminated water supplies. Any serious epidemic disease would have been fatal for the group as they would no longer have been able to hunt. Sick individuals would have died if they could not keep up with the clan whilst moving and survival of the fittest would have occurred. Although many authors extrapolate from the few remaining hunter-gatherer societies today to those of 10-12,000 years ago, it must be remembered that Mesolithic hunter-gatherer societies would have been living in a resource-rich environment, unlike these societies today which have been pushed onto marginal land, such as deserts, by more "successful" groups[74]. In addition, not all hunter-gatherer societies would have been identical, different groups would have evolved different survival strategies depending on the food and prey species available. Research on modern hunter-gatherers, living in the tropics and sub-tropics, shows that they derive more calories from collecting vegetable materials such

---

first cousins, and these marriages are thirteen times more likely to produce mentally and physically disabled children than are found in the rest of the community. The Pakistani community in Britain produces three per cent of births in the UK, but approximately one third of children born with recessive genetic illnesses, and it is placing a huge liability on the medical resources of those areas where the Pakistani communities are concentrated.

The question of how to deal with this problem is obviously a political one as well as a medical one. Approximately half of the states of the USA ban marriages between first cousins but most countries do not. A similar problem occurred in Orthodox Jewish communities with Tay-Sachs disease, a recessive neurological disease that kills children by about the age of four years. The problem was solved by creating a genetic register and ensuring that individuals who are carriers are not introduced and matched.

74   Diamond has asked the question, why didn't the aborigines of Northern Australia use the farming techniques of New Guinea as they had trading links across the Torres Straits and must have been aware of them? He has suggested that the hunter-gatherers were just too well-off. The question, therefore, may not be why had certain groups of hunter-gatherers failed to "progress" to farming, but what forced the others to do so?

as nuts, seeds, fruits and tubers than they do from hunting. However, by the end of the Ice Age, humans were formidable and efficient co-operative hunters with an advanced weapons technology. Over time this led to the serious reduction of many big game animals in the temperate zones forcing the hunters to use alternative sources of food.

Whilst edible seeds would always have been collected, such sources of food would have become more important as animal sources of food vanished. Seeds ripen over a period of time and collection therefore involved being in the right place at the right time and staying longer. This would have generated bigger middens harbouring more parasites capable of causing disease, and also attracted pests such as rodents and flies, which carry a number of diseases that can be transmitted to humans. At this point, social not biological evolution started to direct human development. Ultimately, the collection of seeds and domestication of animals led to farming[75], and activities such as fishing led to the use of rafts and boats that encouraged trade.

Excavation of rubbish tips of Mesopotamian communities shows food sources changing over time; initially the bones of gazelles are widespread but these have disappeared by about 7,500 BC. They have been replaced by the bones of sheep and goats, animals that we would consider domesticated. Archaeology of the villages of this period shows they had a population of a few hundred and the middens contain the remains of shellfish, fish, fruit, nuts and wild cereals.

---

75   The distinction between hunter-gatherers and agriculturalists is not always a clear-cut either/or situation. Examples during the last couple of hundred years suggest that farming and hunter-gatherer life-styles were intertwined in some areas. Some hunter-gatherer communities were sedentary, but did not grow crops. The Indians of the North West Pacific coast of Canada lived by fishing (mainly salmon), frequently in large villages of a thousand or more individuals. Although they were hunter-gatherers they had hereditary chiefs, land ownership, lived in large cabins and supported craftsmen, especially wood carvers, specialising in the production of artefacts such as large elaborate canoes and totem poles.

The excavation of Göbekli Tepe, a site in modern-day Turkey on the northern edge of the Fertile Crescent, has caused considerable interest in recent years and raises more questions than it answers. The site has been dated to approximately 9,500 BC and is thought to have been a temple for sky burials. It consists of a number of large buildings constructed of dressed stone blocks. Monolithic upright pillars, weighing up to fifty tons in some cases, are found that have been moved approximately five hundred metres from the quarries where they were excavated. Some of these pillars have carved reliefs of human arms, whilst others are carved with a variety of animals, birds, insects and reptiles. To date, only about five per cent of the complex has been excavated.

Göbekli Tepe pre-dates Neolithic culture in the Fertile Crescent and many aspects associated with this period, such as pottery, wheels, writing, metalwork and agriculture. There is also a level of organisation not previously found in Mesolithic culture. It has been estimated that the complex would have taken a work force of at least five hundred labourers to build it with all the supporting logistics such as shelter and food supply. The quality of the stonework, reliefs and sculptures strongly suggests the existence of specialist artisans. It obviously involved a hierarchical society, probably controlled by a priestly caste, and at least one archaeologist has suggested that slavery may have been involved, something that has not previously been associated with Mesolithic hunter-gatherer groups.

The size and quality of Göbekli Tepe suggest a society with a complex level of organisation several millennia earlier than previously suspected, and it means that we may have to re-think our theories on the length of time that some crowd diseases may have been evolving.

By 5,000 BC, towns containing populations of several thousand people living on sites of thirty to forty acres are found, cereals were grown, sheep and goats were kept, and there is evidence of trade over considerable distances. One town, Catalhoyuk in Turkey, is on the northern edge of the Fertile Crescent and has been investigated intensively since its discovery in the 1950s. It is dated to the period 5,500–3,700 BC and is thought to have contained up to ten thousand inhabitants, The final stages in this development were ploughing, irrigation, the use of draught animals for transport, pottery, the development of large walled cities for protection and ultimately metallurgy and writing.

Numerous factors would have influenced the development of crowd diseases in the populations of these towns. These would have included density of population, availability of fresh water, trade, agriculture and the keeping of livestock.

TRADE

There is considerable evidence of widespread trading networks developing at a very early stage of our social evolution. Archaeological investigation of numerous Mesolithic sites in Europe and the Near East reveal seashells hundreds of miles from the nearest coastline. Holes have frequently been bored in them so that they can be strung and used for decoration. Similarly, the point of origin of obsidian, which is a volcanic glass, can be determined by its chemical signature. This also travelled great distances and was a highly prized trade item because of the extremely sharp edges that can be obtained by working it.

Mummified bodies dated to 6,000 BC have been found on the edge of the Taklimakan desert on the Chinese border, these are Caucasian or Indo-European rather than Mongoloid, and suggest trade links between China and Europe at this early date. Some of the items traded may have been unusual. Botanists have always assumed that the domestic apple, *Malus domestica,* was a hybrid of wild species found in northern temperate climates. This has been challenged recently, and it is now suggested that the ancestor of all eating apples is *Malus sieversii,* a species found on the border of north-west China and Kazakhstan that was introduced into Europe by early Neolithic traders around 4,000 BC.

Spices were transported over great distances at least as early as 3,000 BC and their use for cooking, medicine and magic was widespread. Although some spices came overland from China, most were traded by sea in a series of short coastal voyages, presumably increasing in value every time they changed hands. Many spices were assumed to come from Arabia or East Africa. They did not, these were just the last ports of call before they reached Egypt and the Mediterranean.

The evidence for these trade links is considerable. Cities such as Sumer were using cardamom, imported from India, as early as the third millennium BC, and typical Harappan seals of steatite (soapstone) from the Indus civilisation, dated to around 2,000 BC, have been found in Mesopotamian sites. Many of these seals appear to have been labels attached to trade goods. Cloves dated to approximately 1,720 BC have been found in Syria, the only source of cloves at the time being the Moluccas (Spice Islands), whilst traces of pepper, native to the Malabar coast of India, were found in the mummy of Rameses II (Rameses the Great), who ruled Egypt from *ca* 1,279-1,212 BC.

Black pepper was also a major Roman import from India. The Greek historian and geographer, Strabo (*ca* 64 BC-23 AD), mentions over one hundred and twenty ships per year trading between the Red Sea ports and the Malabar coast for pepper, and a contemporary Tamil account writes of *"ships arriving with gold and departing with pepper"*. Strabo also mentioned a seaman, Eudoxos of Cyzicus, who sailed repeatedly to India around 110 BC, but disappeared whilst attempting to circumnavigate Africa.

Rome also imported vast amounts of frankincense and myrrh for use in cremation ceremonies. These are products of trees and shrubs that only grew in the Arabian Peninsula and Somalia, and Egyptian expeditions to obtain them are mentioned as early as 2,800 BC. The amounts of money Rome spent on spices and incense were huge, Pliny complained in the first century AD that Rome was beggaring itself to pay for them. They had to be paid for in cash, not trade goods, and the figure mentioned by Pliny is about ten tons of gold per annum, a claim substantiated by the large number of Roman gold coins still found in India today.

Trade in spices continued throughout the centuries; the Venerable Bede (*ca* 673-735) was aware of pepper and its properties, and claimed it combated colds and plague. For Bede to have known of pepper at this date would have required trade routes stretching between Northumbria and India.

The search for spices led to the voyages of Christopher Columbus (1451-1506), and Vasco da Gama (1460-1524). By the fifteenth and sixteenth centuries, the Ottoman Empire controlled the eastern Mediterranean and the western end of the Silk Road, thus controlling the trade routes for silk and spices. Both the Spanish and Portuguese were desperate to break the Ottoman stranglehold and in 1494, they signed the Treaty of Tordesillas, which agreed to divide the Atlantic, and any new lands found to the west, between them.

The Spanish monarchs, Ferdinand and Isabella, financed Christopher Columbus on a series of four voyages to discover a route to India by sailing west; one of his backers mentioned "*ad loca aromatic*" (to the land of spices) in a letter. On his first voyage in 1492, Columbus discovered the islands of Cuba and Hispaniola (Santa Domingo) and was convinced he had reached Cathay (China). He did not reach the mainland of the Americas until his third voyage in 1498, when he landed in modern day Venezuela. Whilst in Hispaniola in 1492, Columbus captured some of the local Taino tribe, who were taken back to Spain as slaves. It was the capture of these slaves that led to the theory that the epidemic of syphilis that started in 1493 in Europe, had originated in the Caribbean (Ch 14).

The price the Taino paid for their "discovery" was very high; it is estimated that there were approximately two million of them in 1492, but by 1520 they had been reduced to a few thousand by disease and slavery and had vanished by 1550.

The Portuguese prince, Henry the Navigator, sponsored three voyages starting in 1497 by Vasco da Gama around the coast of Africa. These were intended to reach India and gain control of the spice trade. A supplementary aim of these voyages of discovery was to reach the kingdom of the legendary Christian monarch, Prester John[76], and enlist his aid against the Muslims. The result was a series of Portuguese trading posts around the coast of Africa, and the establishment by the Portuguese of the colony of Goa, on the west coast of India. A secondary result was the transmission of syphilis to Africa and India, where it was known as the Frankish disease.

It was not only spices that encouraged trade, but also jewellery. Necklaces containing lapis lazuli have been found in Egyptian tombs dated as early as 3,300 BC. The only source of this material were the mountains of the Hindu Kush, and excavations in Pakistan suggest that there was trading in lapis as early as the seventh millennium BC. Lapis lazuli was also ground-up to produce the intense blue colours found in many early European manuscripts, such as the Book of Kells and the Lindisfarne Gospels. The Sutton Hoo treasure contains gold jewellery set with garnets that came from either India or Afghanistan. The ship burial in which they were found is thought to be that of King Raedwald of East Anglia who died around 626 AD[77]. Similarly emeralds can be traced to specific mines by analysis of their chemical signature. Emeralds from mines in the Peshawar region of Pakistan have been found in Celtic grave goods in Western Europe, dated to pre-Roman

---

76   The legend of the fabled kingdom of Prester John is probably due to garbled accounts reaching Europe of a Christian kingdom in Ethiopia.

77   Raedwald is one of the Saxon kings who are referred as "Bretwalda" or Overlord of Britain. The Venerable Bede lists seven Bretwaldas in his *"Historia ecclesiastica gentis Anglorum"* (Ecclesiastical History of the English People) written about 731 AD.

times, and cornelian jewellery from Harappa in the Indus Valley, dated to about 2,500 BC, has been found in the royal tombs of Ur.

Other major trading items included metals. Herodotus writing around 430 BC mentions the Phoenicians, who were based in city states such as Tyre and Sidon, in modern day Lebanon, trading for tin as early as 1,250 BC to the Cassiteirides (The Islands of Tin). These are thought to be Cornwall, although no Phoenician artefacts dated to this period have been found in Britain. Phoenician metalwork and carved ivory has been found in both Egyptian and Assyrian excavation sites. Cyprus was also trading in copper; a shipwreck off the Cypriot coast, dated to the second millennium BC, was carrying nearly eleven tons of high quality copper ingots. The name Cyprus is derived from the Greek word "Kupros" meaning copper. Tin and copper are the two ingredients of bronze, the amount of copper varying between about seventy and ninety-five per cent, although there are also various trace ingredients, such as arsenic, that would have influenced the behaviour of the bronze[78].

Olives, olive oil and wine were also traded widely, and numerous early shipwrecks in the Mediterranean contain amphorae, chemical analysis of the residues in them shows they were used for these items.

It is obvious from the number and variety of examples that there were extensive trading networks at a very early date, and these were sufficiently robust to survive major problems such as the collapse of the Western Roman Empire in the fifth century AD.

THE RISE OF AGRICULTURE

Diamond (1997) discusses the rise of agriculture, the acquisition of crops and domesticated animals in some detail in *"Guns, Germs and Steel"*, and this account uses that as a

---

78   The Bronze Age lasted from roughly 3,000-1,000 BC.

framework. The acquisition of crops and animals is considered later.

Agriculture originally developed in a number of areas independently, these include the Fertile Crescent, China, Meso-America (central southern Mexico and adjacent areas of Central America), the Andes and the eastern USA (Mississippi Valley). The Fertile Crescent is the area that runs from the eastern coast of the Mediterranean Sea (modern day Southern Turkey and Lebanon), through Syria and Iraq down to the Persian Gulf, including the area known as Mesopotamia or the Land between the Rivers (the Tigris and Euphrates).

A number of other important centres of origin of domesticated plants also existed in addition to those listed above including India and Ethiopia. Many crops are found originating in more than one centre of origin. Wheat (*Triticum*) is a classic example, and different species of wheat are found in the Fertile Crescent, Asia Minor, central Asia and Ethiopia. In many plant genera when this happens, the number of chromosomes varies widely from area to area, and, in the case of *Triticum*, species with the haploid (7), diploid (14), triploid (21), tetraploid (28) and hexaploid (42) number of chromosomes are found. The result is an extremely versatile cereal, ideal for genetic manipulation, that has spread world-wide. A second example is cotton, at least four different species were domesticated independently at various times in different parts of the world, the earliest around 5,500 BC.

Agriculture probably evolved in the Fertile Crescent first. It is thought that plants were starting to be domesticated around 8,500 BC, and animals slightly later. The evolution of agriculture in China was around the same time or possibly slightly later, but agriculture only appeared in the Americas around 3,000-2,500 BC, and with one or two exceptions, animals were never domesticated in the New World.

Agriculture on a large scale did not appear in some very suitable areas with a Mediterranean type of climate until relatively modern times, these include California, parts of Australia, and the Cape region of South Africa. This is usually due to a lack of suitable indigenous crops for domestication. Some early sites such as the Sahel in Africa, much of Iran/Iraq, and parts of China where substantial agriculture was once found are now degraded by over-cultivation and erosion.

Diamond considers that there are a number of reasons for thinking that agriculture in Eurasia started in the Fertile Crescent, and then disseminated outwards.

- The Fertile Crescent has a very high diversity of plants and animals, considerably higher than any other area in the world with a Mediterranean type of climate. These include a number of species that spread worldwide such as wheat, barley, chickpeas, flax, sheep, goats and cattle.

- There is a considerable temperature and rainfall variation due to the number of mountain ranges. The altitude changes produce a wide range of environments encouraging diversity, which led to the evolution of large numbers of species of annual plants. The different altitudes also meant staggered harvests, and people could therefore follow crops up into the hills as they ripened.

- The seeds of wild grasses in the Fertile Crescent are generally larger than elsewhere in the world. The Fertile Crescent has about thirty of the top fifty seeds world-wide in terms of size. Barley and emmer wheat (the wild ancestor of domesticated wheat) are both native to the area and are in the top dozen. Grasses use a type of photosynthesis known as C4 that is considerably more efficient than the C3 form of photosynthesis used by most plants. As a result, grasses are able to convert sunlight energy into plant chemicals, such as sugars, much more efficiently and grassland produces a higher yield than a similar area growing crops carrying out C3 photosynthesis.

- The fourth advantage was a diverse population of large animals capable of domestication including sheep, goats, pigs and cattle. Cattle and horses both need richer pastures than sheep or goats, and the rise of cattle, and especially horse-based economies, are closely associated with the quality of pasture available.

The dispersion of different crops and animals and the ideas and technologies associated with them from the Fertile Crescent was also helped by the fact that the main axis of Eurasia is East/West. This means that crops and animals can disperse along similar latitudes (same lengths of day), similar climates and probably similar diseases, which obviously creates less stress for them as they disperse. Both crops and animals are subject to disease gradients in exactly the same manner as humans.

By comparison, a map of the world shows that the long axis of the Americas is North/South, and North and South America are separated by the Isthmus of Panama. This area of dense jungle isolated the civilisations of Mexico from those of the Andes to the south, whilst to the north the Mississippi Valley was separated from Mexico by deserts. These geographical barriers were in addition to the latitude gradient that meant that there were already considerable problems to the diffusion of crops and animals.

Because of the problems of traversing jungles, the use of llamas as pack animals did not spread outside the Andes, and the Olmec, Aztec, Maya, Toltec and other Meso-American civilisations remained without any large pack animals or edible domesticated animals. This not only caused a lack of easily available meat protein, but also the protein derived from animal milk. There were obviously no problems with East/West trade in the Americas, as obsidian weapons have been found in North America at least a thousand miles from their point of origin, and the Clovis culture spread across the Great Plains very rapidly.

The main axis of Africa is again North/South, and some authors have claimed that sub-Saharan Africa was cut off from North Africa by the Sahara desert and early crops and technology could not diffuse into sub-Saharan Africa. However, much of the Sahara was a rich region of Mediterranean flora in the Neolithic period supporting a varied wildlife, including many of the large Africa fauna[79] and substantial areas were being farmed and grazed as recently as 4,000 BC. This is obviously considerably later than the diffusion of crops and technology from the Fertile Crescent, which is thought to have occurred into the Nile valley before the sixth millennium BC.

The scale of the diffusion of crops was considerable, at one archaeological site near the Nile Delta, over 160 silos for storing cereals were found, dated to before 5,000 BC. It was not just crops that were imported from the Fertile Crescent, the tools and weapons found at the site are also very similar to those found in the Fertile Crescent.

It is more likely that the spread of crops, tools, animals and technology into tropical and Southern Africa were stopped by jungle diseases such as yellow fever and malaria, in the Congo and Cameroon in West Africa, and also by diseases on the East African plains. Once south of the Sahara, domesticated animals such as horses and cattle are subject to the protozoan disease, trypanosomiasis, carried by the tsetse fly, and other animal diseases such as rinderpest. These render large swathes of sub-Saharan Africa no-go areas for domesticated animals and humans (the human form of trypanosomiasis is also referred to as African sleeping sickness [Ch 16]).

Crops migrated from the Fertile Crescent over considerable distances. Emmer wheat is found in archaeological sites as

---

79   This is substantiated by numerous rock carvings and paintings in the present day Sahara showing large animal species normally associated today with the game parks of Kenya and South Africa.

early as 9,000 BC in the Fertile Crescent and had spread to north and western Europe by 5,000 BC. A number of modern cereal crops such as oats and rye were originally weeds associated with various species of wheat. As the cultivation of wheat moved northwards, oats and rye that are hardier increased in significance and, today, both of these are grown widely in colder northern areas where wheat is on the margin of viability.

It was not only food crops that were grown, crops were also grown to provide fibres for the manufacture of cloth, thread, nets ropes and various other items. These would have included cotton, flax, and hemp. Flax has a dual purpose in that as well as producing fibres, the seeds can be crushed to give linseed oil, a useful waterproofing agent, and it has been suggested that it was initially grown for its oil content rather than its fibres.

The technologies required to process crops spread at the same time as the plants, these would have included harvesting and storage techniques. Other technologies followed agriculture such as the use of wheeled transport and draught animals, milking of domesticated animals, beer and wine fermentation, pottery, metallurgy and writing. Many people think that these technologies would have spread one at a time, but obviously if a whole village or tribe moved for some reason, they would have taken a complete package with them.

Other areas of similar climate throughout the world lacked the wide range of potential starting materials available in the Fertile Crescent. For example, the eastern USA had no cereals worth domesticating and no domesticated animals except dogs. The result was that the Mississippi mound builders did not start to develop their civilisation until maize and other crops were introduced from Mexico.

Although the Americas had far fewer potential crops than the Old World (it is estimated that some 85% of cultivated crops today originated in the Old World), several crops imported into Africa from the Americas have become more important than some indigenous crops. These include maize, sweet potatoes, tomatoes, sunflowers, peanuts and the important cash crop, tobacco. They also included the cacao plant whose pods are used to make chocolate and vanilla, grown by the Maya, whose pods provided the flavouring for chocolate. Cacao is now grown widely in sub-Saharan Africa as a cash crop.

ACQUISITION OF CROPS

The amounts of wild cereals available were very substantial in the Fertile Crescent; work by botanists has shown that crops were so heavy that it is possible to harvest up to eight hundredweight per acre annually (one tonne per hectare), using stone-age technology such as flint and obsidian-edged sickles. The other technique, still used by hunter-gatherer groups, is to beat the cereal with a stick whilst holding a basket underneath. Whilst it obviously comes from a later date, black-figure pottery from Greece, dated to the sixth century BC, shows farmers beating olive trees with sticks and holding baskets underneath to catch the falling fruit.

It is probable that some hunter-gatherer societies had already settled close to this food source before they started cultivating plants, and these groups probably supplied the manpower for the construction of Göbekli Tepe. In the initial stages, agriculture was basically a form of plant collecting but it is possible that hunter-gatherers replanted some of the seeds, bulbs or tubers they had collected in a more convenient spot and fenced them off to protect them from wild animals such as deer and pigs. This obviously represents a major step on the road towards becoming farmers.

The development of an agrarian as opposed to a hunter-gatherer society was marked by considerable changes in the types of plants and animals found in archaeological sites. Plants were domesticated at different times. Excavation of archaeological sites suggest that varieties of wheat were domesticated around 9,000 BC, rice around 7,500 BC, whilst many soft fruits were not domesticated until well into the second millennium AD. The domestication of plants can be defined as growing a plant and changing it either consciously or unconsciously.

All crops arose from wild plants, which raises the question of why some wild plants became crops, whilst others did not. The reasons are numerous and complex, but one example is the production of bitter or poisonous leaves and fruits that protect the plant from browsing animals and insects. Occasionally, a non-bitter or non-poisonous mutant is formed, and Diamond quotes almonds as one of the better known examples. These produce a chemical known as amygdalin, a cyanide derivative of sugars. It is also found in the kernels of a number of stone fruits such as cherries, peaches and apricots. Amygdalin breaks down to form the extremely poisonous chemical, hydrogen cyanide (prussic acid), but the loss of a single enzyme results in plants that cannot synthesize amygdalin, and therefore do not produce cyanide. Presumably early humans saw animals eating non-poisonous almonds and tried them, and as a result, almonds became cultivated. This is a relatively simple example of a single mutation involving the loss of a single chemical, the effects of which are immediately obvious. A modern day example of the same type is the discovery of naturally occurring, caffeine-free, coffee plants in Ethiopia.

Other types of genetic changes would have involved a series of mutations that might not have become apparent for many generations, but, over a period of time, selection of plants producing certain advantages to humans would have occurred. The first farmers were not consciously carrying out plant breeding, they would have merely been selecting plants with certain characteristics that made their lives easier. Some of the changes are obvious; higher-yielding varieties, larger seed size, seeds clustered on the stalks instead of individually, plants that held the seeds firmly and did not disperse them (allowed easier collection), and longer stalks (did not have to bend over so far).

Cereal crops produce a huge number of seeds, which germinate at different times, enabling some seeds and plants in each generation to survive prolonged wet and dry periods, and early or late frosts. This type of behaviour represents an important survival strategy for the plant. Over generations, the collection of seeds at a specific time, and saving a portion of the seeds collected to form the seed stock for the following year, would have established synchronicity in the germination of the crop. This allows it all to be harvested simultaneously, obviously to the great advantage of the farmer.

A major factor would have involved dormancy. The factors influencing this vary widely from plant to plant, and the breaking of dormancy by the plant does not always correspond with the farmer's view on the optimum time. Practical experience handed on from one generation to the next, over a long period of time, would have been essential to optimise the crop.

Plants need to spread their seeds over a wide area and they adopt a number of strategies to do so which includes fruits being eaten and the seeds spat out or passing out in faeces. In many cases the seeds must pass through the gut of an animal or bird, with the seed coat being subjected to partial digestion or abrasion before they can germinate. Passing out with faeces also gives the new plant a kick-start as it comes with its own ready-made bed of fertiliser.

Larger fruits would have been chosen for consumption and seeds from these fruits would be more likely to produce larger fruit and over numerous generations, small wild fruits would evolve into the commercial varieties found today. One farming technique that had been developed by Roman times was the grafting of fruit trees onto root stock, a technique widely used today in commercial orchards and vineyards and plant breeding is mentioned by several Roman authors. Cato Marcus Porcius (Cato the Elder, 234-149 BC) wrote *"De Agri Cultura"* which is the oldest complete surviving prose work in Latin around 160 BC. It provides us with a wealth of information on the transition of Roman farming from smallholdings to large-scale farming and deals especially with the cultivation of olives and grapes. Cato is perhaps better known as the politician who preached against the resurging power of Carthage and finished every speech with the phrase, *"Delenda est Carthago"* (Carthage must be destroyed)[80].

Another important Roman author is Publius Vergilius Maro (70-19 BC), the poet Virgil[81], who wrote the *"Georgics"*, four books of poems on farming and rural life in Italy. He mentions grafting as a technique essential for the cultivation of crops such as apples that do not breed true when grown from seed. Much of his work is a political plea for the restoration of agricultural life after the rural depopulation following the civil wars of Pompey and Caesar, and Anthony and Octavian (Augustus).

One important example of a large increase in size is maize (*Zea mays*) whose wild ancestor is teosinte *(Euchlaena mexicana)*, a type of Mexican grass[82]. Genetic studies suggest that modern maize may have been domesticated by 7,000 BC. Maize cobs from early settlements dated to around 3,500 BC are about 1.5cm in length (a little over half an inch) but by the time of Columbus, the Amerindians were growing maize 15cms long (six inches) and modern varieties are frequently 50cms (twenty inches) long.

Various types of seed dispersion are found and these

---

80   He got his wish in 149 BC when Rome provoked Carthage into the Third Punic War by making impossible demands designed to curb the growing mercantile power of Carthage. The war lasted until 146 BC and at the end of it Carthage had been destroyed and razed to the ground. Only twenty per cent of the estimated 250,000 inhabitants survived. They were all sold into slavery and the territory previously ruled by Carthage became a Roman province. As he watched the city burn, the Roman general, Scipio Africanus the Younger, pondered on the ultimate fate of Rome, perhaps a prophetic foresight given the epidemics that ravaged Rome in the second to fourth centuries AD and the collapse of the Western Roman Empire that followed.

81   He is better known for writing the epic poem, the *"Aeneid"*.

82   Maize is not found in the wild and the evolution of teosinte into maize is controversial.

can also be subject to mutational changes. Many plants have specialised mechanisms for dispersing seeds when ripe, and whilst these dispersal mechanisms do not prevent humans from harvesting the seeds, they make harvesting very labour intensive. Obviously bending down to collect individual seeds that have been spread over several square metres is significantly more difficult and time-consuming than picking them off a stalk, a handful at a time. Mutant plants producing seeds that do not disperse would therefore have been harvested preferentially, and when sown, these seeds would have given rise to a higher percentage of the same mutant. Eventually over a period of generations, the mutant would have become the dominant cultivated type. Some wild cereals are an example of this. The seeds are scattered when mature by the disintegration of the stalk and the loss of a single gene stops the stalk breaking up. In the wild, this mutation is lethal as the seeds are left dangling in mid-air where they rot or germinate; the seeds from these mutant plants however are the ones collected by humans. This was probably one of the earliest human "improvements" (selection) of any plant, and has been called the "*wait for the harvester*" mutation. Other mutations involving different features would also have been selected over time. Repeated sowing and harvesting would select these changes over years, and it has been estimated that wheat would have required approximately two hundred harvests to become domesticated as we would recognise it today.

Modern requirements for cereals are driven by the milling and baking industries that obviously operate on a vast scale compared with antiquity. High yields are essential, as also are varieties that do not mutate easily. Further requirements are ease of milling, production of flour that bakes well, high protein levels, awnless (beardless) varieties, drought, disease and frost-resistance, plus various other features. Modern varieties of wheat are usually sub-divided into hard and soft wheat, hard wheat such as *Triticum durum* requiring special milling. In the case of barley, the brewing industry dictates major requirements for the crop, one of the most important being the levels of nitrogen required.

As mentioned at the beginning of this chapter, evolution involves both mutation and selection. It is obvious in the cases mentioned above that human selection has replaced natural selection, and many modern varieties or cultivars of these crops would not have "evolved" if left to their own devices, they would have been eliminated very quickly. They would not survive today and if left to nature would rapidly disappear.

Crops such as wheat and barley grow quickly, from sowing to harvest is only a few months and such a harvest is still compatible with a hunter-gatherer lifestyle. On the other hand, crops such as olives, dates, figs, and grapes require several years to start fruiting, and also, in a number of cases require annual pruning. This suggests that the people harvesting them are staying in one place for a prolonged period of time. This was recognised by the early Greek city-states whose code of warfare required them to *"spare the olive and spare the vine"*. This was recognition that annual crops, such as cereals, could easily be replaced if destroyed, but if olive trees and grape vines were destroyed, the land would be devastated for years. Thucydides states that the olive groves at Delphi were sacred and if destroyed, the result would be a *"sacred war"*. This was all-out war with no prisoners being taken. The same prohibition is found in the Bible, The Book of Revelation contains the verse, *"See thou hurt not the oil and the wine"* (Revelation 6.6).

Although the number of plant species worldwide has been estimated at around 450,000, only a few hundred have ever been domesticated. Today, only a small number of food crops, less than about twenty different species of plants, meet approximately eighty per cent of all human calorific requirements. These are wheat, barley, rye, oats, millet, maize, sorghum (a form of millet) and rice, all of which are forms of cereals. The only other significant crops are potatoes, sweet potatoes, cassava (manioc), yams, taro, sugar cane, bananas and possibly crops such as sugar beet, soya bean, chickpeas, oil palms and groundnuts (peanuts) in recent years. Five cereals, wheat, maize, barley, rice and sorghum predominate, accounting for over half of the calories consumed. If one of these twenty or so crops fails due to disease, the effect can be catastrophic. The Irish potato famine in the 1840s was a classic example of this problem (Ch. 13).

One major problem is that many of these crops are high in carbohydrates and calories, but low in protein; maize, rice, potatoes, cassava, bananas and yams are notorious for this problem. The result is that although they allow a high population density to develop, individual members of farming communities have a poorer standard of health than hunter-gatherers. Cereal crops are also low in minerals, and children fed on diets high in cereals and low in vegetables frequently suffer severe mineral deficiencies, rendering them susceptible to numerous diseases. Archaeological investigations in the Yucatan show that the Maya who ate a diet largely composed of maize were particularly prone to this problem. The characteristic lesions of a deficiency of iron, and therefore general anaemia, are found widely in the skulls of young children. This would have been exacerbated by tropical parasites such as intestinal worms removing blood from their victims. A similar situation is found in skeletons excavated from archaeological sites in the Eastern Mediterranean. In this case, the problem is more probably caused by the difficulty of iron absorption in diets high in cereals, legumes and nuts that all contain large amounts of a chemical known as phytic acid, which slows down the absorption of iron from plant sources. The situation is compounded by the combination of the genetic disease thalassaemia and malaria (Ch 16). As a generality, haem iron (iron from meat) is absorbed considerably more efficiently than non-haem iron, i.e. iron from plant sources. It is worth pointing out that humans evolved to be omnivorous, if we had evolved to be herbivorous, we would have larger teeth, much more powerful jaw muscles and a gut the size of a silverback gorilla.

The cultivation of many crops such as wheat, barley, olives and grapes in areas such as Greece, Thrace and modern day Turkey, all of which are adjacent to the Fertile Crescent, caused relatively little damage to the local ecosystem as any introduction of new pests or diseases would have been minimal. The cultivation of some crops however, especially rice, can cause major changes to the ecosystems into which they are introduced.

Rice is the most widely grown of all crops and today it provides the basic cereal for about two billion people or nearly one third of the world's population. It was first cultivated and domesticated by the Chinese in the Yangtse Valley and is not found in India before about 5,000 BC. The increase in the size of cereals can be estimated from the size of phytoliths (phyto meaning plant and lith meaning stone). Grasses are very high in silica, and phytoliths formed from silica are characteristic of grass species. There is a marked increase in the number of phytoliths of wild rice, *Oryzae rufipogen,* in archaeological sites from about 12,000 BC, indicating increased collection of this species. Phytoliths become bigger showing the appearance of domesticated rice (*O. saliva*) around 7,500 BC, and by 6,500 BC most traces of wild rice have disappeared from archaeological sites. The earliest form of rice farming did not involve irrigation, it used wetlands, but over time, irrigation was introduced and this resulted in major changes in the ecology of an area, increasing the range and incidence of a number of diseases such as malaria (Ch 16) and schistosomiasis (Ch 19).

It is interesting that, although humans have been selecting varieties of plants to give improved yields for thousands of years, during this time relatively few new species of food plants have been developed. One of the few examples is triticale, a genetic recombinant of wheat and rye that is very cold-resistant and is used as a fodder crop in northern latitudes.

One problem that arises in the modern farming world, especially in developed countries, is the growth of only a few high yielding varieties of a crop species. Certain varieties are specifically selected for their heavy yields and disease resistance and other varieties are lost either through attrition or deliberate legislation. The result is that the genetic pool of the species is reduced. This causes problems if it becomes necessary to reintroduce genetic variation to the crop because of the development of new strains of a disease. Even the poorest yielding variety of a plant species, one that is totally inadequate for modern agriculture, may be an important source of some disease-resistant feature at some time in the future. European Union legislation in the early 1970s restricted the sale of seeds of certain vegetables and cereals to those officially listed, in order to protect seed companies. Seed companies make profits from competitive markets and will obviously not support old varieties unless there is a significant public demand. The introduction of seed banks in a number of countries in recent years has been made in an attempt to alleviate this situation. Examples are the Heritage Seed Library established in the UK, Arche Noah in Austria, the Svalbard Global Seed Project based in Spitsbergen and administered by Norway, and in Switzerland, an organisation known as Pro Specie Rara protects rare breeds of animals, as well as fruit and vegetables.

The problem raised in the previous paragraph have been highlighted by both bananas and potatoes in the last quarter of a century or so, and there is a serious problem with wheat at the present moment[83]. Bananas are a classic example of the

---

83   Wheat is destroyed by a fungus disease known as Black Stem Rot, caused by *Puccinia graminis*. A new strain of the fungus known as Ug 99 appeared in Uganda in 1999, and is spreading rapidly eastwards towards countries such as Iran and Pakistan. Three anti-rust genes are present in most commercially grown varieties of wheat, but the present strain of rust has mutated to resistance to these. It takes a minimum of five

difficulty relating to the development of new varieties. They are a major crop especially in the developing world, where they are found in a variety of colours and sizes and may be sweet or starchy. Most bananas contain starch, and are grown widely as a staple food in countries such as Uganda. The sweet varieties sold as a fruit in developed countries are usually grown as a cash crop for export.

Bananas are one of the world's oldest food crops, originating in South East Asia at the end of the last Ice Age. They are descended from the wild banana, *Musa acuminata,* which is diploid and forms a large number of hard seeds, making the fruit virtually inedible. Occasionally rare mutants are found that produce seedless, edible varieties of banana. These mutants are triploid, not diploid, that is they contain three sets of chromosomes, not two, and are sterile. They can only be cultivated by cuttings, and each variety of banana is basically an infertile clone producing plants lacking in genetic diversity.

Plants that reproduce sexually show genetic diversity because in each generation the genes are assorted into new combinations. This enables the plant to evolve responses to diseases, edible bananas however lack the genetic diversity to combat pests and diseases. The result is that banana crops have been declining in yields for fifty years, and a situation resembling the spread of potato blight in Ireland is developing.

Until the 1950s, a variety known as the Gros Michel dominated the commercial banana market of the developed world. This mutant was found in the 1820s in Asia, but was vulnerable to a fungal wilt known as Panama Disease. The fungus contaminates the soil, is impossible to eradicate, and infected fields must be abandoned with cultivation being moved to fresh land. This variety of banana was eventually abandoned when suitable land was exhausted.

A new variety, the Cavendish, found in southern China,

years to develop disease resistant strains of wheat adapted to local growing conditions and then produce sufficient seed for planting large areas.

was introduced which is resistant to Panama disease, and this now provides most of the bananas sold in the developed world. Although the original plants were found in China, samples were brought to Great Britain in the nineteenth century, and grown at Chatsworth, the ancestral home of the Duke of Devonshire (the Cavendish family). It was cuttings from these samples that were used to provide plants for commercial trials, hence the name given to this variety. However, a new fungal disease, Black Sigatoka, which first appeared in Fiji in 1963 has now spread world-wide. This fungus attacks the Cavendish variety, causing serious reductions in yield. It is only kept in check by spraying large amounts of fungicides and bananas are one of the most heavily sprayed crops in the world. The fungicides account for approximately twenty-five per cent of the production costs, and it has been alleged that they cause cancer in workers and genetic defects in their children. The latest problem is that a new strain of Panama disease is appearing which attacks the Cavendish. As already mentioned, this is a soil fungus and cannot be controlled by spraying.

Because all the edible varieties of banana are sterile, changing the genetic profile to disease resistance by cross-pollination is impossible. It would be theoretically possible to sequence the DNA of the wild inedible banana, find resistance genes and then use genetic techniques to introduce these into a laboratory tissue culture. These could then be grown into plants using standard plant propagation techniques. The process would be difficult, very expensive, extremely time-consuming and would carry no guarantee of being successful. It is also necessary to produce a variety that is pleasant to eat if it is to be used as a cash crop. Peasant societies, where the crop is being used as a staple food, do not have that option; they either eat it or starve, whether it tastes pleasant or not. The only other option is to hope that a new triploid variety of banana is found growing wild, that this can be propagated and possesses all the attributes needed.

ACQUISITION OF ANIMALS.

In addition to discussing the acquisition of crops, Diamond also discusses the acquisition of animals in some detail.

Some groups of hunter-gatherers would have lived by following herds of wild animals as they moved between winter and summer pastures. At some point, this behaviour would have changed, depending on the animals involved, from shadowing the herd and killing animals to herding them. Once this happened they were moving towards farming. Such behaviour is still seen in cultures such as the Sami in Lapland, some of whom live in the traditional manner following their reindeer herds.

Many animals would have been attracted to the cereals being grown or harvested by early agriculturalists and this would have allowed their capture and domestication, orphaned animals may have been kept as an insurance policy against starvation[84]. Over time there would have been selection towards increased docility, this would usually mean smaller and more tractable animals, especially the males. The reduction in size is probably a result of the selective culling of young, large adult males for meat over a long period. This would have been very common in northern latitudes as it was not possible to grow sufficient fodder crops to keep all the livestock through winter.

One marked example of the changes caused by domestication is the small horn size in modern domesticated male goats compared with the huge curved horns of wild males. Another is the loss of the ability to moult in modern breeds of sheep. Ancient varieties of sheep lose their wool over a wide area by moulting in late spring, modern breeds have to be shorn so the fleece comes off in one piece.

---

84   At one early archaeological site in North Africa, there is evidence that wild sheep were kept penned at the back of caves, and given fodder which included one plant known to act as a soporific. Homer records sheep being kept in a cave in the *"Odyssey"* when Odysseus and his men are trapped in a cave by the cannibalistic giant, Polyphemus.

These changes are reflected in the archaeological differences found in various sites. In hunter-gatherer sites, the distribution of bones shows that they would have killed any animal that could be caught. Therefore bones from a wide range of species, old and young, male and female animals are found. In farming sites however, there would only be a limited number of domesticated species and there would be a preponderance of bones from young males which had been slaughtered as being non-essential for breeding stock. The results are not completely clear-cut, as many early farmers would have supplemented their diets with the occasional hunting expedition.

A similar situation to crops arose with animals. Only a very small number of larger animal species have ever been domesticated, in this context, the word domestication means animals that are bred in captivity. These animals included the dog that was the first animal to be domesticated from the wolf *(Canis lupus)*, probably at least 15,000 years ago[85]. Dogs were probably domesticated in several different areas and generally used for hunting, guard duties and herding. With the exception of parts of Asia, Mexico (Aztecs) and Polynesia where dogs were bred for food, they were normally only eaten when other sources of protein and meat were lacking, indeed in most hunting communities eating the dogs is a last resort to avoid starvation.

Other animals domesticated across the Euro/Asian landmass for the purposes of food, skins and transport were cattle, sheep, goats, pigs and horses. The available evidence suggests that the goat was probably the first species to be domesticated. Although goats are important as they can survive on very marginal land, they are also, by far, the worst species in terms of causing environmental damage. Evidence from the Fertile Crescent shows that goats and sheep were being domesticated by 8,000 BC, and one site in Iran suggests that goats may have been kept as early as 10,000 BC.

---

85 This date is controversial. A number of experts consider that dogs were domesticated thousands of years earlier than this.

Ancestors of the five main groups of domesticated animals were all found in Eurasia, but not the Americas. Sheep and goats are descended from wild ancestors found in the Fertile Crescent. Cattle descended from the wild aurochs of Europe and India and pigs descended from wild boar that are widespread throughout Eurasia. The ancestors of horses were related to Przewalski's wild horse, still found in Central Asia, and were probably first domesticated somewhere in the region of Kazakhstan.

A few other species were domesticated in relatively localised areas, for example, different species of camels in desert areas, reindeer in Lapland and water buffalo in South East Asia. Other domesticated animals included donkeys descended from the wild ass found in Ethiopia and Somalia. These were domesticated about five thousand years ago and have spread worldwide. A number of birds were also domesticated, the most important being the chicken, a descendant of the jungle fowl of South East Asia[86].

All the groups domesticated are herbivores, with the exceptions of pigs that are omnivores and regarded as unclean by a number of religions and dogs that are carnivores. All species capable of domestication, with the exception of dogs, were domesticated between approximately ten thousand and five thousand years ago.

The same species might have been domesticated independently in different parts of the world. It is probable that pigs were domesticated in more than one centre as they appear in both the Fertile Crescent and China at a very early stage. Cattle were also domesticated in at least two centres. European cattle that have no hump are descended from the European aurochs whilst the humped cattle of India are descended from the Asian aurochs. Genetic analysis shows that the two groups separated long before they were domesticated and therefore must have been domesticated independently.

86   The one item of livestock that originated in the Americas, and then spread worldwide, is the turkey, introduced into England in the seventeenth century.

Many domesticated animals differ markedly from their wild ancestors, their body shape is different, they have different fur patterns and many of them breed all year round as opposed to annually in their wild relatives. Darwin thought that the process of domestication would have been extremely slow but experiments by the geneticist Dmitry Belyaev in Russia suggest that species change very rapidly once selective breeding is started. He found that within twenty years it was possible to turn wild silver foxes into a domesticated fox with a greatly altered appearance and behavioural characteristics similar to those of a pet dog. Similar experiments were carried out on other species, including rats. One curious feature was that the animals were only selected for their docile temperament, all the other changes such as shape and colouring came as part of the package.

Domesticated animals are in the same position as cultivated plants, they would not survive in the wild. One only needs to consider the possibility of the modern ungainly dairy cow, with its huge udder, attempting to evade predators such as a wolf pack.

The question arises: why were only some large species domesticated and always the same or similar species across the Eurasian landmass? There are a number of reasons and Diamond summarises these under several headings.

- It is not easy to domesticate an animal whose diet is too specialised.
- It is not economically or practically viable to domesticate an animal whose growth rate is too slow. In addition, these species tend to be very large and handling them (especially the males) causes major problems.
- Many animals have highly specialised breeding requirements, and difficulties arise when attempting to breed them in captivity. Classic examples of this problem were the hawks

> and cheetahs used for hunting in many early cultures.

- Many animals closely related to domesticated species are not suitable because of their unpleasant temper and unpredictability. Examples include the African buffalo, zebra, and the onager (the wild ass of Asia), whose temper was so notorious that the Romans called one of their military catapults an onager, because of its kick when fired.
- Other reasons include the disposition of the animal involved. Obviously a tendency to run or jump fences, at the slightest provocation, does not lend itself to easy herding. This rules out many species of deer and antelope, some of which can accelerate from 0-50 mph in a couple of seconds and jump a high fence with ease.

Virtually all species of domesticated large animals have certain social characteristics. They live in herds or large family groups, have a well-established hierarchy of dominance and occupy overlapping territories instead of mutually exclusive ones. This type of social behaviour is necessary for herding as the hierarchical structure allows coexistence without fighting. The human herder effectively takes over the position of the dominant animal. Animals with an exclusive home range cannot live as large herds as dominant animals are always fighting. Some animals including many species of deer and antelope live in herds for part of the season, but the males become highly territorial during the breeding season.

No large animals were domesticated in the New World, with the exception of llamas, vicunas and alpacas in a relatively small area of South America. These are varieties of the same species of camelid and do not live in large herds. In addition, they were not kept indoors in byres as were many of the farm animals in the Old World and the local people did not drink their milk. This is of considerable importance to the development of tuberculosis (see Ch. 11) in humans, and also exposure to several other diseases. The consequences of this for the inhabitants of the New World are discussed elsewhere.

A similar situation is found in animals as occurs in plants. Many old breeds are becoming extinct in areas such as Europe, as they do not conform to modern ideas of farming (e.g. putting on weight quickly), even although we are realising, rather belatedly, that they may possess many desirable qualities such as producing very lean meat, or have the ability to thrive on marginal land[87].

In addition to providing meat and hides, livestock also furnish milk and fertiliser, animals that can be milked supply several times more calories over their lifetime than a one-off slaughter. The production of milk led to one interesting difference in the genetics of various groups of people. A large majority of the world's adult population is intolerant to lactose (milk sugar), and cannot use milk or its derivatives as food. All children possess the enzyme lactase, which allows the lactose in breast milk to be utilised. As most children are weaned, this ability is switched off genetically and lost. In farming communities where large quantities of milk were available, it was obviously an advantage to retain lactase activity, as it meant an additional food source was available. Children who had this ability had a genetic advantage, and the result is that lactose tolerance became widespread throughout Europe, where dairy farming was common.

Animals can also be trained to pull ploughs, allowing heavier land to be cultivated and the use of the plough was another item of technology that originated in Mesopotamia and diffused out to other areas. Cultures that used digging sticks

---

87   The Soay and North Ronaldsay sheep found on some of the islands off the west coast of Scotland are well-known examples. Dry stonewalls have been built around the islands, not to keep the sheep in, but to keep them out and away from the fields of the islanders. The result is that the sheep are confined to the foreshore, where they live on seaweed, frequently wading out belly-deep into the sea to obtain it.

could only cultivate light sedimentary soils in river valleys and flood plains. In North America, the heavier soils of the prairies with prairie grasses that formed root systems as deep as six feet or more were not farmed until draught animals and ploughs were introduced by the pioneers. However, once these deep root systems were destroyed by ploughing, massive erosion followed, resulting in the prairie dust bowls of the 1930s.

Large animals, specifically horses, oxen and camels were also used for transport. The use of horses allowed the expansion of the Indo-European peoples westwards from their original homelands in the Hindu Kush, displacing all the earlier cultures and their languages throughout Europe except the Finnish, Hungarian and Basque languages that belong to the Finno-Ugaric group of languages. Once linked to chariots, horses revolutionised warfare in Europe and the Near East (although the earliest chariots were drawn by asses). The classic example of the new technology was the use of chariots by the Hyksos (Shepherd Kings) to conquer Egypt around 1,650 BC. Horse technology was late coming to Egypt, as war chariots were being used in Mesopotamia at least five hundred years earlier. Chariots have been referred to as the *"world's first war machine"* and the numbers involved in battles can be substantial. It has been estimated that in 1,274 BC, the Battle of Kadesh between the Egyptians and Hittites involved approximately 5,000 chariots.

Further technologies related to horses were the invention of stirrups and saddles. These allowed successive invasions by the people from the steppes, such as the Huns in the fifth century AD, to sweep across Europe. Those with horses, saddles and stirrups had a huge military advantage over those without. The development of saddles and stirrups made the mounted warrior, especially the horse archer, supreme. The first indication of what we would recognise as modern paired stirrups is found in an early fourth century Chinese tomb and they were widespread in China by the fifth century.

The military use of horses however should not be over-rated as is frequently done when considering the conquests of Cortés and Pizarro in the New World. Horses only have a limited military value in areas such as jungles, mountains and street fighting. There were far more effective reasons for the total defeat of the inhabitants of Meso-America and the Andes at the hands of the Spanish conquistadors.

THE CONSEQUENCES OF FARMING

Farming probably arose as a response to the extermination of wild game over large areas. The development of agriculture caused a huge increase in human numbers over a relatively short space of time in evolutionary terms, and concentrated the population into much larger communities than had been the situation previously. Typically one acre of crops will feed 10-100 times as many people as a hunter-gatherer life style.

A sedentary farming mode of existence means more children. Hunter-gatherers carry all their weapons and possessions and a mother can only carry one baby. The first child must be able to keep up with the clan, on the move, before the mother can have a second. In practical terms this works out at one child about every four years, and family size is regulated by several methods. In sedentary farming communities, individuals did not need to carry all their belongings from place to place and women were able to have a child every year. Each additional child is more help with the harvest and other chores such as herding once it is big enough, and over several generations this obviously results in a much higher population. The rise in population requires more food, those who produced more food had more surviving children, and the increased population required more food. The whole process rapidly becomes autocatalytic[88].

One of the advantages of a hunter-gatherer mode of existence is that by moving frequently, humans would have left parasites and pest species such as rats and mice and

88   The efficiency of biomass conversion is generally considered to be 10 to 1, i.e. 10 pounds of plant food is required to produce 1 pound of meat.

contaminated water behind. A settled farming mode of existence however greatly increases the risk of contaminated land and water and results in a significant increase in the number of intestinal parasites such as worms. The farmers must have been able to cope with the increased parasitism as their numbers rose over time, allowing them to displace the hunter-gatherers to increasingly marginal land.

The increased number of children explains the paradox that although farming produces increased calories/acre, food producers are less well fed than hunter-gatherers because the increase in population outstrips the food supply. This is still a common problem today in countries such as the Philippines where there is strong religious opposition to birth control. In many cases, farmers are also less fit and well fed than hunter-gatherers, because much of the food consumed has a high calorific value, but is low in protein.

The discussion above also raises the chicken-and-egg question of whether a rise in population forced humans to develop different methods of obtaining food, or did the change to farming allow the population to rise because extra food was available?

In addition to the increased population produced by a sedentary life style, farming also allows the accumulation of non-portable possessions that ultimately produce significant advances in technology. In a static society, possessions do not have to be carried everywhere, and the production of excess food allows the development of a class of craftsmen, specialists and technologists who can barter or sell their expertise for food and other items. This cannot happen in a hunter-gatherer community where everybody is involved in finding food, and possessions are kept to essentials such as clothes and weapons.

A settled existence also allows food to be stored and the storage of food is pointless if it is not stored safely. Stored food is obviously essential for the development of towns, and also to feed the artisans and specialists. Once food is stored, it is necessary to keep track of it, and a tally system develops, which evolves into writing. This probably involved notched tally sticks originally, although the cultures of Meso-America used coloured cords knotted at intervals. Notched sticks as a form of writing (Ogham) were still being used in Ireland as late as the third or fourth century AD. Clay tablets with a single symbol on them have been dated to approximately 3,000 BC in China, and are considered to be seals, whilst the earliest writing in Sumer has also been found on clay tablets. These have been translated as lists of food and supplies being kept in various storerooms. The existence of such seals implies that some form of controlled storage is being used. Once writing has developed, full-time bureaucrats and scribes appear who eventually dominate the system and this evolves into a hierarchy of hereditary leaders who levy taxes.

In addition to feeding other full time specialists, stored food will also support a professional army that will usually defeat any society not able to support an army. The development of armies occurred at a fairly early stage, the Stele of Vultures, dated to *ca* 2,525 BC, shows a Sumerian army with standardised equipment. The warriors appear to be arranged in a military formation similar to the Greek phalanx, which strongly suggests a professional army, as this formation implies a high level of co-operation, training and discipline. The stele also shows that the city-states had groups of artisans and manufacturing bases large enough to produce substantial quantities of standardised equipment even at this early date.

There are numerous common features in early civilisations throughout the world. They had an elite who in most cases were literate and numerate, had an advanced knowledge of mathematics, the solar system and calendars, large-scale architecture and in the Old World, metallurgy[89]. Large-scale

---

89   Metallurgy probably developed first in the Fertile Crescent. Large deposits of malachite (copper carbonate) are found in this area, and the ore is easily recognisable as it is coloured bright green. Presumably the earliest

architecture requires division and specialisation of labour, a practical knowledge of mathematics and meticulous, large scale planning and organisation. This cannot be done by consensus, it requires a powerful ruling class, as does the use of irrigation systems, which require corvées to keep them in good repair. The Athenian philosopher, Plato (428-348 BC) makes the point in *"The Republic"* that democracy and consensus politics are very inefficient methods of government. Although Athens was nominally a democracy, much of its wealth and power were based on silver mines worked by a slave population.

In comparison, hunter-gatherers exist in small communities with a minimal social hierarchy. Leaders of the group are chosen for their knowledge and hunting skills, but everyone is involved in acquiring food and non-productive passengers are too great a drain on the system. Bureaucrats therefore do not appear and gain control.

The general influence of farming is to reduce both animal and plant diversity, make the biological population more uniform, and reduce the complexity of food chains. This generally destabilises the ecosystem and requires a great effort on the part of the farmer to be profitable. In addition to causing a shortening of the food chain and a reduction in the number of species, farming also causes an increase in the number of individuals of each species present. Numerous pest species such as insects benefit from this change, including

copper smelting occurred when someone used rocks containing malachite as hearth stones for a fire, and made the correlation between fire, malachite and copper. Wood fires (700°C) do not burn hot enough to smelt copper from malachite and the process would have involved the use of charcoal that burns at 1,100°C. It would probably also have involved a windy day producing a blast furnace effect. Archaeological investigation suggests copper was being smelted in Jericho possibly as early as 7,000 BC, a date considerably earlier than that generally accepted for the Bronze Age (3,000-1,000 BC). It is also not obvious how the use of copper developed into the use of bronze; presumably some early smith was experimenting mixing metals, and realised that if tin was added to copper, the resulting product was harder than either of the ingredients. After that it would have been a case of adjusting the quantities of each ingredient to obtain the optimum mixture.

those carrying human, animal and plant diseases. Cultivated fields are effectively a monoculture of a single species of plant, and once a microbial disease or an insect infestation has gained a good foothold, it is virtually impossible to eradicate it and extremely difficult to control it.

Effective crop farming requires the control of weeds. This may be done by hand and the use of digging sticks in small communities, but it is extremely inefficient, and other methods were developed. One control method is the regular flooding of land through the use of sluices as few weeds can survive flooding at regular intervals. This allows the cultivation of rice, one of the crops mentioned earlier; the downside is that it also encourages mosquitoes to breed.

Agriculture based on irrigation developed in Egypt, Mesopotamia, the Indus Valley, the Yellow River Valley and parts of Meso-America. Irrigation societies need a high level of social co-operation, specialisation and forced labour to maintain the necessary infrastructure of dams, canals, ditches and waterwheels necessary to raise water to higher levels, and an autocratic and authoritarian leadership to organise and control the distribution of water, and hence society. The development of the priesthood in the Nile Valley, with its specialised knowledge of the timing and extent of the annual flooding, is the best-known example. Large-scale irrigation started to appear about the same time that states started to appear, but whether states predated irrigation systems, or vice versa, is debatable. The use of canals for irrigation would also have allowed the use of small boats for the transport of goods.

Irrigation farming in a warm climate approximates to tropical conditions as far as parasites are concerned. The water is usually stagnant or slow flowing, allowing the breeding of mosquitoes carrying malaria and various other diseases. It also allows the existence of blood flukes causing schistosomiasis, which involve humans and water snails as alternate hosts.

Diseases of this type cause the human host to become seriously anaemic, and the general listlessness of agricultural workers may have helped a hierarchy and different social castes to develop. This situation occurred even in relatively temperate countries such as Japan, where worm and fluke infections were widespread until well into the 1950s, and the southern states of the USA, where hookworm infections, caused by *Necator americanus* were notorious until the start of World War II.

One widely used and effective method of weed control was ploughing, which allows indefinite cultivation of land. It also changes the physical structure of soil, allows heavier soil to be used and leads to increased yields as destruction of the weeds allows crops to be planted into an empty ecological niche. Recent research however, suggests that ploughing, by destroying the weed cover and breaking up the soil structure, increases the rate of erosion and degradation of the soil. The use of the plough allows the permanent settlement of a village, which increases the probability of disease due to contamination of water by both animal and human sewage. The use of human sewage as a fertiliser in countries such as Japan also contributed to the problems of increased disease. Practices such as these led to a considerable rise in intestinal parasites, problems of food poisoning and water pollution.

A third method of controlling weeds still used in some parts of the world is the primitive slash-and-burn technology. This has been blamed for many of the problems of deforestation and soil erosion, but it also creates a problem in that the felling of trees destroys the forest canopy displacing the vertical ecosystem. In a number of cases, this is known to have caused an increase in the incidence of malaria, changed the type of malaria found locally and also initiated numerous local epidemics of yellow fever.

Even with all of these problems, as already mentioned, agriculture allows population densities to develop which are much greater than those arising from a hunting mode of existence.

The protection of animals and crops from disease and pests requires great efforts by the farmer, but protection from human predators requires even more effort. The organisation of this protection provided a major stimulus to the social, political and military development of many societies.

THE FORMATION OF STATES

There is an interesting discussion between Socrates and two of his followers, Glaucon and Adeimantus, related by Plato (427-347 BC) concerning the *"First Principles of Social Organisation"* in *"The Republic"*. This dialogue discusses the minimum size of a community and the necessary social interaction required to make it function.

It starts by assuming that the community needs farmers to produce food and continues by agreeing that a number of specialised craftsmen are required such as weavers, shoemakers and smiths. From this point, it develops by considering that merchants and traders are needed and that seamen and shipwrights are essential (the discussion was taking place in Athens, a city-state based on sea-trade). The end of the first section concludes by deciding that it would be good to have a few luxuries as well as the necessities of life.

The next section, *"Civilised Society"*, decides there is no point in having a few luxuries at a feast if there are no poets and musicians to provide entertainment. The discussion then expands to include a wide variety of other individuals with specialised skills, and concludes by deciding that the territory available is no longer large enough to provide for such a community. The logical extension is then made that it is necessary for the community to have a standing army of professional soldiers to *"carve off a slice of our neighbours' territory"* which will obviously lead to war.

States may be formed by a number of different processes, one of which is communities amalgamating as protection in the face of a stronger enemy. The amalgamation of different states to form the USA, as protection against Great Britain, in the late eighteenth century, is a classic example of this process. A similar situation may well have occurred in many early civilisations, as most of them give detailed and graphic accounts of battles and conquest in their art, writing and sculpture.

A second method of states forming is by conquest. Early civilisations consisted of a dominant group taking food and resources (taxes) from subordinate groups, whilst leaving enough food for the subject group to survive for the rest of the year. In return, the dominant group usually provided some form of protection from more dangerous enemies (predators). It obviously made sense for the dominant group to only take a portion of the resources, and come back for more in subsequent years, rather than take the lot in a one-off attack. Similarly, it made sense for the subordinate group to hand over any surplus as an annual tax, rather than have everything destroyed in a single raid. The balance was presumably worked out by trial and error over a period of time. This can obviously be regarded as a form of parasitism, albeit macro-parasitism, rather than parasitism caused by microbes. The result is the same however, the removal of resources from the host community.

The production of food surpluses and other resources allowed many early civilisations to develop politically, and acquire powerful armies of well-armed, professional warriors, which obviously made the subjugation of less organised neighbours relatively easy. Organised specialists in violence (i.e. professional soldiers and armies) will normally defeat a civilian militia more usually engaged in agriculture.

The fate of the conquered people varied; if plenty of space was available they moved further away from the conquerors. If there was nowhere for the defeated tribe to move, then several scenarios were possible. The victors could exterminate the vanquished and confiscate their land, or kill the men and enslave the women and children. A further possibility was to let the defeated tribe live, but exploit them in one of several ways. States are specialised and society is stratified, so the defeated community could be used as slaves and forced labour. The Roman Empire made frequent use of this policy. There were exceptions, although the Romans used slaves extensively for construction purposes, they were never trusted with constructions used for military purposes. Hadrian's Wall, for example, was built entirely by the Roman army.

Alternatively the defeated tribe could be left *in situ*, but as mentioned earlier, tribute (taxes) could be exacted and the losers would eventually be incorporated into the victorious state. This type of policy initially prevailed in the early Roman Republic when Rome was conquering the cities and tribes of Italy. Men from the defeated tribes were incorporated into the legions and offered citizenship. The Romans however only gave them one chance. If the defeated city or tribe revolted, they were destroyed. One example was an Alpine tribe of north east Italy, the Salassi, who revolted, were destroyed in battle and the next day the local slave markets were saturated with 25,000 slaves for sale. The Romans returned to this type of policy later in the Empire when various Germanic tribes were offered land within the Empire and their men were expected to serve as auxiliaries to the Roman army.

In many cases, the amalgamation of the defeated peoples into the victorious tribe or state led to the development of castes, or a social stratification with well-fed ruling classes, warriors and priests, and poorly fed peasant and slave classes. This could cause problems if the system became top heavy when it could collapse, a situation thought to have happened to the Mayan civilisation of Meso-America around 1,100 AD. It could also be dangerous if the slaves became too powerful. Many of the Arab caliphates and later the Ottomans recruited slaves as soldiers, forming the Mamelukes and Corps of Janissaries. Both groups became very powerful and frequently engineered palace coups, in some cases replacing the ruler with one of their own leaders.

Urbanised conquerors did not always succeed in imposing their presence on tribal societies. In countries such as India, tribal societies lived in the jungle, were protected by jungle diseases and attempts to conquer or integrate them into the urban society were unsuccessful. The result is that India is a country with a large number of castes and sub-castes, and a plethora of languages (over 140 are recognised officially). This was not found in countries where tribal societies were not protected by jungle diseases. It is estimated that before the expansion of Rome, some forty languages were spoken in the Italian peninsula but by the time the Empire was founded, Latin was the only language remaining. Today we cannot even decipher Etruscan, one of the most important languages of early Italy after Latin.

The logical conclusion of this evolution of states is the development of what have been termed the *"Gunpowder States"*, leading ultimately to the modern super-power. After about 1,600 AD, governments became able to control large areas due to the development of more powerful weapons such as warships and cannon[90]. Such states included the English,

---

90   There were major developments in the manufacture of cannon between the reigns of Henry VIII of England (*r* 1509-1547) and his daughter Elizabeth I (*r* 1558-1603). At the start of Henry's reign, cannon were made by welding strips of metal together to form a hollow tube closed at one end. This was reinforced by forcing red-hot hoops of metal over it that shrank as they cooled. By the reign of Elizabeth, cannon were being cast in one piece, and the English foundries making cannon were years in advance of any in Europe. There were also major developments in warships. The great warship of Henry, the *Mary Rose,* which sank off the English coast in 1545, carried a crew of hundreds of men, mainly archers and men-at-arms, and would have expected to board, or be boarded by, the enemy. She also carried a motley collection of cannon of a wide range of calibres. One can just imagine the confusion trying to find the correct charge of powder and the correct sized cannonball during the heat of battle. By contrast, by the last two decades of Elizabeth's reign, English warships had evolved into relatively small, fast and highly manoeuvrable ships manned by a small crew of trained seamen. One

Dutch, French and Spanish/Portuguese in Western Europe, all based to a large extent on sea-power. In each case, the state was controlled by a centralised hierarchy employing a relatively small number of state employees in professional navies and armies. Weapons such as warships and cannon became so expensive that only governments could afford them, but they allowed governments to centralise control. As a result wars became fewer, as rebellious nobles could no longer afford to equip an army. The downside was that wars generally became more bloody and prolonged as they were fought between states with a greater access to resources.

THE DEVELOPMENT OF CIVILISATIONS

In the Bronze Age, a number of Old World civilisations[91] developed which would have been the focal points of different disease pools, the Nile Valley, the Indus Valley, Mesopotamia and the Yellow River Valley being amongst the most important. All were based on fertile plains with adequate access to drinking water and also with access to rivers or the sea for transport and trade. The civilisations of Meso-America and Peru appeared at a later date, and have been omitted at this stage for reasons that will become obvious in later chapters. The excavation and interpretation of archaeological data from these early cities is frequently very difficult, as more recent cities are usually built on top of ancient ones, resulting in numerous layers of civilisation.

The population explosion of approximately 6-4,000 BC caused many cities such as Ur in Sumer (Southern Iraq), and Memphis and Thebes in Egypt, to rise above a critical population threshold. The size of towns would have been limited by the

wreck of a pinnace, about seventy feet long, from the coast of Alderney in the English Channel, shows that she was carrying twelve cannon, all the same calibre, mounted on an advanced form of gun-carriage. Within a couple of generations, English warships had become a mobile fighting platform, with a coordinated weapons system, capable of destroying an enemy at long range.

91 The definition of the word "civilisation" may be contentious as to many people it implies a cultural superiority over the barbarian. It is however, being used in this context in the sense of living in a city, with an organised society, and having a social division of labour controlled by the state.

fertility of land surrounding them and the distance food could be transported before it rotted. If the town was on a river, then food could obviously be transported over a greater distance, and the same was true if irrigation canals were constructed. A similar situation was seen in numerous countries in the nineteenth century with the construction of the railways. The result of these transport systems was that the size of towns and cities was no longer constrained by agriculture and the fertility of the land in the immediate vicinity.

By 6,000 BC, numerous agricultural communities were appearing in southern and western Mesopotamia, and excavation suggests widespread trading networks judging by obsidian found a long way from its point of origin. Sumerian tradition claims the first city is Eridu, and excavation dates this to around 5,000 BC, by which time signs of artificial irrigation are starting to appear. On the basis of archaeological investigations, Uruk (Erech in the Bible), a city of Bronze Age Sumer, is estimated to have been nearly ten kilometres in circumference with walls fifty feet high, and a population of approximately fifty thousand. The epic of the semi-legendary ruler, Gilgamesh, dated to the early part of the third millennium BC, contains the passage, "*Look at the walls of Uruk, gleaming like polished bronze, inspect the inner wall, the like of which no man can equal*".

Cities of this size are large enough to support several crowd diseases, including most of the present day diseases, if they are relatively close to, and in regular contact with other large cities through trade. By the third millennium BC, there were a considerable number of independent city-states on the Babylonian plain, some of them with populations of over one hundred thousand. Excavations suggest that there were well-established class divisions, with a ruling elite controlling much of the wealth. There was a considerable amount of trade, and writing was developed in Sumer before 3,000 BC. Large numbers of tablets have been found of which the majority are bills, accounts, inventories of various types and lists of food stores.

All of the cities were based on irrigation canals, and there appears to have been constant warfare between them when they were not trading, in spite of interdependence on water supplies and irrigation. One of the problems with continuous irrigation is that it produces a build-up of salts, especially in areas of poor drainage and high evaporation, and the land eventually becomes barren. By 2,000 BC, much of the area was suffering from salinisation, and around this time there is a switch from growing wheat to barley, which is more salt resistant.

Organised warfare appeared at an early stage, and after many hundreds of years of campaigns, the city-states of Sumer were united around 2,300 BC by Sargon. Sumer was finally destroyed as a separate entity around 1,900 BC by the Amorites, and all its cities were sacked. One of the re-occurring problems for the cities on the Babylonian plain was that there were no natural frontiers that could be defended easily and they were therefore always open to attack.

Excavations suggest that Jericho, which is also in the Fertile Crescent, was a walled city with a population of about three thousand before 7,000 BC, and recent excavations in China have also indicated that there may have been significant concentrations of people considerably earlier than 4,000 BC. If correct, these earlier dates could have considerable implications for the length of time that crowd diseases may have been evolving.

Other major civilisations include that of Harappa, based around the River Indus, which covered an area the size of Western Europe and included most of modern day Pakistan. Early archaeological sites have been dated to around 6,000 BC, and their civilisation flourished from *ca* 3,300-1,700 BC, reaching its height between 2,600-1,900 BC. The largest city was Mohenjo-Daro with a population of about eighty thousand, and the whole area had a population estimated at five million. About fifteen hundred settlements have now been identified. Their culture was very advanced for the period, Mohenjo-Daro was laid out on a grid system by 2,500 BC with running water and sewage disposal. There appears to have been a uniformity of writing[92] and technology, including a standardised weights and measures system, over the whole area. Rice, wheat and barley were grown using widespread irrigation systems, and they were probably one of the earliest civilisations to cultivate cotton, which requires very large quantities of water. Cornelian jewellery from Harappa and seals unique to their culture have been found in cities such as Ur, indicating they were part of a widespread trading network. Sargon, who ruled Akkadia from 2,334-2,279 BC, claimed in a cuneiform inscription that ships from a wide variety of places including the Indus were bringing trade goods to Mesopotamia. The Harappan civilisation, which appears to have been Dravidian, collapsed around 1,700 BC due to a number of factors, including serious droughts linked to a weakening of the monsoons and a major river system changing course. Mohenjo-Daro was attacked and destroyed, and the Dravidians were driven into areas of southern Indian, such as Tamil Nadu, by the invading Aryan Indo-Europeans. Several authors have suggested that the origins of the caste system may date back to this period.

Once urban society had evolved, disease probably became the major cause of death, although famine and inter-tribal and inter-community warfare would also have played a role in limiting the population. The early Israelites were certainly aware of the problem; as the Old Testament puts it (Ezekial 7; 15), "*The sword is without and the pestilence and famine within;*

---

92   Their writing has not been deciphered; most of the seals found contain only four or five characters, some of them accompanied by carvings of real or mythical animals. These are too short to apply decipherment techniques, such as frequency analysis, to them.

he that is in the field shall die by the sword, he that is in the city, famine and pestilence shall devour him".

Each civilisation had its own climate and ecosystem and micro-organisms would have developed within these ecosystems producing a distinct set of diseases and immune responses for each community. A brief examination of the Egyptian dynasties based on the Nile Valley probably provides the best-documented example of the development of a civilisation, and provides a useful model for the interactions between civilisations. It also makes us realise that although different diseases may have arisen in different civilisations, the interaction between these civilisations meant that these diseases had probably spread considerably earlier than we realise.

Changes in the flood patterns of the Nile around 12,500 BC appear to have caused considerable tension between the various groups inhabiting the Nile Valley. Excavation of one group of burials dated to this period shows that at least forty per cent of the inhabitants had died violently, with arrow or spear heads embedded in their bodies, and cuts and fractures to skulls and hands (typical defensive injuries).

The first irrigation canals appeared in Egypt in the third millennium BC, and Egypt was unified by Menes to form the Old Kingdom that lasted from *ca* 2,700-2,100. During this period the population is thought to have reached about three million. The Old Kingdom broke into two (the First Intermediate Period) around 2,100 BC. Archaeology suggests that the break-up corresponds to a severe drought lasting about thirty years, during which the annual flooding of the Nile appears to have been greatly reduced. Egypt became two warring states, Upper and Lower Egypt, that were finally reunited by Mentuhotep II, (the king of Upper Egypt around 1,960 BC), to form the Middle Kingdom.

These states traded with the African interior for items such as ivory and slaves[93], and had probably come into contact with many diseases from sub-Saharan Africa at an early date. By 1,900 BC, the reunited Egyptian kingdoms were campaigning into Nubia, and many Nubians were being conscripted into the Egyptian armies. The impetus for these campaigns probably came from the desire to control the gold mines of Nubia (the name Nubia is thought to be derived from the Nubian word for gold).

Between approximately 1,630 and 1,520 BC (the Second Intermediate Period), Lower Egypt was ruled by the Hyksos (the Shepherd Kings), whose capital was at Avaris in the Nile delta. Contemporary accounts state that they came from the East, although their origin is in dispute. Many authors suggest that they migrated down through modern day Lebanon and Israel, but some think that they came from Saudi Arabia. Native Egyptian kings ruling from Thebes in Upper Egypt finally expelled them to form the New Kingdom.

By *ca* 1,450 BC, the Egyptians were campaigning under Thutmose III into northern Israel with major battles at Megiddo, and sieges at Joppa (modern day Jaffa). By the time of the nineteenth dynasty, which included powerful kings such as Seti I and Rameses II (Rameses the Great), the Egyptians had been in major confrontations with the Hittite Empire of northern Anatolia. This culminated in a series of battles, the major one being the Battle of Kadesh (*ca* 1,274 BC) in modern Lebanon. The result was a series of treaties between the Egyptians and the Hittites and Mitanni. At this time the Egyptian empire stretched from the mouth of the Nile in the north, to between the fifth and sixth cataracts in the south (modern Sudan), and from Libya in the west, whilst in the east

---

93   Frequent references are found in Egyptian records to trading with the Land of Punt, and the constant supply of items such as slaves, ivory, rare woods, spices and exotic animals. The Land of Punt is generally considered to be the Horn of Africa, i.e. modern day Somalia.

Babylon on the Euphrates was paying tribute and so were the Assyrians in Northern Iran.

During the eighth century BC, Egypt was ruled by Nubian kings (the Black Pharaohs), and there then followed several centuries of confusion. Firstly, the Assyrians gained supremacy, but were forced to withdraw after a short period to protect their home territories from the rising power of Babylon, thus allowing native Pharoahs to regain control. These retreated up the Nile valley after their defeat by the Persians under Cambyses in 525 BC. They took numerous aspects of Egyptian culture with them and formed a new kingdom between the fifth and sixth cataracts with a capital at Meroë. This was finally destroyed in 350 AD by Rome, some four centuries after the destruction of dynastic Egypt.

The Persians ruled Egypt for approximately two centuries (with a short intermission), until Alexander the Great destroyed the Persian Empire. After his death, one of his generals, Ptolemy I, seized Egypt and established the final dynasty that culminated in the death of Cleopatra (30 BC) and Egypt ultimately becoming a province of the Roman Empire.

In addition to these activities that were mainly land based, Egypt had boats large enough to carry troops and cargo as early as 4,000 BC, suggesting that trade along the Nile Valley and coastal regions was widespread[94]. They would have

---

94   Until recently, the earliest evidence suggesting sea-going canoes or rafts dated back to the human occupation of Australia, estimated to be around 40-50,000 BC. Australia and New Guinea were isolated from Indonesia, even at the height of the Ice Age, by a number of deepwater channels, the widest being about 50 miles across. The implication is that there must have been vessels capable of surviving this journey, even if they were only blown off course accidentally. This theory, however, received a major shock with the recent discovery of the bones of a dwarf human species, just over one metre tall, on the Indonesian island of Flores. This has been named *Homo floresiensis* and is believed to be a descendant of *Homo erectus* (it has also been nicknamed "the hobbit" after the characters in *"Lord of the Rings"*). One near complete skeleton and bones from about six other individuals have been found. Flores lies to the east of the Wallace Line (a hypothetical line separating the flora and fauna of Asia from that of Australia), and is separated from other Indonesian islands by

come into contact with numerous peoples based around the Mediterranean through the trading empire of the Cretans based at Knossos, which was destroyed, around 1,500 BC, by the explosion of the volcano, Thera (Santorini). Further contact with other Mediterranean peoples came with the attacks by the People of the Sea as the Egyptians named them. These were a confederation of Aegean tribes who attempted to invade Egypt, during the reign of Rameses III (*ca* 1,184-1,153BC). This occurred whilst they were migrating into the Near East, possibly because of climate changes leading to drought and poor harvests.

Athens had also established a large sea-going trading empire by the fifth century BC, with numerous satellite cities throughout the eastern Mediterranean, and was importing and exporting goods to and from Egypt. Thucydides claimed the Plague of Athens (430 BC) started in Egypt (Ch 8).

Given the levels of interaction between the various societies and civilisations as described above, it is reasonable to assume that by 2,000 BC, and probably considerably earlier, Egypt, various Near and Middle Eastern kingdoms and a number of

---

approximately fifteen miles of a deep-water channel with dangerous currents. It was previously thought that humans had not crossed the Wallace Line until the human occupation of Australia. However, the finding of *H. floresiensis* and stone tools dated to 94,000 years ago on Flores, shows that they must have had the ability to cross this dangerous waterway. Much older stone tools have also been found at a different site, which have been controversially dated to 840,000 years ago. If this is correct, it means that *H. erectus* also crossed to Flores, although no *H. erectus* remains have been found. *H. floresiensis* is the most extreme form of adaptation of the genus *Homo* ever discovered and it suggests that the genus *Homo* is more subject to evolutionary forces than some people may care to think. It is an example of *"island dwarfing"*, what is occasionally called by biologists *"shrink to fit"*. This theory considers that when a species is isolated on an island, it becomes smaller as resources are limited; numerous examples of this occurring are known. The most recent remains were dated to around 18,000 years ago, and were found beneath a layer of volcanic ash, dated to 10,000 BC, suggesting that as a species, they were probably wiped out by an eruption about that time.

early Mediterranean civilisations had developed a more or less common disease pool.

A similar situation probably occurred with other empires and cultures. Further east, civilisations and empires based on Mesopotamia also had sea-going boats as early as 3,500 BC. The various civilisations of India, China and South East Asia were in contact with each other through trade over the Silk Road and along coastal routes at an early date, and Mesopotamia (Persia) is known to have been trading with the civilisations of the Indus Valley.

As these civilisations interacted, diseases would have passed from one to the other and caused epidemics of various types. This process continued with the development of new civilisations, especially around the Mediterranean as these foci were linked closely by sea trading routes. Overland trade routes such as the Silk Road would have been less effective at spreading disease. The time involved in journeying from one centre to another allowed the disease to attack all the susceptible individuals, and either kill them, or, if they recovered, they had high levels of immunity. Sea routes, where possible, would have been chosen due to the larger amounts of cargo that can be carried, the lower cost involved and the speed. Overland routes require a large number of pack animals. A train of at least five hundred animals would be needed to move thirty to forty tonnes of cargo, an amount that could be carried in a medium sized sailing ship with a crew of twenty men. The overland route would also require the employment of herdsmen to tend the animals, pack animals to carry fodder and act as spares, guards to protect against bandits and payment of taxes or bribes at various customs posts. Pack trains are also slow compared with sailing ships that could travel a hundred miles a day, with favourable winds and currents, even allowing for the fact that they would have stopped and anchored somewhere safe for the night. A large pack train negotiating difficult conditions such as mountain passes would do well to travel ten to fifteen miles per day. Until the nineteenth century, with the development of initially the canal system and then railways, overland transport has been so difficult that most big cities were either near a river or the sea enabling ships to bring in food and other commodities.

In the Bronze and Iron ages, communities had to deal with a stream of new diseases with little or no respite. Cities could not sustain their numbers from their own resources, but they still grew in size because of the influx of migrants from the countryside. The growth of cities required rural peasants to produce an excess of both children and food. Many of these child migrants would have died relatively quickly as they would not have had the levels of immunity enabling them to deal with the urban diseases. A similar situation was seen in nineteenth century France, with army conscription; young men from rural areas were bigger, stronger and fitter than young men from cities, but they were also far more likely to die during the epidemics generally associated with campaigns.

The situation has changed in the last hundred years or so. The migration of the rural population into cities still occurs as can be seen from the many shanty towns in the developing world, although the effect now is to greatly increase the urban population, as disease is not a major corrective factor (at present).

The transmission of diseases from one centre of population to another had probably been going on for centuries in humans. The Plague of Athens has already been mentioned and numerous examples occur over the next thousand years or so. Another well-known example is the Antonine Plague (Plague of Galen) of 165 AD (Ch 10), generally considered to be the first appearance of smallpox in Western Europe.

The Late Roman Empire was overpopulated, the degree of overpopulation can be seen by the fact that Rome (the city) needed to import approximately 6,000 tonnes of grain per week, much of which came from North Africa through the port of Ostia. The population had expanded massively over several centuries, and eventually there was a series of epidemics causing a population crash that culminated with the advent of the Dark Ages.

These epidemics were exploited by the Christian religion that promises an afterlife. If half the population is dying from something unknown and unseen, then any religion promising life after death has a considerable advantage over those that do not. Similarly, Islam, which also promises paradise for the faithful, arose in the aftermath of the great epidemic known as The Plague of Justinian (Ch 9), which swept the Near East and Western Europe in the sixth century AD.

Moral reasons, not biological ones, were used to explain these epidemics. The early Christians believed that God was punishing Roman decadence and this is still widely believed today, especially by the Catholic Church and many fundamentalist denominations. The moral reasons today may not include gladiatorial contests, but they certainly include premarital sex, birth control, homosexuality, drugs and divorce. All are seen as agents of the moral decay and degeneration of society, and the Catholic Church has used these examples at regular intervals, over hundreds of years, to argue against the introduction of various social changes, the most important one in recent years being birth control. However, the great epidemics of Rome in the three or four centuries after Christ were a biological response to overpopulation, and provide a useful model for what happened in the Americas in the sixteenth and seventeenth centuries.

POPULATION CONTROL

Three major factors control the populations of all species, famine, disease and predation, and these factors apply to human populations in the same way that they apply to animal populations. In the case of humans, birth control can also be added to the list of population control methods. Natural disasters can be added to the list, for example, a population at risk because it is forced to live in an area prone to serious flooding, on the sides of a volcano, or in an earthquake-prone area by population pressures on more desirable land. Unfortunately for humans, areas prone to flooding and the sides of volcanoes also tend to be highly fertile, and the temptation to exploit rich farmland frequently overcomes natural caution and common sense.

As humans are the dominant species (at the present time), we do not generally suffer from predation by other large animals, however, in the human species, war may be regarded as the ultimate form of predation (and as a species we are extremely good at it). The three natural major controls on the human population, disease, famine and war are frequently closely inter-related, as events in Africa and other parts of the world demonstrate at regular intervals.

The first person to suggest the relationship between overpopulation and disease was the economist, sociologist and clergyman, Thomas Malthus (1766-1834), in his *"Essay on the Principle of Population"* published in 1798. He argued that unlimited population growth outstrips the supply of food and other vital resources, *"the power of population is infinitely greater than the power of the earth to produce subsistence for man"*. When this happens in an animal species, the birth rate falls, the death rate rises and the number of predators increases. In humans, death occurs from overcrowding, poverty, famine, war and disease. As Malthus put it, *"Sickly seasons, epidemics, pestilence and plague advance in terrific array and sweep off their thousands and tens of thousands"*. Malthus later added moral restraint to his other factors for controlling the size of human populations. We would interpret this as birth control today, although Malthus was suggesting marriage at a later date and a limited number of children, especially amongst the poorer classes. The implication is that if moral restraint does not prevail, then one or more of the other three will take over. His work had a considerable influence on Charles Darwin's theories about competition being the driving force of natural selection and evolution.

Darwin refers to this in *"The Descent of Man"* suggesting that medical advances such as vaccination meant that, *"weak members of civilised societies propagate their kind"* and commenting that no farmer or breeder of domesticated animals would allow such poor specimens to breed. Herbert Spencer coined the phrase, *"Survival of the fittest"* in his book *"Principles of Biology"* in 1864 and Darwin used this phrase, equating it to natural selection, in later editions of his work.

There are regular increases in various animal species leading to epidemics, and/or increases in the predator population, which ultimately cause a crash in numbers. Well known examples are the periodic increases in various rodent populations such as lemmings, causing increases in diseases such as tuberculosis amongst the lemming population and large increases in numbers of predators such as foxes, wolves, owls and hawks. Studies of these types of inter-relationships show that different species are inter-dependent upon each other, right to the top of the food chain. The relationship between species is extremely complex, and events changing the numbers and behaviour of one species frequently impinge on other species in a totally unexpected and unforeseen manner. It is not only the influence of one animal species on another that is of importance, but also the effect of plant species on the availability of food and habitat.

Research using rats shows that Malthus was correct in some of his ideas, and rat populations under stress mimic many of the problems of human populations under stress. Rat populations allowed to increase in numbers without a concomitant increase in area and food (resources) start fighting, ignore their young and show many of the medical problems associated with human populations under similar conditions of stress.

Malthus was right in asserting that the Four Horsemen of the Apocalypse were not supernatural apparitions as had been generally supposed until then, but an ecological response to a population imbalance[95]. Many people were critical of his work during the twentieth century, and his views were not popular with many liberal and social reformers, who regarded his work as politically incorrect, mainly because he suggested that the restraints should apply to the poorer classes. A major criticism was that he assumed that the population would increase geometrically, i.e. 1,2,4,8,16,-,- whilst the food supply would only increase arithmetically, i.e. 1,2,3,4,5,-,- leading to widespread starvation.

The human species generally lacks natural large predators (except ourselves), and as a result it has expanded in a similar manner to the rabbit population of Australia. The main reason the human species as a whole has managed to avoid the Malthusian solution so far, is that as a species, we are extremely inventive. Until now we have managed to find and exploit (and overexploit) new resources faster than we have depleted the old ones. The obvious example was the so-called Green Revolution, in the 1960s and 70s, which negated Malthus's calculations on the supply of food. Whilst this exploitation of new resources works in the short term, it will not work in the long term (i.e. centuries or millennia), and it is reasonable to predict that the longer it is before the correction factor is applied, the more draconian the correction factor will be when it does occur. Unfortunately, the human race is extremely arrogant, and large

---

95   The Four Horsemen of the Apocalypse as described in the Bible, in the Revelation of St John, are the red rider and red horse, the black rider and black horse, the pale rider and pale horse, whilst the Fourth Horseman is the white rider on a white horse. The interpretation of these riders varies from one academic or cleric to another. The pale horse and pale rider depend upon which version of the Bible is being read. The original version of the Book of Revelation was written in Greek in the first century AD, and uses the word *"chloros"* meaning green. However when this was translated into Latin in the early fifth century, by St. Jerome, to give the Vulgate version of the Bible, *"chloros"* was mistranslated as *"pallidus"* meaning pale.

numbers of otherwise intelligent people (including many who should know better), assume that *H. sapiens* is a special case, and that the Laws of Nature do not apply to us.

Over the last decade or so, some authors are starting to consider that the theories of Malthus may have a considerable element of validity in them, and it is worth pointing out that just because the proofs of a theory are not as comprehensive as they might be, it does not necessarily mean that the theory is wrong. In spite of the controversy that the work of Malthus raised and is still raising, there was one positive benefit. It led the government of the day to realise that it had no knowledge of the total population of the country and its make-up; the result was the first national census of 1801.

Some authors (including Malthus) have suggested that the defeat of various diseases, especially smallpox, removed one of the factors controlling the size of the human population and this has allowed numbers to increase greatly over the last two centuries (Ch 10). The extension of this idea is that, over time, other diseases will take the place of smallpox and become corrective factors in their own right. We are already starting to see this with HIV and AIDS greatly reducing the average life span in many African countries. If this suggestion is correct, then HIV/AIDS may be the shape of things to come, and it is interesting to note that HIV attacks humans in a different manner to any known disease that has previously attacked our species. As such, it represents an evolutionary challenge that *H. sapiens* has not faced before.

If we reinterpret Malthus and replace the word "famine" with "shortage of resources" and extend this to include food, clean fresh water, land, oil, energy and minerals, and replace "predation" with "war", then the predictions of Malthus become significantly more ominous.

As a final note, it is reasonable to assume that if the human population as a whole does not start to practise population limitation by birth control, then famines, epidemics and wars will become more numerous and serious as resources are depleted. An example of such a situation occurring in a closed society is Easter Island that is discussed very briefly in Chapter 20, as also are the other pressures on our society.

CHAPTER 6

The Evolution of Disease

WHERE DID DISEASES ORIGINATE?

Some authors divide diseases into two types, ancestral diseases and crowd diseases. Ancestral diseases are those that have afflicted humans for many millennia, and include diseases such as the various parasite worm infections and malaria. A common feature of many of these ancestral diseases is that they do not produce a strong immune response from the host.

Many diseases are of a type known as crowd diseases and these require a population of a critical size before an epidemic can occur. There must be a minimum number of susceptible people to allow the disease to spread. The minimum number required to sustain a disease varies from disease to disease, but is usually in the range of one hundred thousand. Some, such as chickenpox, can survive with smaller populations whilst a few diseases (e.g. measles) require a much larger population. Statistically, measles requires approximately 7,000 susceptible people at any one time to produce an epidemic. The minimum population required to allow the virus to circulate is approximately 3-500,000 people; if the population is below this figure, the virus dies out locally and must be re-introduced. This can be shown by the behaviour of the measles virus in island communities, above and below the critical population mass.

A classic demonstration was provided by a study of measles in the Faroe Islands in 1864, at a time when the population was just below 8,000. The Danish physician, Peter Panum, was able to track the epidemiology of the disease following its re-introduction to the islands. He showed that it was contagious by droplet infection before the symptoms appeared, and also demonstrated that Faroe islanders, who had lived through the previous epidemic of 1781, were still immune, the first documented evidence that immunity to measles was lifelong.

The majority of bacteria and viruses with the potential to cause epidemics leave the survivors with varying degrees of immunity. Once the disease starts, most susceptible members of the population are infected rapidly, and either recover with a high degree of immunity, or die. Therefore a village or small community rapidly runs out of new hosts, and the disease disappears for a smaller or larger number of years until a new, sufficiently large, susceptible generation develops; even then, the disease must be re-introduced to the community. An epidemic disease can be compared to a fire, too little fuel or fuel too thinly scattered, and the fire goes out. The population therefore needs to be dense enough to keep transmitting the disease, and big enough to keep producing a new batch of susceptible individuals. As a generality, these will be the children born since the last epidemic, or immigrants into the community from an area that has not experienced the disease. A stable new disease pattern arises when both pathogen and host survive the first few encounters, and eventually reach a mutually tolerated co-existence.

Many of these crowd diseases in humans are related to diseases in animals. We share a large number of parasites and diseases with dogs, cattle, horses and poultry. Some of these diseases are identical across host species, for example, influenza causes very similar problems in all host species. However, a number of disease-causing organisms, that jumped the species barrier from animals to humans, became specific to humans over a period of generations[96].

---

96   The suggestion has been recently made that the term *"species barrier"* should be replaced by *"species hurdle"*. The implication of the word barrier is that it brings something to a halt, the implication of hurdle is that it can be crossed if sufficient energy is expended.

The relationship between many human and animal diseases are still obvious, for example, the measles virus in humans is similar to rinderpest in cattle and distemper in dogs. Similarly, horses, pigs, poultry and many marine mammals are excellent hosts for influenza, bubonic plague is found in rodents, colds occur in horses, smallpox is related to a wide variety of pox diseases found in animals and most recently, HIV is closely related to viruses found in other primates. It is probable that most crowd diseases of humans were caused by disease agents that made a species jump from an animal to humans at some time in the past. The huge numbers of animals, such as cattle and horses in wild herds, would have allowed the disease to effectively become a childhood disease of the herd. However, once the disease made the species jump into humans, it would have been attacking a immunologically naïve population and would have become deadly.

A documented example of the devastating effects of a new disease on an immunologically naïve society can be seen in the major epidemic of measles that reached Fiji in 1875. It is estimated to have killed over 40,000, out of a population of approximately 150,000, and many cases were reported of people dying from starvation, because everyone in the village was ill at once and too sick to obtain food. This contrasts with the measles epidemic in the Faroe Islands mentioned earlier; although over 75% of the islanders caught measles, the mortality rate was only about 1.5 %. The difference, between the Faroes and Fiji, was the fact that the Faroe islanders had experienced measles previously. The inhabitants and their descendants must have had some residual immunity to the disease and therefore were not affected as severely.

The first cases of disease causing organisms making a species jump probably happened when hunters killed game. Sick animals would have been easier to catch than healthy ones and therefore the risk of acquiring the disease would have been greater. These diseases would probably have subsided rapidly, as the hunters would have lived in small communities. The disease would have either destroyed or seriously damaged small communities of susceptible humans but would then have died out before it could spread to other communities. A hunter-gatherer type of existence means that communities are at a considerable distance from each other, so each outbreak of an infectious disease would be isolated. However because of the close proximity of animals, there was always a focus for re-infection.

THE DISEASE PROCESS

The first stage in the disease process is the entry of the pathogen into the body. Nearly all pathogens must enter the body before they can replicate and spread although there are a few exceptions. Some pathogens of the gut, such as the cholera causing bacterium, do not actually invade the body although most people would consider this to be a technicality.

The body has a number of barriers to prevent the entry of pathogens, some of which are physical and some chemical. The skin and mucosal surfaces provide physical barriers as long as they are intact, whilst cilia in the respiratory tract expel foreign bodies by wafting them up to the throat and mouth, where they can be removed by swallowing, spitting or coughing. Mucus is secreted by the cells of the respiratory system, the gastro-intestinal tract and the urino-genital system; it is sticky and is able to trap and immobilise invading micro-organisms.

Chemical defence systems include hydrochloric acid in the stomach which kills most but not all bacteria, and would have been a very effective defence against food poisoning organisms when our ancestors were scavenging carrion. Other defence mechanisms include the bacteria in the vagina that produce acids protecting this organ against pathogenic bacteria, whilst the enzyme lysozyme occurring in tears and sweat destroys many bacteria found in the eyes and on the skin.

Fever and inflammation are a common response when the body is infected. The normal temperature of the human body is 37°C, which is close to the maximum temperature at which many pathogens will grow. Elevating the temperature a few degrees slows down the growth of the pathogen thus allowing human hosts extra time to marshal their immune defences.

Very few pathogens are able to penetrate unbroken skin. A few metazoan parasites are able to achieve this feat, examples include the American hookworm (Ch 4) and the cercaria of schistosomes (Ch 19). Most pathogens that invade through the skin require it to have been damaged by a bite, cut or burn. In the case of humans, some of these types of injuries may be self-inflicted, such as the puncture wounds from injecting drugs. Mucosal surfaces are much easier for pathogens to penetrate, and numerous parasites are able to cross the surfaces of the respiratory, gastro-intestinal and urino-genital systems. The pathogen normally gains entrance to the body at a single point such as an insect bite or a particular mucosal surface, and the initial infection is usually local. The primary defence is the localised inflammation process (Ch 7) that works by concentrating host proteins with anti-bacterial properties in the area where the invading micro-organism has penetrated the skin.

Pathogens can live either inside host cells (intracellular) or outside them (extracellular). Viruses by their very nature are intracellular, whilst metazoan parasites are extracellular by virtue of their size compared to the host cell. Bacteria and protozoa may be either extra- or intracellular depending on their identity. An intracellular mode of existence may cause problems for the host, as it might enable the pathogen to evade the surveillance of the immune system.

Although the initial infection is local, many pathogens then spread throughout the body and there are a number of ways of achieving this. The first is by cell-to-cell contact and these organisms tend to remain localised, even although the symptoms, such as fever, are widespread throughout the body. The most common method for pathogens to spread is via the blood and lymph systems as all the tissues of the body require a blood supply and are drained by the lymphatic system. Some spread via the nervous system; this is common in the viruses, and allows *Herpes simplex* (the virus causing the cold sore), to become established throughout the body. Sometimes other organs are infected, for example, the rabies virus travels from the point of entry (bite wound) via the nervous system to organs such as the brain and the salivary glands.

How do Micro-organisms Cause Disease?

There are several methods of causing disease, one of the most common being the secretion of exotoxins. Many bacteria produce exotoxins that have a very specific effect on the host. Exotoxins are poisons secreted by the bacteria that are able to diffuse through the surrounding tissue or medium. They include the powerful neurotoxins released by the bacterial genus, *Clostridium,* which cause diseases such as tetanus (lockjaw) and botulin poisoning. Botulin is one of the most deadly poisons known, less than 1μgram (approximately one thirty-millionth of an ounce) is sufficient to kill an adult when given by injection. Other bacteria producing powerful exotoxins include *Shigella* (dysentery), *Vibrio cholerae* (cholera), *Streptococcus pyogenes* (scarlet fever) and *Corynebacterium* (diphtheria).

Some bacteria from the genera, *Staphylococcus* and *Streptococcus,* may produce toxins known as super-antigens that cause excessive stimulation of the immune system leading to a toxic shock syndrome and certain types of food poisoning.

Many bacteria, especially some of the Gram negative rods, produce endotoxins. These are components of the bacterial cell wall and are not released from the bacterial surface; they act on the host to produce a variety of symptoms including fever and a fall in blood pressure.

Intracellular pathogens may or may not function by killing the host cell. Some multiply inside the host cell and leave it by a process known as budding (a process analogous to blowing up novelty balloons with more than one compartment), whilst others multiply and cause the host cell to burst (lyse) releasing the micro-organisms.

A few pathogens such as *Entamoeba histolytica* are predatory, and eat (graze) on the host cells, and a very small number, such as some of the filarial worms, cause a physical blockage of the lymph system.

How do Diseases Spread?

Diseases can be spread by a variety of methods with some diseases having more than one mode of transmission. Four different types of transmission can be distinguished.

- Person to person contact with no intermediate host. Diseases of this nature include the sexually transmitted diseases or infections (STDs or STIs). These are spread between adults by genital, anal or oral sex (horizontal transmission) but may also be transmitted from mother to baby *in utero* or at birth (vertical transmission)[97].

- Diseases transmitted by some common factor (fomite). By far the most efficient fomite is contaminated water, followed by contaminated food (a poor second). Diseases spread by these two fall into what is known as the oral/faecal group. This includes cholera and food poisoning, both caused by faecal contamination of water, or some food item that is then consumed. Fomites may also include some non-food object contaminated by the victim, and then handled by a second person who contracts the disease. The general group also includes HIV (usually regarded as an STI), when it is spread by drug addicts sharing hypodermic syringes. A number of diseases of this type have been spread by the multiple,

---

97   Vertical transmission implies transmission from one host generation to the next, horizontal transmission is transmission between members of the same generation.

medical use of non-sterile syringes in developing countries. Some cases of AIDS and malaria are known to have been spread in this manner, and it has been a major factor in at least one epidemic caused by the Ebola virus.

- Airborne or droplet infection. These are diseases in which the infected person coughs or sneezes out infectious particles that can frequently travel several metres, before being inhaled and infecting a susceptible person. A well-known poster in the UK during the twentieth century publicised the fact that, *"Coughs and sneezes spread diseases"*, and urged people suffering from flu to stay at home. The size of the particles is of considerable importance, and once particles enter the respiratory system, larger ones will settle first and smaller ones travel further into the lungs. Diseases in this group include colds, influenza, smallpox, tuberculosis and pneumonic plague.

- Vector borne diseases involving some intermediate host. The vector is frequently an arthropod or insect, such as fleas, ticks, lice, flies or mosquitoes. Typical of these diseases are malaria, yellow fever, sleeping sickness, bubonic plague and typhus. Other vectors are occasionally found, for example, snails are involved in the transmission of schistosomiasis (bilharzia), and pigs in the transmission of trichinosis. Vectors involved in the transmission of various worm infestations include fish and household pets such as dogs and cats. Some vector borne diseases may involve more than one vector, this is considered later in this chapter.

Epidemics spread by different means also produce different responses within the community in terms of the number of people infected and the speed with which the epidemic spreads. Epidemics spread by droplet infection, such as influenza, rise and decline relatively slowly, whilst diseases such as cholera spread by a fomite such as a contaminated water supply, rise very rapidly, but also fall rapidly once the source of the infection is removed.

Host/pathogen relationships may also behave rather differently depending on the method of transmission. An example is the *Variola* virus, which causes smallpox if contracted by droplet infection, but if applied to abrasions of the skin usually produces variolation (Ch 10) and immunity to the disease. A further example is the bacterial genus *Shigella* that typically causes dysentery when occurring in food or water, but may become a sexually transmitted disease involving homosexual men.

PARASITISM

Many parasites require more than one host to complete their life cycle. When this occurs, the host in which the sexual phase of the parasite's life cycle is completed is known as the definitive host; all other hosts are known as intermediate hosts.

Several different forms of parasitism can be defined, based on the method of transmission of the parasite between hosts. These include passive transmission, active transmission and vector transmission.

Passive transmission is commonly found in parasites of the gut such as tapeworms (Cestodes). The eggs of the parasite pass out in the host's faeces onto the soil, and are eaten by the intermediate host, the eggs hatch and undergo further development in the intermediate host. The parasite will undergo no further development unless the intermediate host is eaten by a suitable definitive host, higher up the food chain. There are several variations on this theme; there may be no intermediate host or there may be more than one intermediate host. The no host situation is found in amoebic dysentery, caused by the protozoan *Entamoeba histolytica,* in which a highly resistant cyst passes out of the infected host and contaminates a food plant, which is then eaten by a new human host. Once inside the gut of the new host, the cyst is dissolved, releasing the protozoan. Passive transmission is shown in Figure 6.1.

Figure 6.1. Passive Transmission

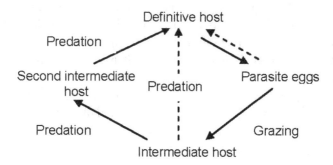

Active transmission occurs in parasites that have a motile phase in their life cycle, enabling them to swim and seek out a new host. There may be more than one intermediate host. Active transmission is found in the blood flukes of which Schistosomes (Ch 19) are an important example and is shown in Figure 6.2.

Figure 6.2. Active Transmission

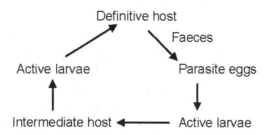

Vector transmission is found in numerous human diseases, including those caused by viruses (yellow fever), bacteria (bubonic plague), protozoa (malaria and sleeping sickness) and metazoan (filarial worms). In all of these cases, the disease is transmitted by a blood sucking insect, or arthropod acting as a living syringe (Figure 6.3).

Figure 6.3. Vector Transmission

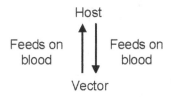

One feature of parasitology that has only been recognised recently is that in many cases, the parasite manipulates the behaviour of the host(s). A number of examples are known. Perhaps the most easily understood is that found in passive transmission where the parasite changes the colour or behaviour of the intermediate host, thus rendering it more conspicuous, and therefore more likely to be eaten by the definitive host.

Examples are also found in the vector transmission of parasites, one of the best studied probably being malaria. Studies show that mosquitoes infected with the malarial parasite produce a reduced amount of an enzyme (catalyst) known as apyrase. The effects of this are discussed in Chapter 16.

THE EVOLUTION OF EPIDEMIC DISEASES

Epidemic diseases attacking humans generally have a number of common features.

- They spread quickly and efficiently from an infected person to a healthy person, and the whole population is exposed relatively quickly.
- The disease is frequently acute, the victim either

dies within a short space of time, or if they recover, the recovery is usually complete.

- Those victims who recover generally develop antibodies against the disease, and usually have long term or life-long immunity.

Microorganisms causing human epidemic diseases are frequently confined to *Homo sapiens* and are not found in other animals. Smallpox, measles, chickenpox and mumps are typical examples. Studies in molecular biology show that many of these human diseases are related to those found in social animals, i.e. the ones humans domesticated.

Evolutionary trends in diseases can be seen if a number of diseases of different types are examined.

The first type are diseases which humans still catch from animals. These include psitticosis caught from pet birds, leptospirosis from dogs and rats, tularaemia from rodents such as rabbits and foot and mouth disease from cloven-hoofed mammals. All these diseases are at an early stage of evolution in humans, it is unusual for humans to catch them from animals and they are not transmitted directly from human to human.

The second type are diseases that have infected humans, been unable to establish themselves, and have died out. One example mentioned earlier was sweating sickness in the fifteenth and sixteenth centuries (Ch 1). A more recent example in the twentieth century is O'nyong-nyong fever, found in the late 1950s in East Africa. This was a viral disease of monkeys, involving mosquitoes as vectors, that infected several million people, generated very high levels of immunity amongst those infected, and then disappeared. A small number of cases re-appeared in the late 1990s, presumably when human herd immunity had fallen to a low level.

The third type of diseases are those which have an animal host, but have established themselves in humans in small localised areas, and may progress to an epidemic disease or die out. Examples of this type are Lassa fever, Ebola, and Marburg disease. A further recent example that is more established than these is Lyme disease. This was recognised in the early 1960s in the USA and UK, but is now reaching epidemic proportions in the North-Eastern USA. An example of a relatively recent disease that has obviously established itself in humans on a large scale is HIV, which is now causing a major pandemic. In all of these cases the pathogen may have made more than one attempt to jump species, causing a small-scale epidemic on each occasion.

The final stage is the long established epidemic disease, found only in humans, which passes directly from person to person, without the involvement of animals. These are the evolutionary survivors of numerous diseases, which over many generations have jumped from animals to humans. No doubt many of the viral or bacterial species that attempted this jump failed, but diseases such as smallpox and measles succeeded, and are now no longer capable of infecting animals.

Not all diseases are known to science, new ones appear regularly; it has been estimated that some thirty-five new diseases have appeared in the last three decades. Whilst some of these are localised, esoteric diseases occurring in only a few victims and known only to specialist doctors, others, such as Ebola and AIDS, have become notorious world wide in the last two or three decades. We have no reason to be complacent about these localised, esoteric diseases; some of them may well have the potential to become the next pandemic in the same manner as HIV.

One of the latest of these new diseases is SARS or Severe Acute Respiratory Syndrome. This appeared in Guangdong province in China in late 2002, and from there spread to numerous countries, including Hong Kong and Canada. The disease is caused by a member of the Corona virus group, so-called because when seen in the electron microscope, it has a series of spikes on it that resemble a crown. The virus is related to the cold viruses, although it is sufficiently different to the other corona viruses to be placed in a new sub-group. It is one of the largest single stranded RNA viruses known, causes an atypical form of pneumonia with symptoms similar to influenza and is spread by droplet infection, but is also capable of surviving in faeces for several days. It does appear to be relatively difficult to catch it compared with many other airborne viruses.

This is another example of a virus that has made the species jump from an animal to humans. In the early stages of the epidemic, it was believed to be a virus found in chickens or pigs, but has now been shown to have originated in the masked palm civet, a relative of the mongoose bred for food in this part of China. The epidemic was not a major one compared with many other epidemics of the past, only about 9,000 cases were identified, with a death rate of about ten per cent.

It did however illustrate several important features. Firstly, initial attempts to limit the epidemic were difficult because the Chinese authorities would not accept that they were dealing with a new disease, within their borders, that was out of control. The second important feature was the speed with which it spread from China to Hong Kong, and from Hong Kong to Toronto, Canada, where it caused over thirty deaths. In both cases one infected person, travelling to the new location by air, was responsible.

The final interesting factor was the public reaction, which bordered on hysterical at times, especially in view of the fact that this was only a minor epidemic. One wonders what the reaction would have been if it had been a major outbreak of something such as smallpox, or a reoccurrence of the Black Death or Spanish Flu. Given the behaviour of bird flu over the last few years, we may find out in the not too distant future.

CHAPTER 7

The Human Response; The Immune System and the History of Immunisation

The human race has evolved over thousands of years in the presence of a continued assault by dangerous micro-organisms of various types. When our ancestors caught an infection, some of them lived and some died, those who lived had an immune system that was able to cope with the infection and the survivors would have passed this immunity onto their descendants. The process would have been repeated with every succeeding generation and eventually humans with a very sophisticated immune system would evolve. This immune system is still evolving as it is being constantly challenged by exposure to new diseases and variations on old ones.

The human immune system is a complex array of organs, cells and proteins. Its importance can be seen from the fact that babies born with a serious defect in their immune systems usually die in infancy from an infection that a normal child would survive easily. Over the last few decades the importance of the immune system has been brought home to the public at large by the advent of AIDS (Acquired Immune Deficiency Syndrome Ch 18) and increasing levels of cancer.

The function of the immune system is to defend the body against infectious diseases, and its most important problem is to recognise the difference between self and non-self (foreign), and then destroy non-self. Occasionally it malfunctions and causes problems. The most common of these malfunctions are conditions such as hayfever and food allergies that occur when the system produces an inappropriate over-reaction to some harmless material, such as pollen or certain types of food. In extreme cases, it over-reacts to the point of causing anaphylactic shock that may kill some individuals. Other problems occur from auto-immune diseases such as lupus, rheumatoid arthritis and various forms of colitis. These are caused when the immune system attacks the body's own tissues, that is, it has failed to distinguish between self and non-self.

By the second decade of the twentieth century it was obvious that the immune system was extremely complex, at first examination perhaps over-complex, but harmful parasites and pathogens come in many disguises and life styles, and it has to be capable of dealing with these. In most cases it is extremely successful.

It can be broadly divided into two components, the innate or natural immune system, and the specific immune system. The innate system exists in the body before it is challenged by an infection, and because it is pre-existing, it produces an immediate response to infection and tissue invasion. The second component is the specific immune response, which as the name suggests, is produced as a specific response to a specific challenge. As such it is a reactive force rather than a proactive one and it takes some time to respond. Both of these components are essential and so is communication between them. Zinsser showed in the 1920s that any infection mobilises the whole defensive system, and the various components reinforce each other, not compete with each other.

The description that follows is simplified considerably, but an account of the minutiae of the system is unnecessary for the purposes of this book.

THE INNATE IMMUNE SYSTEM

There are several defensive features in the innate immune system. One group of cells found in blood are the white blood cells that are an integral part of the body's defensive system. Several different types of white cells are found, the first of these are the macrophages that are made in the bone marrow. These carry out phagocytosis (from a Greek word meaning *"to eat)*, that is, they can engulf and destroy invading micro-organisms and also dead host cells. They do this by differentiating between live host cells, dead host cells and invading micro-organisms by means of different chemical receptors on the surfaces of various types of cells.

The concept of cells defending the body against an invader was first proposed by Elias Metchnikov (1845-1916) in Russia in 1884. He observed cells ingesting and engulfing foreign particles and referred to the process as phagocytosis. In 1888, Metchnikoff went to Paris to work at the Pasteur Institute, where he studied macrophages and developed the theory of phagocytosis. He received the Nobel Prize for medicine (as did Ehrlich, Ch 3) in 1908, for studies on immunity.

When a pathogenic micro-organism invades a tissue following a wound, the tissue macrophages may not be sufficient to deal with the invader, and they therefore respond by sending chemical messages to summon more macrophages to help them. This is known as the inflammatory response and during this process a battery of different chemicals is released which includes several groups of proteins known as cytokines. Some cytokines act locally; they are formed by cells in tissues, and act on cells in that tissue, thus enabling those cells to communicate with each other. These cytokines stimulate features such as vasodilation (expansion of the blood vessels). This causes increased blood flow to an area, thus increasing the supply of macrophages. They also alter the permeability of blood vessels making it easier for macrophages to pass through the walls of blood vessels and enter the tissue.

One group of cytokines released are the interferons, which amongst their several functions include the inhibition of protein synthesis by viruses. Other cytokines influence the brain causing fever, tiredness and loss of appetite that are all common responses to infection. Fever causes a rise in body temperature which inhibits the growth of certain pathogens, tiredness causes the host to sleep thus conserving energy to combat the infection, and loss of appetite reduces the urge to go looking for food which also reduces energy consumption.

Opsonins are another group of protein molecules found in the innate immune system. These function by binding a phagocytic cell to a foreign cell, and preparing the process of phagocytosis. Wright (see later) showed that, *"body fluids modify bacteria in a manner which renders them ready prey to phagocytes"*, and called this the *"opsonic effect"* from the Latin word "opsonare" (to buy provisions). The opsonins of the innate system only recognise a limited number of pathogens. Antibodies (see later) that are part of the specific immune system can also act as opsonins, and because of their high specificity, they recognise pathogens that have avoided the innate immune system.

Another defensive feature is the blood clotting process. This limits the entry of pathogens into the blood stream and therefore the spread of pathogens throughout the body. Some of the proteins released during the clotting process also attract phagocytic cells to the site, thus reinforcing the number of phagocytes at the point of a wound.

The final feature is the population of natural killer (NK) cells that make up about 1-5% of the white blood cell population. These cells are able to recognise and destroy infected host cells without being damaged themselves.

The encounter between the innate immune system and the pathogen has one of two outcomes, either the pathogen is destroyed or it survives. There are two reasons why the innate immune system may not be able to deal with the infection, either the pathogen was present in overwhelming numbers, or it was able to evade the initial recognition process. Pathogens that have not been destroyed by this initial encounter are then subjected to attack by the specific immune system.

THE SPECIFIC IMMUNE SYSTEM

This consists of a group of cells and proteins able to recognise the different chemical signatures of various pathogens. Pathogens produce large molecules known as antigens, and it is these antigens that are recognised by the specific immune system. This responds by producing antibodies that bind to, and neutralise the antigen. The antigen is usually, but not always, a protein and may be held on the surface of the pathogen when it is known as an endotoxin, or it may be secreted by the pathogen into the blood stream when it is referred to as an exotoxin.

When a person is subjected to a prolonged or severe attack by a pathogen, the white cell (lymphocyte) count in their blood rises significantly. There are a variety of different lymphocytes, one of the most important groups being the β-lymphocytes that produce the proteins known as antibodies. As mentioned above, antibodies recognise the antigens produced by the pathogen and react specifically with them neutralising them. It is this antibody response by the host that is the scientific principle for the production of vaccines against many diseases.

Antibody structure is complicated, one end of the molecule is known as the variable domain and differs from antibody to antibody. The other end, known as the constant domain, remains relatively stable from antibody to antibody. The variable domain contains a number of hyper-variable regions and the molecule is folded so that these are in close contact with each other, forming a single surface. Antibodies do not bind to the whole antigen, the single surface on the variable end of the antibody recognises a small portion of the antigen molecule known as the antigenic epitope, and binds to that.

Five different classes of antibody can be recognised, all having different functions. These functions are dictated by the chemistry of the non-variable domain that differs from class to class.

ANTIBODY PRODUCTION

Antibodies are highly specific and are produced in response to a highly specific stimulus, the antigen. As a result, an antibody is only made **after** exposure to an antigen. Therefore antibodies to measles are made in response to an infection of measles and not in response to influenza, chickenpox or any other disease.

As mentioned earlier, the antibodies are produced by β-lymphocytes. These cells have certain types of antibodies present on their cell surfaces, with different individual β-lymphocytes having antibodies specific to different antigens. When a human is first exposed to a pathogen, most β-lymphocytes will have a surface antibody that does not recognise the antigens belonging to that pathogen. However, a small number of β-lymphocytes (perhaps one in a hundred thousand) will have a surface antibody that does recognise the antigen. This β-lymphocyte binds to the antigen, and is stimulated to undergo a period of rapid replication to produce a large population of β-lymphocytes with the same antibody specificity as the parent. The process is known as clonal expansion.

The time required for clonal expansion explains why a person becomes ill after first exposure to a pathogen, and why there is a time lag, frequently as long as ten days or more, before the specific antibody to that pathogen is produced. After exposure to the antigens of a pathogenic organism, the β-lymphocytes producing antibodies specific to that pathogen enter one of two pathways. Most become plasma cells and produce large quantities of antibody and these cells have life spans varying from a few weeks to months. A small number of β-lymphocytes however, become what are known as memory β-cells. These cells survive in the body for a very long time after the pathogen has been eliminated, and if the person encounters the same pathogen (antigen) a second time, then the memory β-cells initiate a response that is both massive and rapid. The pathogen is swamped before it can obtain a toehold. This is the reason why it is unusual for a person to become ill from an attack by the same pathogen twice, and if they do, then the second experience is generally considerably milder than the first one. The first exposure to the pathogen may either be an attack by the disease-causing micro-organism or by vaccination against that disease.

The β-lymphocytes are not the only cells involved in antibody production, a further type is known as the helper T-lymphocyte, (T stands for thymus, one of the organs of the body). These regulate antibody production by the β-lymphocytes, and are produced in the bone marrow, but migrate to the thymus to complete their maturation. Mice from which the thymus has been removed are seriously immuno-deficient. These T-lymphocytes have a receptor on their surface, either one known as CD4 or alternatively CD8. The possession of these receptors is of considerable importance when HIV and AIDS (Ch 18) are considered.

When proteins from pathogens, such as viruses, break down in living cells they migrate to the exterior of the cell, and if the fragments of protein appearing on the exterior are recognised as foreign by the killer T-cells, the infected host cell is destroyed. The dead cell then shrinks and is engulfed by phagocytes without the virus being released. Obviously, if the virus is not released, then it cannot infect new host cells, and the infection is limited.

There is still a great deal to learn about the immune system. Whilst it has been obvious for many years that it can be influenced by factors such as age and nutritional status, a growing body of evidence shows that immune responses are also influenced significantly by behavioural factors such as stress.

GENETICS OF IMMUNITY

Antibodies are produced by a large group of genes grouped together on a single pair of chromosomes to form what is known as the Major Histocompatibility Complex (MHC). The number of genes present in this complex varies in mammals from species to species, but in humans it is over one hundred. Most of the genes in the complex show a very high degree of polymorphism, with numerous alleles (Ch 5) for each gene, in some cases over one hundred. The result is that the spectrum of different antibodies that can be produced by a large human population is extremely varied. The large number of alleles shows that these polymorphisms are extremely old and have been evolving within the population for millions of years.

As humans are diploid, each individual possesses two copies of the MHC, one inherited from their father and one from their mother and therefore two alleles coding for antibodies for each gene. If both alleles are the same (homozygous), then the person involved will have a high level of resistance to the disease specific to that antibody. If they have alleles coding for different versions of the antibody (heterozygous) then they will have a reduced level of resistance to two diseases. The question of whether it is better to have a high level of resistance to one disease, or a somewhat lower level of resistance to two diseases, depends to a large extent on the nature and severity of the diseases involved, and of course whether the individual is actually attacked by the disease(s) in question[98].

When a pathogen attacks a disease-experienced community, it is a reasonable probability that a number of individuals will have encountered the pathogen before, and will have some degree of immunity. Because of the wide range of variations between each persons MHC, each individual will present a different, if not unique, problem to invading micro-organisms.

---

98   Recent research has suggested that animals may choose their mates on the basis of smell, and the characteristic smell of each animal is linked to the production of pheromones controlled by the immune system. The animal can thus recognise the immune system of potential mates, and can choose a mate to optimise the immune response of any offspring. Whilst humans obviously do not have such an acute sense of smell as rats or dogs, research indicates that the smell of a member of the opposite sex is a definite factor in our "switch-on" or "switch-off" reaction.

Members of the same family do not present as many differences as members of different families, hence the fact that diseases such as measles are able to infect a family of siblings rather more easily than a similar group of non-siblings.

The MHC complex is also involved in tutoring the immune system to distinguish between self and non-self. This tutoring occurs in young babies still protected by antibodies from their mother's milk. Some genes from the MHC complex present proteins from the child's own cells (self) to the T cells and any T cell responding to these host cell proteins is immediately destroyed. This modifies the T cell system, destroying all those that recognise self, and enhancing those that recognise non-self. By the time the child becomes an adult, the only T cells left are those that recognise non-self and therefore attack invading micro-organisms.

It is not surprising that such a complex system can occasionally go wrong. If any T cells recognising self are left, then it can cause a variety of auto-immune diseases such as those mentioned earlier.

The sophistication of the immune system places severe pressure on an infecting micro-organism, and many pathogens have evolved different methods of dealing with this problem. These include hiding inside the host cells; viruses by their very nature infect host cells, but so do larger parasites such as the *Plasmodium* causing malaria (Ch 16). Once inside the cell, the pathogen is difficult to find and destroy. Some pathogens change their surface proteins by mutation at regular intervals to avoid recognition and many of the protozoa use this method of evading host defences.

Mutation by the invading micro-organism puts the immune system under pressure, whilst mutation by the immune system puts the micro-organism under pressure. The result of these interactions is a biological arms race between predator and prey or parasite and host. The stakes are high, the winner takes all.

HIV differs from the other pathogens in that it destroys the host immune system, the only organism known to do so, although a number of other pathogens depress the level at which the host immune system is expressed.

ANTIGENS

The antigenic profile of a bacterium is frequently used by epidemiologists to track down the origin of a disease such as an outbreak of food poisoning. Recent outbreaks of *Escherichia coli* O157 food poisoning are classic examples of this. Bacteria possess a wide variety of different proteins known as the O antigens attached to the outside of their cells. A further group of proteins found on the flagella of motile bacteria are known as the H antigens.

E. coli O157 causes infections that may lead to the death of the victim or severe kidney damage and these infections are usually caused when raw meat contaminates cooked meat, although the outbreak in the UK in September 2009 involved pet animals at a children's farm. Inaccurate or incomplete press reports are a source of great confusion in these outbreaks as they frequently report that *E. coli* was found. *E. coli* is found everywhere, approximately fifty per cent of the dry weight of faeces is *E. coli*. Even although *E. coli* may be found in a suspected source of food poisoning, if it does not have the same antigenic profile as the strain isolated from the sick person, then it was not the source of the infection. Antigenic profiling is therefore of great importance in tracing the source of food-poisoning bacteria during an epidemic.

THE HISTORY OF IMMUNISATION

Technically one immunises against every disease except smallpox, and vaccinates against smallpox after the *Vaccinia* virus used in the process. However, the terms are now used more or less synonymously following a recommendation from Pasteur that the term vaccination should be used for all immunisation processes in honour of Jenner.

Possibly the first reference to immunisation in history is Mithridates VI (the Great), King of Pontus, who deliberately ingested small quantities of toxic compounds to immunise himself against the larger doses that would be used by an assassin. Pontus was a kingdom on the southern shores of the Black Sea, and in the first century BC it became involved in a series of wars with the late Roman Republic over spheres of influence in Asia Minor and Greece.

Mithridates was paranoid about being poisoned and some accounts claim he tested potential antidotes on prisoners who had been poisoned. Other versions suggest he was sent a recipe for a toxic cocktail by a Persian physician, Zopyrus, along with a prisoner to experiment on. Whichever version is correct, the final concoction had over fifty ingredients mixed in honey, and Mithridates took a dose daily to immunise himself against any poison a potential assassin might use.

In 63 BC, Mithridates tried to poison himself after his final defeat by the Roman general, Pompey the Great, but had immunised himself so successfully that he was unable to do so. The historian, Cassius Dio, wrote, *"the poison although deadly, did not kill him, since he had inured his constitution to it by taking precautionary doses every day"*. One of his bodyguards finally ran him through with a sword so that he would avoid the ignominy of being paraded in chains in Pompey's triumph. The progress of Mithridates is described in the poem by A.E. Housman ("Terence, This is stupid stuff", from "A Shropshire Lad").

> *There was a king reigned in the East:*
> *There, when kings will sit to feast,*
> *They get their fill before they think*
> *With poisoned meat and poisoned drink.*
> *He gathered all that sprang to birth*
> *From the many-venomed earth;*
> *First a little, thence to more,*
> *He sampled all her killing store;*

And easy, smiling, seasoned sound,
Sate the king when healths went round.
They put arsenic in his meat
And stared aghast to watch him eat;
They poured strychnine in his cup
And shook to see him drink it up:
They shook, they stared as white's their shirt:
Them it was their poison hurt.
I tell the tale that I heard told.
Mithridates, he died old.

Pompey is alleged to have found the recipe and taken it back to Rome where it was mentioned by Pliny the Elder, and described by Celsus in *"de re Medicum"* as *"Antidotum Mithridaticum"*. The recipe was later "improved" by Andromachus, physician to the Emperor Nero, who had a vested interest in poison (it was one of his favourite methods of assassination). One of his improvements was to add vipers' flesh on the assumption that it must contain something that stopped the snake poisoning itself. He claimed that the final version would not only counteract all poisons and cure the bite of poisonous creatures, but also cure a wide variety of diseases. Andromachus's theriac (treacle) was endorsed in the second century AD by no less than Galen himself, who claimed that, *"whoever took a dose in the morning was protected against poison for the day".*

The recipe spread throughout Europe, being seen as not only a protection against poison, but also a cure-all against numerous diseases. Theriac was compounded mainly in Venice, as it was considered that Venetian vipers were the most poisonous and therefore the best ones to use. The trade became so important commercially that the Venetian authorities supervised all stages of production to stop sub-standard (and cheaper) ingredients being used. Theriac was used widely as a protective in fifteenth and sixteenth century Italy during the period when the Borgias were in power, who were notorious for using poison to achieve their political ends. It was also used in France during the period of Catherine de Medici, another ruler alleged to have used poison as a weapon. The theory of using small doses of poison as a protective against large doses was obviously well understood; the author Alexandre Dumas uses the theme in his novel, *"The Count of Monte Cristo"*.

Theriac was always in short supply in England, and apothecaries started making *"English Treacle"* substituting English herbs and poisons for exotic ones from southern Europe. Mediterranean suppliers retaliated by reducing their prices and a trade war started. In 1585, English apothecaries complained, *"Strangers do daily send into England a false and naughty kind of Mithridatum and treacle in great barrels"*, and in 1612, *"Genoese treacle"* was castigated as rubbish. In 1745, *"An Essay on Mithridatum and Theriaca"* was published by a London doctor, William Heberden. He stated that the most that could be said of it was that it would make the sick sweat, *"which is commonly the virtue of a medicine which has none"*. In spite of this, Mithridatum remained in some European pharmacopoeias until the late nineteenth century.

Immunisation has been one of the most significant developments in the prevention of infectious diseases over the last two hundred years, and is the cheapest and easiest way to have a major impact on public health. Over eighty percent of children world-wide are immunised against one or more of the common childhood diseases, and in North America and Western Europe, the deaths of children from infectious diseases such as measles and diphtheria are now rare.

Less than 100 years ago, these diseases caused major epidemics in the United Kingdom with measles killing fifty to one hundred children a year. In addition, about one child per thousand developed inflammation of the brain, whilst one in four thousand developed permanent brain damage. The figures supporting immunization speak for themselves. Both measles and diphtheria are notifiable diseases in the UK, that is, the doctor must report them to the appropriate medical authority. In England and Wales in 1940 there were over four hundred thousand cases of measles peaking at nearly eight hundred thousand cases in the early 1960s. Immunisation was introduced in the late 1960s, and in 1997 less than two hundred cases/year were reported. Similar figures are found with diphtheria, over forty-six thousand cases in 1940 and four cases in 1997, whilst whooping cough (pertussis) had over fifty-three thousand cases in 1940 and less than three thousand in 1997.

The first person to use an immunisation process in England was Lady Montague, the wife of the English ambassador to the Ottoman Empire, who had suffered from smallpox in 1715, and had been badly disfigured by it. When her husband was posted to Turkey in 1716, she saw the process of variolation and had her own son treated successfully in 1718. Lady Montague introduced the process to England in 1721 when she had her daughter variolated by Charles Maitland, who had been the embassy doctor in Istanbul. Variolation and vaccination are described in detail in Chapter 10.

The second vaccine that came into common use was developed by Pasteur against rabies, a disease still causing an estimated fifty-five thousand deaths every year in India and Africa. Rabies is a viral disease caused by the bite of an infected animal such as a dog, although the natural host appears to be the bat. There are references to Spanish soldiers in South America contracting rabies in the sixteenth century after being bitten by vampire bats. Bats are now known to carry a number of viruses resembling rabies and it has also been claimed that they may carry the Ebola virus. The only case of human rabies originating in Britain in many decades was recently caused by a bite from an infected bat.

The large number of rabies cases in India appears to be a classic example of the law of unintended consequences. The drug, diclofenac, is used for veterinary purposes to treat cattle, but this is highly toxic to the vultures that feed on the carcasses of dead cattle. It causes irreversible kidney damage, vulture numbers crashed and the carcasses were eaten instead by feral dogs whose numbers rose dramatically. It has been calculated that between 1992-2006, an extra five to six million feral dogs appeared, many of them carrying rabies, and these dogs were responsible for approximately thirty-eight million people being bitten. National statistics in India show that for every one hundred thousand dog bites, one hundred and twenty-three people die of rabies, suggesting that over the fifteen year period approximately forty-seven thousand people died of rabies as a result of the reduction in vulture numbers.

Rabies is one of the oldest documented diseases about whose identity there is little or no argument, and it is also one of the most feared. The symptoms are spectacular and once they appear the disease is invariably fatal. They include fear of water (hydrophobia) and madness (the French name for rabies is la rage). It was well known to the Greeks (being described by Hippocrates) and the Romans (Plutarch), who were both aware that it could be caused by the bite of an infected dog. It was also described by the Chinese, and in early Mesopotamian scripts, dated to around 2,300 BC, the law prescribed a large fine for the owner of a rabid dog that killed someone.

The historical treatment was varied although the Roman physician, Celsus, who gave a very accurate description of it in 30 AD and thought that the poison was contained in the saliva of the infected animal, advocated cauterising wounds with a red-hot iron. This might have worked if carried out sufficiently quickly after exposure (i.e. whilst the virus was still in the wound), before it had become disseminated throughout the body.

There were several outbreaks in England in the first half of the eighteenth century and in one major outbreak in London in 1752 orders were given that all dogs should be shot on sight, a bounty being paid for each dead dog. A number of serious outbreaks in the second half of the nineteenth century led to regulations controlling the importation of dogs and other livestock from Europe. A rigid six-month quarantine was imposed for all dogs imported into the UK. This was very effective and Britain was free of rabies from 1922 onwards. The six-month quarantine has now been lifted as long as the dog is in possession of a valid rabies vaccination certificate.

Rabies was a major challenge to Koch's work as the virus could not be shown to obey Koch's postulates (Ch 12), mainly because the technology for studying viruses was not available at this time.

The incubation period in humans is variable and may be as long as a year, but once the symptoms appear it is fatal. It is however, possible to immunise a person who has been exposed to the disease during the incubation period. Pasteur was the first to treat a human patient successfully in July 1885, a nine-year old boy, Joseph Meister, who had been savaged by a rabid dog. Contemporary medical opinion considered he was certain to develop rabies. A second, fifteen-year old shepherd boy was treated successfully, later the same year, after being bitten by a rabid wolf. In later years, Meister became the concierge of the Pasteur Institute in Paris; he committed suicide in 1940 when he was unable to stop the Nazis entering the crypt of the institute where Pasteur is buried.

Pasteur began his work on rabies in 1880 using rabbits as a model system, and in 1881, he showed the spinal cord and brain tissue to be the main sources of infectious material. In 1884, he found that if rabbits that had been deliberately infected with rabies had their spinal cord removed and dried, it gradually lost its virulence over two weeks to form an attenuated virus (one that is still alive, but has reduced virulence). He prepared a series of spinal cords, dried for different lengths of time, which had varying degrees of virulence, and initially tested these using dogs. If this attenuated material was injected into a dog starting with the least virulent and progressing to the most virulent, it was possible to immunise the animal against rabies.

Pasteur progressed from these initial experiments with dogs to people. Joseph Meister who started treatment within sixty hours of being bitten, received a series of injections at daily intervals and on the fourteenth day he was injected with fully virulent material. The treatment was successful, and formed the basis of an immunisation system that became used worldwide. In common with many of the treatments developed in the nineteenth and early twentieth centuries, a similar course of action would not be possible in the present day due to the various health, safety and ethical regulations.

Over the next year Pasteur immunised a large number of people, some of them coming from as far away as Russia. Out of 350 people immunised, only one developed symptoms and died and she was treated very late, some thirty-seven days after being bitten. We now know that it is necessary to treat the person at risk before the virus reaches the brain, the time that takes being determined to some extent by the proximity of the infected wound to the head.

Pasteur was heavily criticised at the time and it was strongly suggested that people who had been bitten would have recovered anyway. However, a major study in 1916 showed that Pasteur was correct. Out of six thousand people treated, only 0.6% died of the disease, whereas when people who had been exposed to rabies were not treated, there was a 16% mortality rate.

The vaccine was modified slightly in the 1920s by treatment with phenol. A live vaccine was developed in the late 1940s and early 50s from an attenuated virus passed through fertile hens eggs. This proved more effective and fewer injections were needed. Over ten million people per year are now treated using this vaccine.

Rabies is spreading across Europe at present, and attempts to halt this spread by creating a buffer zone of immune animals involves baiting chicken heads with oral vaccine and leaving them where they will be eaten by foxes, which are the main carriers of the disease in Europe.

These experiments by Pasteur initiated the development of vaccines for immunisation against a wide range of serious diseases. He also worked on a number of commercially important diseases, developing vaccines against anthrax in farm stock and chicken cholera.

In 1897, Sir Almroth Wright (1861-1947) and a number of his colleagues successfully immunised themselves against typhoid, a serious water borne disease, using heat-killed bacteria. Wright was director of the inoculation division of St Mary's hospital in Paddington, London and whilst there, he suggested a disease therapy based upon general immunity. He attempted to get his methods of typhoid vaccination introduced into the British Army, but was refused because of inter-departmental feuding. The result of this refusal was the deaths of about thirteen thousand troops from typhoid during the Boer War in South Africa. The Army finally insisted on compulsory typhoid immunisation for soldiers in 1913, before the start of World War I. The figures speak for themselves. In the Boer War the incidence rate of typhoid was 105/1,000 soldiers, with 14.6/1,000 dying from the disease. In World War I, the corresponding figures were 2.35/1,000 and 0.14/1,000.

Wright also developed a diagnostic test for brucellosis, a serious bacterial problem occurring in unpasteurised milk, and attempted to develop a vaccine against this disease. In the best traditions of early bacteriologists, he injected himself with the vaccine his team had prepared, then dosed himself with *Brucella*, but this time it did not work and he got a severe dose of brucellosis. As a result of this, Wright was rather cruelly nicknamed *"Sir Almost Right"* by his contemporaries.

Wright was joined by Fleming (of penicillin fame), and they were able to show that Lister's technique of using strong antiseptics to clean wounds killed phagocytes and prolonged the healing process. Wright and Fleming recommended removing foreign bodies and washing wounds clean with sterile saline, which accelerated the mobilisation of phagocytes and antibodies to the area of the wound. Again the British Army did not accept these methods until World War II, resulting in a large number of unnecessary deaths from gangrene.

A major development in the control of one of the most serious diseases was the preparation of a vaccine against tuberculosis by Calmette, one of Pasteur's protégés, and his co-worker Guérin. This vaccine, known as BCG (Bacille Calmette-Guérin), was an attenuated bacterium unable to revert to the infectious form, and was first used in 1921. It is still used today but its efficacy is very variable, the possible reasons are discussed in Chapter 11.

There are several modern day techniques for producing vaccines. Production of vaccines against diphtheria and tetanus use an extract of the inactivated protein exotoxin causing the disease symptoms. Whooping cough makes use of a killed suspension of bacteria, whilst measles, mumps, rubella, and the oral polio vaccine all use an attenuated virus grown in tissue culture. Smallpox is rather unusual in that the vaccination process uses a living related virus that does not cause a serious disease in humans but which offers cross immunity. The variolation technique, which used live smallpox virus, was successful because the virus was introduced into the human by an unusual route, i.e. through the skin instead of the inhalation of infectious particles into the lungs.

A recent development is the use of polysaccharide antigens (compounds based on sugars); these do not normally stimulate immunity, but will do so if attached to a suitable protein. One of the bacterial meningitis vaccines is of this type.

Two vaccines were introduced against the disease polio in 1935. Brodie used a virus inactivated by formaldehyde, and Kolmer used a vaccine of live attenuated virus. Neither of the vaccines was tested adequately, and both were a disaster causing numerous vaccine related cases of poliomyelitis and a number of deaths. They were both withdrawn after heavy criticism. In the early 1950s, there was a polio epidemic in the USA causing over fifty thousand cases per year. The disease mainly affected children under the age of five, entering the body and multiplying in the intestines, with one case in every two hundred progressing to paralysis.

Jonas Salk (1914-95) headed a team developing a vaccine using a virus killed with formaldehyde, but much more carefully prepared and tested than the 1935 version. The Salk vaccine was given to children in an initial test in 1953, and in 1954 over 400,000 were treated. The main problem with this vaccine was that it had to be given by multiple injection and boosters. There were serious problems when a faulty batch of vaccine caused over two hundred cases, in which eleven people died and seventy-five per cent were paralysed.

At the same time, Albert Sabin (1906-1993) was leading a second group preparing an alternative vaccine. The Sabin vaccine used live attenuated virus, could be given orally in one dose and was more effective. In addition to the above advantages, it was also cheap, and because live vaccine was used, it spreads to non-vaccinated children by the oral/faecal route. One disadvantage was that it was inactivated by heat making storage difficult especially in the tropics. The use of live attenuated virus can also cause problems with the reversion of the virus to the wild type capable of causing disease. There have been cases of attenuated poliovirus being given to young children, and when this passed out in their faeces, it had been modified to a form capable of infecting their non-immune parents and causing polio.

The Sabin vaccine was introduced for general use in 1960, and by the mid 1960s, the number of cases of polio in the USA was down to less than six hundred per year. One problem that did not arise until the 1990s was that this vaccine was passed through monkey cells at one stage in its preparation, a fact that caused considerable suspicions when the origin of HIV was initially considered (Ch 18). When this suggestion was first mooted, many hospitals responded by destroying their records of immunisations carried out using the Sabin vaccine to avoid possible litigation if the suggestion proved to be correct.

The WHO was aiming to eradicate polio by 2005 but has failed to do so; the original target for elimination was the year 2000. One of the main problems has been in countries such as Nigeria, where a number of Muslim areas, in the north of the country, greatly distrust the central authorities, government officials and foreign health workers distributing the vaccine. The refusal to be immunised has frequently had religious overtones. The Chairman of the Supreme Council for Sharia in Nigeria (who is also a doctor) stated, *"We believe that modern-day Hitlers have deliberately adulterated the oral polio vaccine with anti-fertility drugs and contaminated it with viruses which are known to cause HIV and AIDS"*. The result was a large increase in the incidence of polio in northern Nigeria that then spread to a number of neighbouring countries in the region.

Immunisation programmes have recently become the target of a vocal minority questioning universal immunisation against diseases that do not currently pose a public health threat in developed countries. Pressure groups of this type ignore the fact that these diseases are not currently a threat precisely because they are controlled by immunisation.

Vaccines are given to healthy people to prevent disease, not sick ones to cure them. It is very easy to find someone who would have died (or think they would have) without medical intervention, such as antibiotic therapy or surgery. It is impossible however to find someone who would have died if they had not been immunised. There are two reasons for this, firstly they might not have contracted the disease, and secondly, even if they had, they might have recovered. It is however, easy to find individuals who were adversely affected by the immunisation process (or think they were, which in public opinion comes to the same thing).

If a single child dies as a result of an adverse reaction to vaccination, the anti-vaccination groups create a massive furore frequently fuelled by inaccurate press reports. They totally ignore the thousands of children whose lives have been saved by the vaccination process.

Immunisation therefore requires a much lower level of risk than other medical treatments. If the disease is rare (because of immunisation), an individual might decide that the risk of immunisation is not worth it. However, if sufficient people decide the risk is not worth taking, the percentage of the population immunised against the disease falls, and the level of herd immunity also falls, leaving the non-vaccinated members of the herd highly vulnerable to the disease. It is therefore essential that a vaccination process must have a very high level of efficacy and a very low risk of side effects or complications to be acceptable. In terms of safety, a severe adverse response of less than one in 100,000 is considered the minimum acceptable figure, and in practice this is usually closer to one in a million. The question arises, what is an unacceptable side effect? Obviously Guillain-Barré syndrome (Ch 15) is an unacceptable side effect of flu vaccination, but is a sore arm for a couple of days an unacceptable side effect of typhoid or tetanus vaccination? Some people think so.

There is a long history of opposition to vaccination in many countries. Public scepticism about vaccination is long-standing. A famous cartoon in 1802 by Gilray shows cows growing out of human bodies as Jenner vaccinated people against smallpox using the cowpox virus. Numerous pressure groups, many of them supported by various religious factions, sprang up in the nineteenth century and attempted to get smallpox vaccination banned, especially after it became compulsory. Whooping cough vaccine also received a lot of bad publicity after it was alleged that the vaccine had caused brain damage, as also has flu vaccine (Ch 15). The UK is by no means the only country to suffer from a loss of confidence in immunisation. In France, accusations have been made that the use of a vaccine against hepatitis B is linked to multiple sclerosis, and there have been attempts to link various immunisation processes in the USA to increases in the level of diabetes.

There is a major controversy in the UK at present regarding the MMR (measles, mumps, rubella) triple vaccine. Measles is closely related to the virus causing distemper in dogs, and the virus causing rinderpest in cattle. Whether humans caught it from dogs or cattle is irrelevant, as the virus has now adapted to humans in a form that is no longer infective for either of these species. As it no longer has an animal reservoir, it needs a constant supply of new susceptible people to cause an epidemic, at least 7,000 at any one time. These mainly come from the birth of children in Western Europe and North America, but migration into cities from the countryside is an important factor in many developing countries, and was also important in historical times.

It is spread by droplet infection (coughs and sneezes) and has a very high transmission number, that is, the number of people infected by each primary case. This number is much higher than either influenza or smallpox, and the result is that measles is one of the most infectious diseases known. It is now a routine childhood disease, and was almost eradicated by immunisation in the decade 1970-80, but reappeared because of the failure to immunise all children, especially in slum areas of the developing world. It is still widespread in non-Western nations, where because of poverty and malnutrition, it kills approximately ten per cent of its victims. Measles has long been associated with poverty, malnutrition (both low protein and low calorie, which are not necessarily the same thing) and overcrowding. In the early part of the twentieth century, it attacked the working classes much more severely than the middle classes. Indeed the cynical comment was made at the time that the best protection against measles was to catch it young as a member of a well-fed, middle-class family.

The estimated number of deaths in 1970 was eight million[99], but this figure had fallen to about two hundred thousand per year by 2006, the majority of them children. It is still the leading cause of childhood mortality that could be prevented by vaccination, and may also cause problems such as blindness and encephalitis in those it does not kill.

There have been serious problems over the uptake of the MMR vaccine in the UK over the last decade. In 1998, a paper was published in *"The Lancet"*, the premier British medical journal, by Dr. Andrew Wakefield and a number of co-authors. This paper described a case study of twelve (a very small sample in statistical terms) children, and claimed that there was a link between the MMR vaccine, bowel disease and autism. The level of autism has certainly increased, in the 1970s one child in 2,000 was diagnosed as autistic, the figure now is one in 200. This has become a world-wide problem, no rational scientific explanation has been proposed[100] and some experts consider that one major factor is an artificial reporting phenomenon (a medical term meaning doctors are getting better at recognising it). Many children are now also labelled *"autistic spectrum disorder"*, leading one to suspect that the goal-posts of diagnosis have been moved to include mild cases, children who, fifty years ago, would have probably been labelled by a teacher as inattentive or daydreamers.

It has been claimed that many children are normal until they receive the initial dose of MMR vaccine, which is given at the age of about fifteen months, but that they develop autism after this injection. The vaccine is an attenuated virus, and one suggestion was that it caused persistent bowel disease,

---

99   The Arab physician Rhazes, who first distinguished between smallpox and measles, thought that measles was considerably more dangerous than smallpox.

100   A small number of very severe cases of autism have been linked to possible mitochondrial mutations.

food was not digested properly causing the production of toxic chemicals which entered the blood stream and damaged the immature brain causing autism. Another suggestion was that the mixture of three vaccines overwhelmed the immune system of immature children, and a further one was that a very small amount of a mercury based compound used as a preservative in the vaccine was causing the damage. The compound involved, thiomersal, was removed from vaccines in the USA in 1999, but the rates of autism have not fallen, indicating that the low levels of mercury involved were not responsible for the condition.

The argument that the immune system is overwhelmed is also unlikely. Most parents are only too aware that as soon as a small child starts attending playgroup or a crèche, they suffer from a constant stream of colds, sore throats, earache, stomach upsets and other minor ailments. If the immune system of a small child can cope with this continuous assault, it should be able to cope with the MMR vaccine.

Following publication of the paper, public confidence in the triple vaccine declined sharply and parental pressure groups started to demand single vaccines instead of the multiple vaccine. This would require initial injections and boosters for each disease given at the appropriate intervals. The main argument against the use of single vaccines is that it would take much longer, the child would need to be immunised against each disease individually at intervals and then wait for further appropriate intervals before receiving the booster doses. The child receiving this treatment would therefore not be immunised, or only partially immunised, for a much longer period of time than the child who had received the triple vaccine.

The result of this controversy was that the number of children immunised against these diseases fell, herd immunity declined to a dangerously low level and diseases which had been more or less confined to history in the UK reappeared.

The level of vaccination required to give a high level of herd immunity against measles is recommended by the WHO to be ninety-five per cent uptake, with an eighty-five per cent uptake being regarded as dangerously low. In many parts of the UK, the uptake fell to below eighty per cent as a result of the controversy and in inner London it was considerably lower than this. The figures speak for themselves, in 1998 there were 56 cases of measles in England and Wales, in 2007 there were 990 and in 2008 the figure had risen to 1,348, a twenty-four fold increase. The first death in the UK since the early 1990s occurred in 2006, closely followed by a second. There were also three deaths from measles in Dublin in 2000, and in Holland, a further three children died in 2001 amongst a group opposed to vaccination on religious grounds.

Measles has been labelled officially as endemic in the UK, and this country is now regarded as one of the worst five in Europe for measles, along with Germany, Switzerland, Italy and Romania. The WHO had hoped to eradicate measles world-wide by 2010 but this deadline has been missed.

Rubella (German measles) is also a major problem, although it only causes a mild disease in children, it is very dangerous to pregnant women, causing congenital rubella syndrome in the unborn child, leading to problems including deafness, blindness and mental disabilities.

The paper in *"The Lancet"* caused a major controversy and was challenged by many doctors and scientists who raised numerous objections. The conventional medical opinion is that autism is present from birth and only becomes obvious at about eighteen months. The problem is that this is just after the time the MMR vaccine is given. It can be calculated statistically to determine whether this is a chance event, or whether there is a link between the two. The rise in autism in different countries should match the use of the MMR vaccine in that country if the two are linked, but no correlation has been found in any country. In a number of countries, the increase in autism started before the MMR vaccine was introduced, and has continued to rise even in countries such as Japan where the vaccine was withdrawn in 1993. In Denmark, where the public health of all children is tracked very closely, it has been possible to study the behaviour of children who received the MMR vaccine between 1991 and 1998 (approximately eighty per cent of their peer group), and the twenty per cent who did not receive it. The sample involved over half a million children making it highly significant statistically. Comparison between the two groups showed that the rates of autism were virtually identical in both groups, and therefore there was no correlation between the MMR vaccine and autism. Similar statistical surveys have been carried out in some of the other ninety countries where the vaccine has been used since it was first introduced in 1970, and no link between MMR and autism can be found.

The response of the UK government medical advisors and politicians is that there is no statistical evidence to link autism and the MMR vaccine and no need to provide individual vaccines. The problem with statistics however, is that many parents do not understand or believe them (Ch 1). The attitude of many people in Britain, especially following Blair's government, is that the use of statistics is a cover-up for government spin, propaganda and lies. The net result is that there has been a serious loss of public confidence in the UK in the triple vaccine and a substantial fall in the number of children being vaccinated. This was not helped by the refusal of Tony Blair, the former British Prime Minister, to state whether his young son had received the triple vaccine. This compares unfavourably with Queen Elizabeth II, who announced publicly that both Prince Charles and Princess Anne had received the polio vaccine soon after it became available.

A major factor has been that no-one knows what causes autism or why there has been a massive rise in the number of children suffering from it. Psychologically, people like to be able to blame some external factor when things go wrong and blaming the MMR vaccine for autism is an obvious choice given the proximity of the timing.

In 2004, the editor of *"The Lancet"* claimed that the paper submitted by Dr. Wakefield was flawed, and a month later, ten of his twelve co-authors retracted their claims of a possible link. In 2007, Wakefield was summoned to appear before a disciplinary committee of the General Medical Council of Great Britain to answer certain allegations relating to the study. The General Medical Council reached their conclusions in January 2010 and Wakefield was found guilty on numerous counts after the longest running investigation in GMC history. In February 2010, *"The Lancet"* retracted the original paper in its entirety.

In early 2009, the US Court of Claims rejected a test case on behalf of a fourteen year old girl, who sued the US government claiming that her autism was caused by the MMR vaccine. The judge, after reviewing hundreds of medical and scientific papers, ruled that, *"The evidence that I have reviewed makes it appear extremely unlikely that the MMR vaccine can contribute to the causation of autism"*. A further comment was made that a linkage between the two had failed to gain acceptance in the medical community.

In June 2009, there was a large outbreak of measles in Wales involving several hundred cases. The Welsh Minister of State for Health called for compulsory vaccination against measles. This suggestion was supported by a former chairman of the British Medical Association, who also suggested that vaccination should be mandatory for school attendance.

A further twist in this saga in the UK has been the recent suggestion that vaccine against chickenpox should be added to the MMR triple vaccine. Whilst vaccination against chickenpox is common in North America, it is not widespread in Europe where chickenpox is regarded as a childhood rite of passage and relatively harmless, although the occasional child infected with chickenpox does die from secondary bacterial infections causing toxic shock. One major argument against the widespread use of chickenpox vaccine is that if all children are vaccinated, then adults will not be exposed to the virus sufficiently frequently to keep their immunity boosted, and a large number of the adult population will develop shingles in a severe form. It would be necessary to give adults booster doses of chicken-pox vaccine, and once this is factored into the equation, the costs and benefits of chickenpox vaccination begin to look very doubtful. Given the present furore in the UK about the MMR vaccine, any Minister of Health who advocated adding a fourth vaccine to the cocktail would no doubt be told by his Sir Humphrey Appleby that, *"he was making a very brave decision".*

The difficulties of developing and using new vaccines are considerable, they include scientific, socio-economic, religious (thwarting God's will) and ethical problems. In economic terms, the investment required to develop a new vaccine is huge, the price of the vaccine is low and requires a high usage to generate a profit. The cost of developing a vaccine to reach a commercial market has been estimated at US$600 million to $1 billion. No firm going to take a financial risk this big, especially in a litigation prone society such as the USA, unless there is a large and lucrative market. The problems are highlighted in the chapter on influenza (Ch 15). In that case there were not only major financial consequences but also political ones. The fiasco was claimed to have had a significant effect on the US election of 1976.

One major feature of the cost problem is that vaccines for military use against bio-warfare agents are not going to be developed because the military requirements are not big enough. Serious problems arose in the US military in the 1990s, when all American troops were required to be vaccinated against anthrax. The vaccine was obtained from a single company, which was later claimed to be having serious financial problems, and there were also questions over the efficacy of the vaccine at a very early stage. The Pentagon admitted that 0.2% of those vaccinated suffered adverse reactions, but the US General Accounting Office claimed that adverse reactions of varying degrees were suffered by between five and thirty-five per cent of those vaccinated.

The result of all these problems is that there are a decreasing number of vaccine producers world wide, and there is a tendency not to produce a vaccine unless it will be widely used in the developed world at a high charge. The development of a vaccine against HIV may be regarded as a case in point. In relative terms, HIV is still not epidemic in developed countries, where it is generally confined to high-risk groups, although the situation is deteriorating. Anti-*retro*viral chemotherapy is widely available and makes vaccine usage in developed countries less likely, however, vaccine production is the only realistic method of dealing with HIV and AIDS in Africa and Southeast Asia due to the scale of the epidemic and the cost of anti-*retro*viral therapy.

Scientifically, the problems of vaccine production include the necessity of identifying which antigens produce a long-lived response. In some cases, the antigen has not been identified, and may not even exist in a stable form due to the rapidly changing genome of the micro-organism involved. A further technical problem is that the antigen may not be long-lived when introduced into the patient, or may not produce a strong response. This is a common problem with polysaccharide antigens. In addition, to be of any use in the developing world the vaccine must be stable to heat, and be able to survive for long periods of time outside a refrigerator.

ANTITOXINS

An extension of the vaccination principle was the development of antitoxins (antisera) by Emile Roux (1853-1933), one of Pasteur's associates. Roux and Alexandre Yersin used horses for the large-scale production of antitoxin by injecting them with diphtheria toxin to produce a diphtheria antiserum used on a commercial basis during the last decade of the nineteenth century. Roux later became director of the Pasteur Institute and Yersin discovered the role of the organism causing bubonic plague. Kitasato and von Behring in Koch's group also worked on a serum for tetanus at the same time.

Antisera are produced by injecting a horse with the disease-causing organism and then taking blood from the animal. This horse blood now contains ready-formed antibodies to the disease, and can be given to a person who has already caught that disease to counter it. This is a passive immunity, as opposed to the active immunity produced when a person is vaccinated against a disease and primed to form his or her own antibodies. The repeated use of such antisera can cause problems as it contains proteins from the horse, which can act as antigens in their own right and may cause an adverse reaction in humans known as serum sickness.

The same principle is now used to prepare antidotes to bites from snakes and a number of other poisonous species. Calmette, who produced the BCG vaccine against TB, first worked on the preparation of anti-venom against snake bite. This was prepared by injecting animals with increasing doses of snake venom inactivated by heat. In the case of horses, the animal is ultimately being injected with up to 200 times the lethal dose of snake venom.

The Iditarod race held every year in Alaska commemorates the importance of diphtheria antitoxin in an outbreak of the disease in Nome in 1925. There was an outbreak of diphtheria in the winter of that year, and the antitoxin was taken over the Iditarod trail by dog sledge as there was no railroad, ships could not get through the pack ice and it was too dangerous to fly during winter. The race started in 1973, and is over a distance of approximately 1,100 miles from Anchorage to Nome.

ALLERGIES

The history of allergies goes back a long time. Lucretius (95-55 BC), in his poem *"De rerum natura"* (On things natural), recognised that not all foods are beneficial to everybody, and observed that, *"what is good for one may be a fierce poison for others"*. Both Hippocrates and Galen knew that certain foods such as cows milk and goat milk were associated with intolerance. Hippocrates recognised allergies in foods such as cheese whilst Galen also noted reactions to certain plants.

Leonardo Botallo mentioned *"rose cold"* in 1565, i.e. catarrh and asthma near flowering roses and early in the nineteenth century a London doctor, John Bostock, described summer catarrh that corresponds very closely to modern descriptions of hay fever. Bostock also noted that it occurred mainly in urban, educated families rather than rural families, even though these were more exposed.

There has been a large increase in asthma, eczema, allergic rhinitis, allergic dermatitis and food allergies[101] in recent years, but this is mainly restricted to the developed countries, especially amongst the more educated and higher socio-economic groups. It has been suggested that this rise in allergies is linked to cleanliness. In 1989, David Strachan observed that allergies in children correlate with inverse family size, i.e. the bigger the family, the less the allergies, and postulated the *"Hygiene hypothesis"*. This suggested that in small families there is less cross infection from older siblings, and considered that early childhood diseases might tutor our immune systems and prevent the development of allergies. Several studies have now been carried out producing similar results. These also suggest that too hygienic a life style results in increased asthma and other auto-immune problems. Modern surveys of urban and rural children produce similar results to those of Bostock, and also suggest that children exposed to pets at a young age are

---

101   In the UK, between 1989-1996, peanut allergy tripled in some areas, whilst in the USA, it doubled nationwide between 1997-2002.

less likely to develop allergies[102], as also are children living on farms. The hygiene hypothesis put forward by Strachan is controversial and not all doctors agree with these views although few alternative ideas have been suggested.

Whilst there is obviously a genetic component to these allergic conditions, the large and rapid rise over the last two decades strongly suggests that environmental factors play a very significant role in these problems. Severe asthma and various food allergies are uncommon in India and Africa where infections of parasites, such as intestinal worms, are common, however people from these countries moving to the developed world experience increases in allergies. Compared with these countries, the inhabitants of the developed world have a relatively sterile and less challenging life style in immunological terms. There are good (relatively) medical facilities, clean drinking water, efficient sewage disposal, central heating, and air conditioning. This cushioned life-style may however be damaging our immune systems, which depend on the continued stimuli from micro-organisms and diseases to mature and develop. The evidence suggests that it is not just exposure to disease-causing micro-organisms that is essential, but also exposure to those generally considered to be beneficial and "friendly". It is not clear which micro-organisms might be protective, nor whether there is a window in time during which they must be experienced.

The treatment of certain auto-immune diseases of the gut using parasitic worms such as the pig whip-worm (*Trichuris suis*) is a recent development still being evaluated, but doctors using these treatments have reported promising results in a number of cases. Our immune systems evolved at a time when humans were heavily infected with parasites, and because we in the West live such clean life styles, our immune systems now do not have enough work to keep them busy. As the

---

102   As grandmother may well have said, *"A bit of clean dirt never did anyone any harm"* or as my wife's grandmother, in Yorkshire, did say, *"You've got to eat a peck of muck before you die"*.

proverb says, *"The Devil finds work for idle hands"*, and our idle immune systems start attacking self and causing problems such as ulcerative colitis. The rationale behind these treatments is to provide the immune system with its ancestral target, thereby recreating the conditions under which it evolved, and it will become too busy dealing with non-self to turn on self.

Chapter 8

Epidemics of Antiquity

There are a number of references to epidemics in ancient texts. Chinese, Vedic and Sumerian documents of the third and second millennia BC describe numerous diseases, but with the exception of one or two, such as malaria which was obviously a serious problem, most cannot be identified from the descriptions given.

One of the best known early references is in the Bible to the Ten Plagues of Egypt. One of these was an epidemic of boils (Exodus 9, 9) and another was the death of the firstborn (Exodus 12, 29). Amongst the Plagues of Egypt were also the death of cattle (Exodus 9, 3) and the destruction of barley and flax (Exodus 9, 31), both important crops. Interestingly, the Bible claims that it was only mature flax and barley that were destroyed, wheat and rye that were immature were not damaged. The word murrain is used (Exodus 9, 3); this is an archaic word derived from the Latin word "mori" meaning to die. The old sense of the word is any disease of animals, and occasionally crops, however since 1745 it has been used more or less exclusively to describe the important cattle disease, rinderpest.

Although they are not an epidemic disease, red tides were one of the plagues mentioned in the Old Testament, *"all the waters that were in the river turned to blood. And the fish that was in the river died. … and the river stank, and the Egyptians could not drink of the water of the river"* (Exodus 7, 20-21). These red tides are caused by several varieties of microscopic algae growing in vast numbers and producing toxins capable of poisoning numerous other aquatic species (Ch 4).

Other examples of epidemic diseases mentioned in the Old Testament include the destruction of the army of the Assyrian king, Sennacharib (reigned 705-681 BC), at the siege of Jerusalem (Kings II, 19, 35). This event has been graphically described in poetry by Lord Byron *("The Assyrian came down like a wolf on the fold")*. The number of dead quoted for this particular epidemic is probably highly exaggerated. Even a powerful empire such as Assyria would have difficulty producing an army that could sustain losses of *"an hundred four score and five thousand"* (i.e. 185,000) dead. If losses of seventy percent are assumed, which is possible for a new epidemic disease attacking an army with a low level of herd immunity, then this would suggest that the Assyrians possessed the logistical capability of supporting an army of over quarter of a million men, on campaign, hundreds of miles from their own country. If the percentage of dead was lower, then the Assyrian army was even larger. Whatever the losses were, it was obviously a major event as it is mentioned by a number of other contemporary sources, including Assyrian and Babylonian ones.

In Kings (II, 6, 18) the prophet Elisha smites the Syrian army with temporary blindness, when it attacks the Israelites at Doshan, whilst Numbers (11, 33) states, *"The Lord smote the people with a very great plague"*. An affliction of emerods (this is usually translated as a plague of haemorrhoids) attacked the Philistines after they captured the Ark of the Covenant (Samuel, I, 5, 6) and carried it off to the Temple of Dagon. It has been suggested that the haemorrhoids were buboes and that this may have been an early description of bubonic plague. The Philistines were also required to make a trespass offering of five golden mice (rats?); *"images of your mice that mar the land"* (Samuel I, 6, 5) which might also suggest bubonic plague, as contemporary sources generally do not distinguish between different types of rodent.

Golden mice are not mentioned in the Bible in relation to the destruction of the host of Sennacharib, but Herodotus (484-425BC), the Father of Greek History, who wrote the first history of the Persian Wars, claimed that mice also appeared on this occasion. By the first century BC, it had been realised that rodents carry disease as Strabo wrote, "*Pestilential diseases often ensue from mice*".

Whilst diseases certainly appear to have influenced military campaigns, they were obviously not severe enough to disrupt the Assyrian, Persian, Babylonian, Hittite and Egyptian empires from producing sufficient soldiers for a never-ending series of armies. A similar situation was seen later with a constant stream of armies from the Greek City states, Macedon, Carthage, the Roman Republic and Empire, and numerous nascent states and empires in the Middle East and Asia, especially China.

To give just one example quoted by Livy in "*The War with Hannibal*". In 218 BC, when Hannibal marched into Italy at the start of the Second Punic War, Rome had six legions. By 217 BC there were eleven and by 211 BC, there were twenty-three in spite of the fact that the Romans had lost several major battles and had suffered an estimated 50,000 casualties at the Battle of Cannae in 216 BC.

The Jews of the Old Testament may not have realised the cause of diseases due to the small size and thus invisibility of the parasites involved. They probably realised however that some foods were linked with certain diseases such as trichinosis (a disease caused by nematode worms), hence the prohibition on eating pork (Leviticus 11,7), which we now know can carry numerous diseases of this type if not carefully controlled. Muslims also have a similar prohibition. Both of these prohibitions were probably due to observations of pigs, which are omnivorous, scavenging through rubbish tips and eating generally dirty food. In addition, the Jews banned the eating of shellfish that are also scavengers (Leviticus 11, 10). Leviticus lays down a series of rules for ritual hygiene, but these were enforced by priests and not by doctors, a situation already noted in relation to many early civilisations.

Leprosy (Ch 11) is mentioned frequently in the Bible (Leviticus), and lepers were expelled from many ancient communities as the disease was thought to be contagious by skin-to-skin contact, although it is now known that leprosy is one of the least contagious diseases attacking humans.

Parasitic worm infestations may be mentioned in the Bible; some authors consider the fiery serpents mentioned in Numbers (21, 6) are infections caused by the guinea worm, *Dracunculus medinensis* (the little dragon of Medina, [one of the holy cities of Islam]). The worms have been found in Egyptian mummies and are mentioned in Sanskrit literature of the second millennium BC. They are also mentioned by Galen in the second century AD and by Arab doctors of the first millennium AD.

Ritual washing as practised by Muslims and Hindus may reduce disease. However, ritual bathing can also spread diseases when shared with thousands of other pilgrims. Ablution pools in mosques and temples in the tropics frequently harbour schistosomiasis (bilharzia) (Ch 19), which has been found in Egyptian mummies dating back to the second millennium BC. In India, outbreaks of water-borne viral, bacterial and metazoan diseases are notorious in holy cities such as Benares (modern day Varanasi), especially during religious pilgrimages and festivals that frequently involve ritual bathing.

Other examples of epidemics are found in various places; there is a reference (fourteenth century BC) to a disease attacking the Hittites after they captured Egyptian prisoners of war who were used as slaves. Early Indian epics, dated to the second millennium BC, refer to diseases that may possibly have been smallpox or bubonic plague. There are also early oral traditions of disease (possibly smallpox) in India, and many Hindu temples contain carvings suggesting diseases. Scars claimed to be the pock-marks of smallpox have been found on the mummy of Rameses V, dated to the twelfth century BC. A reference is found to the God of Pestilence in the Babylonian Epic of Gilgamesh, written in the third millennium BC, and Chinese texts of the thirteenth century BC mention the rulers consulting soothsayers to determine whether it would be a year of pestilence. The Chinese also had a god dedicated to recovery from disease.

In all of these cases, the descriptions are far too vague to identify the disease involved.

Epidemics known to be important in history include smallpox, measles, influenza, scarlet fever, typhus, plague, syphilis, malaria, yellow fever, schistosomiasis and various others. Some of these appear to have survived virtually unchanged over centuries, but many appear to have been much more dangerous in historical times than they are today due to the lower levels of herd immunity.

A number of early epidemics were recorded by the Greeks, one of the first being the Plague of Xerxes in 480 BC, which afflicted the Persian army attacking Greece and was described in some detail by Herodotus. The identity is uncertain, but it may have been a severe outbreak of dysentery.

Probably the best-documented early crowd disease (the Plague of Athens) was the one that reached the Greek city-state of Athens during the Golden Age (430BC). Athenian political power and influence were at their height, and their navy effectively ruled the eastern Mediterranean which contained numerous Athenian trading colonies on the Black Sea and also on the coast of present day Turkey. Athenian naval power reached as far as Sicily whilst the western Mediterranean was controlled by the rising power of Carthage.

Athens was attacked and besieged by another Greek city-state, Sparta, during the Peloponnesian War (431-404 BC) in an attempt by Sparta to curb the growing power of Athens. The Athenians were only too well aware that they were unable to defeat the Spartans on land, as following their long and arduous training, the Spartan army was dominant throughout the Peleponnese at that time. The Athenians retreated into the city following the advice of Pericles, one of their senior generals. A large number of refugees entered the city raising the population to an estimated 200,000 people. The city became seriously overpopulated with poor living conditions and sanitation during the hot summer months. In ancient and medieval times, military campaigns usually took place in the summer after planting and before harvest; war throughout the winter months is a relatively modern concept.

The Spartans besieged the city but the Spartan fleet was unable to blockade Pireaus (the port of Athens), thus enabling the Athenians to import all the grain and other supplies they needed from their colonies and satellite cities and hence prolong the siege. The disease peaked during the Spartan siege lasting forty days in 430 BC, it then subsided and remained at a low level in 429 BC, but returned in the summer of 428, when the Spartans besieged the city a second time. The total number of dead over the entire period is not known.

The only primary source of our information for the epidemic is the account of the Thucydides (460-400 BC), a member of the Athenian upper class, who wrote about the events some twenty-five years after they occurred. Thucydides, who suffered from the disease himself but recovered, claimed that the epidemic arrived from Egypt by ship, having originated in Ethiopia and presumably travelled down the Nile Valley. It started in Piraeus and spread along the Long Walls, a series of fortifications joining Pireaus to Athens, which is about ten kilometres inland. The Spartan army camped outside the walls mostly escaped the epidemic. Thucydides reported that the Athenians accused the Spartans of spreading the disease deliberately by poisoning the reservoirs. It is not known whether this was true or not but it is one of the earliest suggestions of germ warfare[103]. Many ancient civilisations such as the Greeks, Romans and Persians were well aware of the consequences of poisoning wells and water supplies, especially in desert regions, the generally used method being to dump dead bodies, both animal and human, into a well.

Thucydides claimed that there were outbreaks of the disease in many places including Lemnos, but that it became more deadly when it reached Athens. He also claimed that the doctors had no idea of how to treat it and neither did the priests. It started with headaches, inflamed eyes and the tongue and throat became bloody. These symptoms were followed by sneezing, coughing, vomiting and diarrhoea. The victims then developed a fever and sores appeared on the body that turned into ulcers. They could not bear the touch of clothes or bedding, had a raging thirst and many hurled themselves into public water cisterns. Death usually occurred seven to eight days after the symptoms appeared. Many who recovered were blinded, lost the use of their digits and suffered from total amnesia. Thucydides stated that those who recovered were immune and did not fall ill a second time, or if they did, the second attack was a mild one.

He also claimed that dogs and carrion-eating birds that touched the bodies died, suggesting that it may have been some generalised bacterial infection rather than one specific to the human species. It attacked all the population, irrespective of sex, age or class, lasted several years with a few brief interludes and killed a third of the population. It also killed twenty-

---

103   Aristotle (384-322 BC) emphasised the strategic importance of the water tanks and the necessity of guarding them adequately. Athens was unusual in that it was a city that had not developed on a river and was totally dependent on rainfall collected in large cisterns. All the important posts held by citizens in Athens were selected by lot. Although selection by lot does avoid the problem of corruption, the laws of probability mean that sooner or later the village idiot will be put in charge. The Athenians dealt with this problem by breaking their own rules; the only two exceptions to selection by lot were army generals and the commissioners in charge of the water tanks.

five to thirty per cent of the Athenian hoplites[104] seriously undermining Athenian military power.

Thucydides wrote that people resolved to spend their wealth quickly and enjoy themselves, the *"eat, drink and be merry for tomorrow we die"* syndrome. He stated that there was widespread lawlessness and general anarchy that undermined the moral and civic fabric of Athenian society. He also claimed that no one expected to live long enough to be brought to trial and punished so society broke down, bodies were left to rot in the streets and cremated *en masse.*

The epidemic not only attacked Athens, but the Athenian fleet passed it on to parts of their army besieging Potidaea in Macedonia and twenty-five per cent of the army there died within forty days. At the end of the war, Athens surrendered, the Long Walls were demolished, Sparta became the leading power in Greece and Athens never regained its former dominance. However, Athens did become a leader of the opposition to Macedonian expansion under Philip II (father of Alexander the Great). The dominance of Sparta came to an end in 371 BC when they were defeated at the Battle of Leuctra, by the Thebans, after the Theban general, Epaminondas, revolutionised the organisation of the phalanx.

The symptoms of the epidemic match nothing recognised by the medical profession today. There have been numerous suggestions over the years, such as bubonic plague, smallpox, measles, typhus or a bacterial infection producing a toxic shock syndrome. There has also been a suggestion that it was caused by the Ebola virus and a more recent one that it was typhoid. None of these diagnoses can be authenticated. Zinnser considered smallpox was the most likely suspect for the epidemic with typhus as second choice. However, it may have been the first appearance in Europe of some bacterial disease (such as scarlet fever) that is considered a childhood disease today. In the pre-antibiotic era, scarlet fever killed

---

104   The infantry, literally shield carriers (the mainstay of the phalanx, the fighting formation adopted by the Greek city states).

a very significant percentage of young children in Western Europe. Smallpox is unlikely as Thucydides does not mention the residual pockmarks that are one of the most distinctive features of smallpox; he also mentions the disease killing dogs and carrion birds but smallpox is unique to humans. It is most unlikely that the identity of this epidemic will ever be authenticated beyond dispute. It is however, the first well-documented example of a disease spreading from one centre of civilisation to another.

Although the writings of Thucydides are full of rhetoric (an Athenian literary art form), there is no doubt that his descriptions of the effects of the disease on Athenian society closely resemble those of the Plague of Justinian on Byzantine society in the sixth century AD, and the effects of the Black Death on European society in the fourteenth century. Although there are other descriptions of the Plague of Athens by writers such as Lucretius, the descriptions they give are very similar to those of Thucydides, and it is probable that they were using Thucydides as a primary source. The other surprising fact is that the Plague of Athens is not mentioned by Hippocrates, even although it occurred during his lifetime. We know that some of the works of the *Hippocratic Corpus* have been lost and it is possible that a description of the disease is contained in these lost documents.

In Rome, the historian Livy (59 BC-17 AD), in his account *"The History of Rome"*, listed at least eleven epidemics that had attacked Rome since its legendary date of founding in 753 BC. One of these appears to have been due to Carthaginian intervention in a dispute between the cities of Syracuse and Messina on Sicily, which ultimately led to the First Punic War (264-241 BC) fought between Rome and Carthage. It has been claimed that this epidemic was a crucial factor in the war, causing the Carthaginians to ultimately lose the island of Sicily. This caused them to lose the First Punic War as Sicily was essential for their naval bases. By this time, the growing Roman Republic had colonised Southern Italy, and was regarding Sicily as coming within its sphere of influence. None of the descriptions given by Livy are detailed enough to allow the diseases involved to be identified, although influenza has been suggested as a possibility in one case.

Although Livy mentions a number of epidemics, Italy appears to have been relatively free of epidemic diseases during the period of Hannibal's campaigns (218-203 BC) during the Second Punic War. There is no mention of serious disease in Hannibal's army of about 40,000 men, nor in any of the Roman armies that opposed him, some of which were considerably larger.

Numerous epidemics also attacked Rome and the Empire after Livy's death. In 65 AD, an epidemic occurred that may have been an acute form of falciparum malaria, but the identity is debatable. Another epidemic reached Rome in 125AD that is thought to have started in Africa as an aftermath of a locust infestation causing famine. The estimated number killed was one million, and again the identity is not certain; from the description measles is a possibility.

The Antonine Plague (165-180 AD) (also known as the Plague of Galen), is thought to have been the European debut of smallpox and is considered in detail in Chapter 10. Most of the epidemics occurring up to this point that reached Europe have been described as originating in Africa. The Antonine Plague is the first one described as originating in Asia.

The next major epidemic to reach Rome was dated 250 AD and known as the Plague of Cyprian after Saint Cyprian, the Bishop of Carthage, who first described it. The epidemic apparently started in Ethiopia and although the identity is again not certain, many authors consider it was another epidemic of smallpox. It lasted until 256 AD, and is thought to have killed approximately fifty per cent of its victims. In Rome at the height of the epidemic an estimated 5,000/day were dying, including one of the emperors. This particular epidemic appears to have continued on and off for three centuries and has been credited with causing mass conversions to Christianity.

The seeds of financial instability in the Roman Empire were sown during the German wars of Marcus Aurelius Antoninus who ruled from 161-180 AD and prosecuted these wars at great cost. There were also civil wars involving the first North African emperor, Septimus Severus, during the last decade of the second century AD, and during this period there was a major debasement of the gold and silver coinage with important silver mines becoming exhausted. These wars and the devastating effects of various epidemics caused a serious reduction in the tax base of the empire which was effectively based on a system of import taxes paid at trading centres (mainly ports). These were then used to pay the legions defending the frontiers. When the tax base collapsed, the unpaid legions revolted and a long and bitter series of civil wars followed, in which many generals who could command the following of an army aspired to the purple. Many of these emperors were deposed and murdered within months of taking office. The whole problem was exacerbated by continuous pressure on the frontiers (especially the Rhine frontier) of the Empire by the migrations of a series of barbarian tribes, who in turn were being subjected to pressure on their eastern flanks by the Huns.

By the time of the Emperor Diocletian, who reigned from 285-305 AD, the situation had deteriorated to the point where he passed edicts forbidding farmers from leaving the land. By this time, certain Germanic tribes were being allowed to settle inside the boundaries of the Empire to act as buffer states against more dangerous enemies. This suggests that there was a significant amount of land available due to the reduction in population. Under Diocletian, the empire was split into Eastern and Western parts with co-emperors ruling the two halves, a policy that halted the decay briefly. The Empire was reunited for a short period under Constantine the Great (274-

337 AD), ruling from the Eastern capital of Byzantium which he renamed Constantinople (present day Istanbul). Rome itself however, was sacked by the Visigoths under Alaric in 410 AD.

In 452 AD, the Huns under the command of Attila reached Rome but then retreated, without capturing the city, because of another epidemic, again thought to be smallpox. The Western Roman Empire was finally overthrown by Theodoric the Great (*ca* 454-526), king of the Ostrogoths, in the late fifth century.

During the latter part of the Roman Empire there was a fall in the population of many cities and towns, villages were abandoned, and a general breakdown of the social fabric occurred, with consequent administrative failure and economic decay. After the defeat of the Western Roman Empire, literacy in Europe declined and there was a period lasting for several hundred years, known to history as the Dark Ages.

The Eastern Empire (Byzantine Empire) survived the fall of Rome, and lasted until 1453 AD when it was captured by the Ottomans. It also suffered from epidemics, the most important of these being a massive epidemic that started in 542 AD. This is known as the Plague of Justinian and this, and the attempts of Justinian to reunite the Roman Empire are considered in detail in Chapter 9.

Mesopotamia was relatively stable epidemiologically compared with Europe by the time of the fall of the Western Roman Empire; the serious diseases had subsided to endemic or childhood diseases, suggesting it had a disease-experienced population.

In large countries covering a number of degrees of latitude such as China and India, different disease patterns were found in the north and south. A list of the epidemics thought to have attacked China can be found in McNeill's book, *"Plagues and Peoples"*. China consisted of a number of small kingdoms and suffered from centuries of warfare, known as the Period of the Warring States from 481 until 221 BC, when what is effectively modern China was united under the control of the First Emperor, Qin Shi Huangdi. The victorious Qin dynasty ruled China for less than two decades, falling in 206 BC, and being replaced by the Han dynasty. The power base of the Qin was the upper reaches of the Yellow River Valley. The main factor in the development of this area as a base for further conquests was the building of the Chengkuo Canal which opened in 246 BC, the year the First Emperor acceded to the Qin throne. The canal, which was over sixty-five miles long, linked two of the tributaries of the Yellow River, irrigated nearly six hundred thousand acres of land growing cereal crops, provided food for the victorious Qin army and an income stream for the ruler. It also gave a considerable strategic advantage in the form of improved communications and the ability to move troops quickly.

The Yellow River Valley is hot in the summer but suffers from severe winters that do not allow the survival of tropical parasites. The expansion of the Qin Empire at the expense of the other warring states included the Yangtse valley which is hot and humid throughout the year and supports rice farming which needs irrigation. The boundaries for a number of tropical and sub-tropical diseases occur between these two valleys, including malaria (Ch 16), schistosomiasis (Ch 19) and a number of mosquito-borne diseases such as dengue fever (Ch 17). Malaria and schistosomiasis are both important in that although they do not cause epidemics such as smallpox and measles, they produce a debilitated population unable to resist other diseases.

In the Indian sub-continent, the Indus Valley which is in the north, contained a number of societies such as Harappa. Although the Indus Valley is warm, much of it is also semi-arid and the range of various parasites is limited. The Ganges Valley however is hot and wet, and numerous parasites are found, the range of parasites increasing the further south one moves. The jungles of south and north-east India were inhabited by tribes who lived in small self-contained villages. Although these communities would have probably been destroyed in temperate zones by the diseases of civilisation, in the jungle they were protected by various tropical diseases from the encroachments of urban populations. Instead of being destroyed, they became part of the Hindu caste system. The various rules about contact between castes, and the elaborate purification rites required when this occurs, may be due to an ancestral fear of infectious diseases.

CHAPTER 9

The Black Death: Was it Bubonic Plague?

"Is it possible that posterity will believe these things? We who have seen them can scarce believe them." Petrarch 1350.

The Black Death and the Plague of Justinian played major roles in the history of both Europe and much of the rest of the Old World. An examination of these two epidemics in detail shows how they influenced much of the present day national, political and religious boundaries.

It has been suggested by some authors that there have been four great documented epidemics of bubonic plague. The first of these was the Plague of Athens (430 BC), although most historians would accept that this could have been any one of several diseases and that any link to bubonic plague is tenuous. The Plague of Athens is discussed in Chapter 8. The second was the Plague of Justinian (542 AD) and subsequent epidemics until the middle of the eighth century. The third was the Great Pestilence, which later became known as the Black Death (1347-50), and subsequent epidemics until the mid-seventeenth century. Finally, there was a major epidemic of bubonic plague in China and India in the late nineteenth and early twentieth centuries.

It should be emphasized strongly that the only one of these four epidemics that can be authenticated as bubonic plague, using modern bacteriological techniques, is the epidemic in China and India. Many history texts present both the Plague of Justinian and the Black Death as epidemics of bubonic plague, but this theory is one that is becoming increasingly controversial.

It is probably best to start with a discussion of the epidemiology of bubonic plague, which was elucidated during, and in the aftermath, of the Chinese epidemic that commenced during the late nineteenth century.

Epidemiology of Bubonic Plague

Bubonic plague is primarily a disease of burrowing rodents that are the true hosts and it only infects humans by accident. The epidemiology and inter-relationships of the bacterium and its different hosts are probably the most complex of any disease known. There are five components, the bacterium *Yersinia pestis* (historically this has also been named *Bacillus pestis* and *Pasteurella pestis*), the flea, a rodent host showing a considerable degree of resistance to bubonic plague, a susceptible rodent host, i.e. the rat, and finally humans.

The epidemiology will be examined in some detail as a comparison of the behaviour of authentic bubonic plague and the behaviour of the Black Death highlights some serious anomalies. The assumption made in this chapter is that the Black Death and the Plague of Justinian were the same disease, there is no definite scientific proof but the circumstantial evidence suggests this assumption is correct.

The Bacterium

Y. pestis is a small Gram negative bacterium. A number of different strains are known with varying strains occurring in different rodent species. Analysis of the DNA shows that *Y. pestis* has evolved from *Y. pseudotuberculosis,* a bacterium related to the enteric bacteria causing gut infections. Some experts consider that *Y. pestis* could not have evolved from *Y. pseudotuberculosis* directly, but must have acquired plasmids (Ch 4) or scavenged DNA from other bacteria.

Studies have been carried out on the DNA of the teeth of skeletons who are claimed to have been victims of authentic bubonic plague occurring in the sixteenth century in Southern France. These allegedly indicate that there has been little change in the DNA of *Y. pestis* over the intervening centuries. If correct, this would imply that bubonic plague in the sixteenth century, is similar in behaviour to bubonic plague today in terms of the clinical appearance of the victims and the epidemiology of the disease. The results of this work have been challenged by research carried out at Oxford University on a large number of teeth found in mass graves from the fourteenth century. These included one mass grave from the London area, dug specifically for plague victims. They also studied teeth from mass graves of suspected plague victims in other European countries such as Denmark and France. In all these cases the researchers were unable to detect any DNA sequences from the bacterium *Y. pestis.*

THE FLEA

It has been estimated that at least 30 species of fleas and over 200 species of rodents can carry bubonic plague, and the host/vector permutations are complicated, to say the least. However, it is probable that only one species of flea capable of carrying bubonic plague was present in England in the fourteenth, fifteenth and sixteenth centuries. This was *Xenopsylla cheopsis* (the Oriental rat flea), which will bite humans in the absence of rats, and is generally considered to be one of the most efficient vectors of bubonic plague. The human flea (*Pulex irritans*) is a very poor vector of plague.

The flea (*X. cheopsis)* sucks up blood from an infected host when feeding and the bacteria ingested multiply to form a solid lump in the stomach of the flea. This stops the flea taking up more blood and it becomes increasingly hungry and desperate in its attempts to feed. It sucks blood into its oesophagus, mixes the blood with bacteria, regurgitates it and passes the infected blood back into the host. In effect the flea becomes a living hypodermic needle.

The time required for the bacteria to reach an infective concentration varies from species to species of flea. In *X. cheopsis* it is about twenty-one days from feeding to becoming infectious, but this figure depends on humidity and the external temperature. The flea survives about seventeen days after becoming infectious under optimum conditions. The temperature is also important for egg laying; a minimum of 18°C (65°F) is required.

For the human flea, *P. irritans,* to transmit the disease it is necessary for the flea to bite an infected person and then bite a second person whilst the blood of the first victim is still wet on its proboscis. This implies a very high density of both fleas and humans. The total population of England immediately prior to the Black Death was probably between four and five million, less than one tenth of today's population. Although the density per square mile would have been high in cities such as London, Norwich, York and Bristol, it would have been very low across the rural countryside and any effect of *P. irritans* on the spread of the disease would have been negligible.

THE RESISTANT RODENT HOST

The third factor is a rodent host showing significant resistance to bubonic plague. There are considerable differences in the susceptibility of different species of rodent to bubonic plague. The disease will die out in an area where the rodent host is highly susceptible, for example, the rat, as it rapidly kills large numbers of the susceptible host, reducing the population to a point where the disease cannot spread any further. It will persist where there is a rodent host showing a degree of resistance. In Asia, marmots show some resistance and gerbils are highly resistant, whilst in the USA, resistance is found in ground squirrels.

When bubonic plague is present in the indigenous resistant rodent population, they form a permanent reservoir of bubonic plague that is a potential focus of infection for other rodent species including rats, and ultimately humans. This focus may remain in equilibrium for years, with the bacteria passing between the rodent reservoir and their fleas and only causing a few rodent deaths. It is in effect an endemic childhood infection of the reservoir rodent species. Occasionally the balance of the infection is disturbed, and bubonic plague then spreads throughout the rodent population causing a large number of deaths, a situation known as epizootic plague. The epizootic phase declines again as the number of resistant rodents rises, and the number of susceptible ones falls. If rats are living in close proximity to the reservoir rodent, the epizootic phase may spread to rats by means of fleabites. If these rats come into contact with humans, an outbreak of human bubonic plague may be initiated.

There is no resistant rodent known to be capable of forming a permanent reservoir of bubonic plague in Western Europe.

THE RAT, THE SUSCEPTIBLE RODENT

Only two species of rats are commonly found in Europe, the brown rat, *Rattus norvegicus,* and the black rat, *Rattus rattus.* The brown rat (also known as the sewer rat or the Norwegian rat) spread out from Russia in the early eighteenth century. It did not arrive in Britain until 400 years after the Black Death, and approximately 100 years after the Great Plague of London (effectively the disappearance of this disease from the UK). It is the more hardy and aggressive of the two, is the more common rat in temperate climates, and is the rat that is most likely to be found on farms and moving across country.

The black rat (also known as the ship rat) originated in India and spread along trading routes, especially maritime ones. It is commonly found in towns and in the temperate zone it does not move far from human dwellings, especially during the winter months, as the ambient temperature is too low outside. A variety of dates are given for its arrival in Europe. The evidence from analysis of the bones of rodents in carbon-dated[105] owl pellets, show that *Rattus rattus* was rare in Northern Europe in the fourteenth and fifteenth centuries,

---

105   Carbon dating utilises the rate at which radio-active carbon-14 decays. Living organisms take in carbon-14 during their lifetime. When they die the carbon-14 starts to decay and by measuring the amount of carbon-14 remaining, the length of time that has elapsed since death can be calculated. A number of correction factors are necessary, but the method

and was generally confined to small pockets around seaports and the rivers used for moving trade goods. If black rats and their fleas were responsible for the spread of the epidemic, it would not have spread either quickly or to more remote communities.

The rodents forming the resistant reservoir in Asia (e.g. marmots) have accommodated to bubonic plague and a relatively stable relationship between host and bacterium has developed. This enables the bacterium to survive over a long period and means that when the bacteria infect rats, a stable relationship is not essential to bacterial survival. The result is that epidemics of bubonic plague kill rats very quickly, and in percentage terms, even more rats die than humans.

In a number of recorded, authenticated instances of bubonic plague, mention is made of the large number of rats dying before humans became infected and also during the human epidemic. In both India and China, folklore had made the connection between dead rats and the human form of bubonic plague, and knew that when dead rats started to appear, it was time to flee. In contrast to this, there are hundreds of contemporary accounts of the Black Death in Europe between 1347 and 1500 and there is not a single mention of dead rats in any of them.

The Human

The fifth requirement for a human epidemic of bubonic plague is obviously humans. A human epidemic breaks out when fleas from the resistant rodent host (for example, marmots) attack domestic rodents (rats), and spread to humans when the domestic rodent dies. The rat is not a long-term reservoir as it is so susceptible and dies so rapidly. Occasionally rats are not involved in the process, and in these cases bubonic plague passes straight from the resistant rodent to humans. This has happened on a small scale on several occasions in the USA

---

allows the calculation of the time since death up to approximately 60,000 years. If an artefact is older than this, other methods must be used.

during the twentieth century when campers came into contact with infected ground squirrels. A large-scale example happened in 1910/11 when a large number of hunters, killing marmots for food and skins, caught bubonic plague in Mongolia.

In common with many other zoonotic diseases (diseases primarily of animals), bubonic plague is an extremely dangerous disease in humans causing a high mortality in those infected in the absence of antibiotics. The morbidity, that is the number infected, is however relatively low and typically an epidemic of bubonic plague only kills two to three per cent of the population. Plague can usually be treated successfully with antibiotics such as streptomycin or tetracycline, if it is diagnosed sufficiently early.

There are three classical manifestations of plague in humans. These are bubonic, pneumonic and septicaemic which makes recognition of the disease considerably more difficult. Bubonic and septicaemic plague are not distinct from each other; they differ only in intensity, the speed of infection and the mortality rate. In both cases, humans have been infected by the flea-borne route, and are not infectious to other humans in the absence of fleas. The symptom normally associated with bubonic plague is the bubo (derived from the Greek word for groin). This is a swelling of the lymph glands as they attempt to deal with the infection. Buboes usually appear in the groin, but may also be found in the armpit and on the neck; their size is variable and they generally appear on the second day of the infection. Arab doctors at the time of the Crusades considered that if the buboes were lanced, the patient generally stood a better chance of recovery (if the shock did not kill them).

The bodies of the victims of the Black Death frequently developed purple/black patches, known as *"God's tokens"*, according to contemporary accounts. These are due to the formation of multiple haemorrhages just below the skin. These symptoms are non-specific, being similar in a number of severe septicaemic diseases such as typhoid, typhus, haemorrhagic viral infections and some forms of anthrax. The only distinguishing feature of bubonic plague is the bubo. Contemporary descriptions of victims of the Black Death vary very considerably, with a large majority of them not mentioning buboes.

The incubation period is typically two to six days after exposure to the disease. Approximately fifty per cent of those with the bubonic form of plague will die in the absence of antibiotics within five or six days. Death is caused by the immense number of bacterial cells producing septicaemia and a toxic shock syndrome. If patients are still alive on the seventh or eighth day after the appearance of the symptoms, they have a reasonable chance of recovery.

Virtually everybody suffering from the septicaemic form of the disease will die in the absence of antibiotic therapy. Bubonic plague may become septicaemic, but usually septicaemic plague is present from the onset, and kills the victims rapidly, generally within three days. There are usually no buboes or they are very small, and the victim frequently dies before the symptoms become obvious. The number of cases progressing from bubonic plague to septicaemic plague is normally considered to be less than five per cent.

The third type of plague is the pneumonic form. In this case, the victim is bitten by a flea and initially develops either bubonic or septicaemic plague. In about five per cent of cases, the bacteria invade the lungs and when the patient coughs, the disease is spread to new victims by droplet infection. In this situation, the flea is not an intermediary and the onset of the disease is extremely rapid causing total collapse at a very early stage. The patient dies from respiratory distress within three to six days, usually earlier rather than later, and it is invariably fatal without antibiotic therapy. Pneumonic plague cannot occur in the absence of bubonic plague and cannot exist as an independent form of the disease. It is totally dependent on a primary case of bubonic or septicaemic plague started by the bite of an infected flea, and only appears in the terminal stages of the infection.

The epidemiology of plague is shown diagrammatically in Figure 9.1.

Figure 9.1. Epidemiology of Bubonic Plague

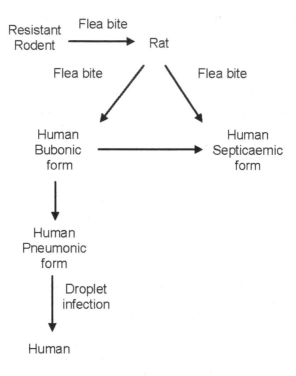

There appear to have been two historical origins of bubonic plague. One was in the foothills of the Himalayas and a second was in either modern-day Somalia or Ethiopia. A third centre developed in the steppes of central Asia at a later date, probably around the time of the Mongol Empire. After each outbreak, the microbe returns to the rodent reservoir but each time the area occupied by the infected reservoir increases, and the epicentre appears to shift slightly, probably due to the migration of the rodent population.

Between 1980 and 1996, over twenty-four thousand cases of authentic bubonic plague were reported to the WHO. This is almost certainly a considerable understatement, and in 1996 the WHO reclassified bubonic plague from dormant to an emerging disease. One recent outbreak in Madagascar involved *Y. pestis* resistant to five different antibiotics and recent outbreaks have also occurred in China and India.

THE HISTORY OF PLAGUE

Plague is buried deep in the psyche of Western Europe, and in England children still sing nursery rhymes about the Great Plague of London in 1665, although some authors claim that the poem was being sung before this date.

> *Ring a ring of rosies,*
> *A pocket full of posies,*
> *Atishoo atishoo,*
> *We all fall down.*

The *"ring of rosies"* is the development of spots caused by the subcutaneous haemorrhages. The *"pocket full of posies"* relates to the belief that the disease could be kept at bay by a pomander of sweet smelling herbs and flowers; *"atishoo"* is the sneezing frequently associated with the disease and *"all fall down"* is death.

The first reference to possible bubonic plague may have been made as early as 1500 BC in Indian epics, although the descriptions are very vague. Much later, Rufus of Ephesus, who was writing at the end of the first century AD, described an epidemic alleged to have been plague that occurred in Egypt and North Africa in the third century BC. There is also a reference in the Bible (1st Book of Samuel) that some authors think may have been plague. However, no Egyptian mummies have been found that show signs of plague, and there is no reference to any disease showing the characteristic features of the Plague of Justinian or the Black Death in any of the Egyptian medical papyri. Hippocrates and Galen do not mention it either.

THE PLAGUE OF JUSTINIAN

The Plague of Justinian, that started in 542 AD and lasted intermittently until the middle of the eighth century, was the first relatively well-documented pandemic of the Old World. The symptoms of the disease started as a slight fever, but progressed to coma and death. The similarity between this and the Great Pestilence (Black Death) have convinced some authors that it was bubonic plague although this of course makes the assumption that the Great Pestilence was also bubonic plague. The little we know about the clinical features of the Plague of Justinian are common to several epidemic diseases, and the very high mortality and rapid spread suggest that it may not have been bubonic plague, but some disease spread from person to person by droplet infection.

Although it is impossible to reach a definitive figure for the number killed by the Plague of Justinian, some authors claim that there were thirty to forty million dead in Western Europe alone, whilst other sources suggest as many as one hundred million died. The generally accepted mortality is towards the lower end of the figures given. Whilst not all authors agree about the scale of the devastation, many historians consider that the demographic effects of the Plague of Justinian, and the epidemics that followed, were greater than those of the Black Death in the fourteenth century. The contemporary sources available suggest that the death toll could have been as high as fifty per cent of the population.

The Plague of Justinian tends to be the forgotten pandemic and relatively few people know about it. Probably the only monument remaining to it is the statue of Saint Michael, the captain of the heavenly host, on top of Hadrian's mausoleum, now the Castel Sant' Angelo in Rome. In 590 AD, there was a massive outbreak of the disease in Rome, and Pope

Gregory the Great led a procession through the city pleading for divine intervention. The Archangel Michael is alleged to have appeared and slain the disease with a sword and is now commemorated by the statue.

Keys has written a very readable description of the historical effects of the epidemic, which the following account draws on. Keys does however make the assumption that it was bubonic plague. A number of historians do not agree with his analysis, much of which they claim is speculation. However, Keys, who is archaeology correspondent for a London newspaper, makes a very creditable attempt to marshal a large number of disparate events, all of them occurring within a relatively short period of time, and link them to a single cause.

By the fourth century AD, the Roman Empire had split into two, the Eastern or Byzantine Empire based on Constantinople (Byzantium) and the Western Empire based on Rome. The Western Empire was overrun in the fifth century by various Central and Eastern European tribes, the Huns, Vandals and Goths being the most important. Rome itself was sacked by the Visigoths under Alaric in 410 AD. By 425, the Byzantine Empire was paying the Huns protection money that, within a decade, had risen to over a ton of gold per annum, a huge drain on the treasury. In 434, Attila, the Scourge of God, became King of the Huns and in 450, he launched an attack on the Western Empire that reached the gates of Rome, but then turned back because of an epidemic that may have been smallpox. The Hun threat effectively vanished with the death of Attila in 453, but the tribes subject to the Huns revolted and destroyed the Western Empire. Rome was sacked again by the Vandals in 455, who also conquered Spain and went on to form a kingdom in North Africa. The Goths finally destroyed the Western Empire in 476, and by the early part of the sixth century, the Ostrogoth king, Theodoric the Great, who died in 526, ruled the whole of Italy, much of the Balkans and also acted as regent in Spain for a young relative.

The Byzantine Empire survived, and prospered under the reign of Anastasius I, who died in 518 without naming an heir. After considerable political manoeuvring, Justin was named emperor, although his nephew Justinian was effectively the power behind the throne. Justinian[106] became emperor on the death of his uncle in 527 and slowly commenced the re-conquest of the Western Empire.

It has been speculated that it was this epidemic which probably prevented Justinian from re-establishing the whole Roman Empire, and which finalised the collapse of the Western Roman Empire and the onset of the Dark Ages in Western Europe. Justinian himself was a victim of the disease but recovered.

The empire's best general, Belisarius, who was born around 505, took command of the Byzantine army and in his first battle at Dara, in 530, he smashed the Persian army which heavily outnumbered the Byzantine one[107] [108]. In 533, his army destroyed the Vandal kingdom in North Africa, capturing their capital Carthage easily. Procopius, in his *"History of the Wars"*, cites it as an example of barbarians being softened and seduced by civilisation and easy living.

By late 535, Belisarius had captured Sicily from the Ostrogoths, and in early 536, he crossed into Italy and besieged Naples, which he finally seized by sending his army into the city through a disused aqueduct. He captured Rome in December 536, and this was followed by the fall of the Ostrogoth capital, Ravenna. Belisarius was forced to return to Constantinople after Justinian became suspicious of his motives and thought he

---

106   Justinian wrote his own constitution *"Deo Auctore"* (By God's Authority) and instigated a wide-ranging code of laws that influenced European laws for centuries. He was also notorious for the ruthless efficiency of his tax-raising bureaucracy.

107   By this time, the Roman army had changed from the traditional infantryman in the legion to heavily armoured cavalry, known as cataphracts, on armoured horses, firing compound bows from the saddle.

108   Persia had been the eastern limit of the Roman Empire for centuries and wars between Rome and Persia were a regular feature of the area.

was conspiring to gain the purple. Given the imperial paranoia of the time, Belisarius was probably fortunate to keep his life. The removal of Belisarius allowed the Goths to regroup, and in 542 they started to reconquer Italy. They were finally defeated by another Byzantine general, a eunuch named Narses, who won a number of battles against them in the 550s.

Our main source of information is Procopious of Caesarea, an administrator in the Byzantine Empire living in Constantinople during the reign of Justinian. He acted as secretary to Belisarius and wrote an account of his conquests known as the "*History of the Wars*" [109]. At one point of his account he states, "*during these times there was a pestilence, by which the whole human race came close to being annihilated...... it started from the Egyptians who live in Pelusium*". Pelusium is close to Alexandria, which at the time was one of the largest ports on the Mediterranean coast and exported huge quantities of grain from Egypt to Constantinople and Rome. As mentioned earlier, diseases tended to move by sea trading routes and frequently appeared first in ports.

Early Arab physicians however, suggested it started in Ethiopia or the Sudan in 540 AD. There are also suggestions that it may have caused severe epidemics in many of the Arab trading ports on the east coast of Africa, and then crossed the Red Sea and caused a serious epidemic in the Yemen, which at that time was a powerful trading empire in Arabia. Once plague reached the Byzantine Empire, it would have caused a major epidemic in an urbanised population with no previous experience of the disease.

When the epidemic started in Constantinople, too many people died for them all to be buried, so bodies were

---

[109]   He also wrote a secret diary, the *Anekdota,* which was not rediscovered until 1683 in the archives of the Vatican. In this, he reveals much of the scandal of sixth century Constantinople, including the fact that the Empress Theodora was a prostitute before Justinian married her. If this diary had been discovered during her lifetime, it is reasonable to suppose that Procopius would have died very slowly and extremely painfully.

thrown into the towers of the city's fortifications until they were full, and finally boats were loaded with corpses, towed out to sea, and the dead were dumped overboard. Procopius claimed that approximately forty per cent of the population of Constantinople died (at the rate of ten thousand per day at the height of the epidemic), out of a total population estimated at half a million.

There are a number of contemporary accounts in addition to that of Procopius. Before discussing these, it is worth noting that neither Procopius nor any of the other writers mention dead rats. John of Ephesus gives rather higher figures than Procopius for the number of dead. He claimed that in Constantinople, officials at the city gates counted the dead as they were removed, reaching 16,000 in a single day. John stated that over 300,000 bodies were removed from the city, and that the official count was abandoned at 230,000. He wrote that the dead were piled up on the seashore like flotsam, boats were filled with corpses that were thrown overboard into the Bosphorus and the Sea of Marmara, and the ships returned to take others. When Justinian ordered the building of mass graves, John wrote that bodies were laid on top of each other like hay in a stack. Another writer wrote of a disease that, *"turned the country into a desert and made the habitations of men to become the haunts of wild beasts"*.

Another contemporary account is given by Evagrius, who was born around 535 AD, and lived through the Plague of Justinian and many of the following less severe epidemics. Evagrius caught the disease and recovered but lost most of his family. He stated that the epidemic started in Ethiopia and wrote that some cities lost virtually all their population. He also left us considerable information about the spread of the disease, claiming that there were many ways of catching it; these included physical contact or being in the vicinity of sick people. Some people (carriers?) remained unaffected in spite of being in close contact with the sick, but passed the disease to others. He also claims that some people caught the disease once or twice and recovered, then caught it a third time and died. If this last statement is correct, it strongly suggests the series of epidemics following the Plague of Justinian were not all the same.

Evagrius suggested the epidemic started in Ethiopia, which at this time was a major trading centre for Yemeni merchants buying slaves and exotic items such as ivory. A number of trading centres are mentioned in Ptolemy's *"Geography"*, such as Opone, Essina and Toniki, whose whereabouts are not known today, but they were probably on the coasts of present day Somalia, Kenya or Tanzania. The trade ceased in the mid-sixth century and the Yemen collapsed as a trading centre around the same time.

Yemen had been a powerful political force in the Arabian Peninsula for about a thousand years until its collapse, making up approximately half of the population of the peninsula. Yemeni prosperity was based on the Dam of Marib, in the interior of the country, which supplied water to a large irrigation system. The dam had been there for a considerable time as it is mentioned by Strabo, writing in the first century AD. Marib was the capital of the kingdom of Saba (thought to be the kingdom of Sheba mentioned in the Bible).

The dam was a major piece of engineering, its dimensions have been given as seventeen metres high, seven hundred metres long and sixty-five metres wide at the base. It was breached several times in the mid-sixth century with large numbers of labourers being required to repair it. Over time there was severe silting up, a reduction in the amount of water retained and hence the area of land that could be irrigated. The dam finally collapsed in 590 AD and was abandoned. This loss destroyed the irrigation system and the agricultural economy, and the local tribes migrated northwards towards Medina. The destruction of the dam came at the same time as a collapse of the trade in frankincense, of which Saba had a near monopoly.

This was due to a rise in the Christian practice of burial rather than the Roman practice of cremation.

The fall of Yemen created a power vacuum in the Arabian Peninsula and political power shifted to Medina and ultimately Islam. There is a reference to plague in the Koran, which describes the fate of a Christian Ethiopian army attacking Medina in the War of the White Elephant during the mid-sixth century. An Arab historian, Ibn Ishaq, who described this war, stated that the enemy perished at every waterhole, and their leader died with sores oozing pus and blood. This is reminiscent of some of the details given by Thucydides in his description of the Plague of Athens. The identity of the disease is not known, although some authors claim it was smallpox rather than plague.

Justinian died in 565, the year that plague returned on a large scale. He was succeeded by his nephew who was mad and a series of weak emperors, the worst of whom was Phocas, whom many historians consider to be as great a tyrant as Nero or Caligula.

During the early seventh century, war broke out between the Byzantine and Persian Empires. The Persians were successful in capturing much of the Empire including Jerusalem, Egypt, Libya and Syria, whilst the Avars and their Slav subjects (nomadic tribes from the steppes) captured the Balkans and Italy was conquered by the Lombards.

The Emperor Heraclius, who replaced Phocas, re-organised both the army and the finances of the empire, and was able to recapture territory in Western Asia and North Africa in 626 AD. By 630 however, the Byzantine and Persian Empires were exhausted, both financially and in terms of manpower. There had been four major epidemics between 542 and the first few decades of the seventh century, plus numerous smaller ones, and the population had been reduced significantly. Disease had reduced the tax base of the Byzantine Empire, and the emperors were also paying protection money to the Avars[110].

110   The silk trade was also costing the Byzantine Empire vast sums

Further revenue losses were due to the loss of land. Over a period of fifteen years it is estimated that the imperial treasury lost seventy per cent of its income. The loss of manpower meant that by 630 AD, the Empire could only field an army of less than forty per cent of its size in the early sixth century.

Within five years of the end of the Byzantine-Persian war, the Islamic religion appeared. Within twenty years its adherents had destroyed the Persian Empire, reduced the Byzantine one to a fraction of its original area, and created an empire stretching from the Atlantic to India. This was ironic considering that both the Byzantines and Persians had trained the Arab tribes in warfare, supplied them with weapons and used them in a series of proxy wars in the Arabian Peninsula.

The prophet Mohammed, the founder of Islam, was born into an influential family in Mecca about 570 AD. At around the age of forty, he had a vision of the Archangel Gabriel as a result of which he started to preach the philosophy of only one God. Mohammed was eventually driven out of Mecca and fled to Medina in 622 AD, where he found support for his ideas. He returned to Mecca at the head of an army in 630 and died there in 632 AD.

The first clashes between the Muslims and the Byzantine Empire came in 629 AD. In 633 the Muslim armies attacked the Persian and Byzantine empires and won a number of battles leading to the temporary occupation of Damascus. In 636 AD, the Byzantine army was effectively destroyed at the battle of Yarmuk. Byzantine power in the Middle East virtually collapsed, and the Muslims occupied Syria and Palestine, and captured Jerusalem.

They invaded the Persian Empire in 637, overran most of Iraq, and by 640 the Persian Empire had been destroyed, and the Byzantine coastal cities of Caesarea and Ascalon occupied. By 642 Egypt had been captured, resulting in the Byzantine Empire losing a major source of its revenue and its main

of money. The western end of the Silk Road was in the hands of Persian middlemen who charged very heavily for Chinese silk passing through their hands. At this time, China was the only source of silk.

source of grain. The Islamic armies reached the borders of India in the east in 652 and had crossed into India by the early eighth century. They also continued westwards from Egypt, through North Africa, and then into Spain, occupying most of it, except the Kingdom of Asturias and the Basque region by 711. Their expansion continued deep into France, until they were defeated at the battle of Tours (732) by the Franks led by Charles Martel (Charles the Hammer), grandfather of Charlemagne. The Muslims suffered further defeats at the hands of Charlemagne who effectively drove them out of Northern Spain in 778[111]. He then defeated the Avar kingdom and inflicted a number of defeats on the Saxons.

Charlemagne was crowned Emperor by the Pope on Christmas Day in the year 800, thus finalising the split between the Eastern and Western Roman Empires, and laying the foundations of the Holy Roman Empire[112]. Some historians are of the opinion that Charlemagne made a serious error of judgement allowing the Pope to crown him, as it led to the subjugation of the secular authority in Western Europe to the church for centuries. Constantine the Great had made the same mistake several centuries earlier and Charlemagne reinforced it.

Reoccurrences of the Plague of Justinian flared up all over the Eastern Empire and Southern Europe at frequent intervals until about 590 AD. There were then small outbreaks for approximately 150 years, compounded by epidemics of other diseases such as smallpox. These small outbreaks occurred at

---

111 The period associated with the legends of Roland, Oliver, the twelve paladins of France, the horn of Roland and the battle at the Pass of Roncevalles. Although *La Chanson de Roland* claims the Moors were the enemy, some sources claim the rearguard of the Frankish army, commanded by Roland, was actually destroyed by the Basques.

112 Voltaire (1694-1778) wrote in 1756, *"This agglomeration which was called and still calls itself the Holy Roman Empire was neither holy, nor Roman and not even an empire"*. Whilst Voltaire may have been correct with these comments, the Holy Roman Empire was effectively the First Reich, and as such acted as a model for much of the Second Reich (Kaiser Wilhelm II [Kaiser Bill]) and the Third Reich (Hitler).

intervals, generally the longer the interval the more serious the outbreak when it occurred, and the greater the mortality rate. The worst attacks appear to have taken place in the Mediterranean, which contained numerous trading centres and it was this area that took the longest time to recover. This prolonged series of epidemics appears to have had a proportionally greater effect on the population of Southern Europe than the Black Death, nearly eight hundred years later. The population died faster than it could be replaced, and it is estimated that the population of Western Europe in 600 AD had fallen by about fifty per cent compared with the population of the Roman Empire at its peak.

Muslim sources gave the series of epidemics that followed the Plague of Justinian names to differentiate them, the Plague of Shirawayh occurred in 627-8, the Plague of Amwas 638-9, the Violent Plague 688-9, the Plague of Maidens 706, the Plague of Notables 716-7 and they regarded the Black Death as the sixth. Some of these were obviously very serious. The Violent Plague was alleged to have killed two hundred thousand people in the Basra area in three days, although the numbers are impossible to verify. One major difference between the Muslim and Christian reactions to plague was that Muslims believed that it was sent to a specific individual by God, and it was therefore useless to flee from an infected area. Because of this belief, Islam also rejected the theory of contagion for the transmission of plague or any other disease, a rejection that later hindered the development of Islamic medicine for centuries.

There were also numerous epidemics of one type or another in Northern Europe. Anglo-Saxon sources mention approximately fifty epidemics occurring in England over a period of five and a half centuries, but their identity is not obvious. In 731, The Venerable Bede (672-735) mentions in his *"Ecclesiastical History of the English People"* an epidemic in the mid-sixth century which *"raged far and wide... and ravaged*

England and Ireland cruelly", and claims that at the time of Vortigen, the King of the Britons, there were hardly enough men left to bury the dead.

Saxon raids on England had started before the end of the Roman era in Britain (which finished when the legions were withdrawn in the first decade of the fifth century). The extent of these raids was such that the Romans constructed a series of defensive fortresses, across South-eastern England from Rochester to Barchester, commanded by a general with the title, Count of the Saxon Shore. The role of these huge buildings has been disputed and it has been claimed that they were fortified granaries for supplying grain to Roman troops operating in Northern France. The main Saxon incursions started between 420-450 AD, when a number of Saxons were initially invited into the country by Celtic kings such as Vortigern, who hired them as mercenaries to defend Northern England against the Picts.

Initially the Saxons were concentrated on the east coast of England, whilst the western side of Britain was occupied by people of Romano-Celtic origin. There was little evidence of trade or any contact between the east and west sides of Britain, which at that time was heavily forested. In his short book, *"De Excidio et Conquestu Britanniae"* (Concerning the Ruin and Fall of Britain), written about 540, the Celtic monk Gildas writes of the Saxons as *"hated by men and God"*. Gildas is one of a very small number of near contemporary accounts that we have of Britain in the early years after the Roman occupation, although even he was writing the best part of a century after many of the events he records occurred. He claimed he was born in the year of the battle of Mount Badon (Mons Badonicus), the suggested dates of which range from 490-520, with most scholars suggesting the year 500 AD[113]. Gildas, who is sometimes referred to as Gildas sapiens (Gildas the wise), unfortunately does not write as a historian, but as

---

113   The site of this battle is extremely controversial. Wales, Scotland and Northern England have all been suggested. The balance of opinion would seem to favour the Scottish Lowlands.

an angry monk with a serious political agenda. His work is mainly an attack on the Celtic kings of Britain for deviating from the path of God, moral laxity, tyranny and inviting the Saxons into the country.

Saxon penetration of England had been stopped by the early sixth century, the period associated with the semi-legendary figure of Arthur Pendragon (King Arthur)[114]. Modern opinion suggests he may have been a Celtic warlord who defeated the Saxons at a number of battles. Nennius, a ninth century monk who wrote *"Historia Britonum"*, links Arthur to a series of twelve battles culminating in Mons Badonicus, a major victory for the Celts. Nennius unfortunately cannot be relied on, one historian describes him as *"unrestrainedly inventive"*, and his account claims that Arthur killed nine hundred and forty Saxons with his own hand. He does however, appear to have had access to fifth and sixth century sources that no longer exist, and as another historian puts it, " *he can neither be trusted nor dismissed"*.

Curiously, Gildas does not mention Arthur; there are several possibilities for this. The most obvious explanation is that Arthur did not exist but twelfth century sources claim Arthur executed Huail, the older brother of Gildas, for refusing to accept him as overlord. It has also been claimed that Arthur levied taxes on the monasteries, presumably to support his war-band. It has to be remembered that the monks were amongst the few people who were literate at this time, and it is possible that Gildas took his revenge in the best way possible; he wrote Arthur out of history.

114　　The legends of King Arthur and the Knights of the Round Table owe their existence to the book *"Historia regum Britannia"* (History of the Kings of Britain), a fictional account written by the cleric, Geoffrey of Monmouth, between 1135 and 1139. Where Geoffrey obtained his material is debatable. Many scholars consider it to be a fictional account based on his imagination, but Geoffrey himself claims it was a translation of a book given to him by his friend, Walter the Archdeacon. Geoffrey describes the book as *"a certain very ancient book written in the British language* (Welsh)" which he translated into Latin.

In the early seventh century, the Saxons started an aggressive expansion policy into western Britain as the demographic effects of various epidemics were felt. The Celts of Britain were trading widely with continental Europe, especially Celtic Brittany and northern Spain, areas suffering from widespread epidemics. Pottery found at Tintagel, the area traditionally associated with Arthur (although the castle is Norman and was built approximately 800 years later), has been shown to have a Byzantine origin, and has been dated to the period 530-560AD[115]. These dates correlate with the appearance of the Plague of Justinian in the British Isles.

The Saxons, on the other hand, were trading with northern Germany and the Baltic region that were initially free of serious epidemics. The result was epidemic diseases that spread from Europe to the Celtic population of western Britain, causing a crash in population in the mid-sixth century. This was approximately two generations before the Saxons started to suffer from a serious loss of manpower due to epidemics. The demographic changes allowed the Saxons to invade western Britain successfully between about 550 and 650 AD, eventually isolating the Celtic kingdoms of Wales, South-west England and North-west England from each other. Wales, for example, was separated from South-west England following the battle of Dyrham (577), about eight miles from Bristol, which allowed the Saxons to reach the Severn estuary.

Evidence for these epidemics comes from both written and archaeological sources. The Plague of Justinian reached Celtic Britain around the middle of the sixth century and both the Annals of Wales and the Annals of Ulster refer to a series of plagues. The Annals of Wales state that in 547, there was *"a great plague in which Maelgwn King of Gwynedd died. Then there was the yellow plague"*. In 682 the entry reads *"A great plague in which Cadwallader, son of Cadwallon died"* whilst in 683 the statement occurs *"a plague was in Ireland"*.

---

115   Some people such as potters have a disproportionally large effect on the archaeological record.

Archaeological evidence shows that many Celtic communities appear to have collapsed in the middle to late-sixth century. Many smaller communities disappeared completely, whilst larger ones suffered a major reduction in numbers. Some authors assume that because small communities disappeared during both the Plague of Justinian and the Black Death, that the inhabitants had been totally destroyed by the epidemic but this is not necessarily correct. It is more likely that many of the smaller communities had been reduced to a point where the settlement was no longer demographically or financially viable, and the survivors just abandoned it.

Returning to Celtic Britain, according to one Celtic source, the capital of Cynddylan, King of Powys was destroyed by Saxons around 642, whilst in the North of England, the Celtic kingdoms of Rheged and Elmet disappeared in the late sixth century, and the Celtic warrior/poet, Aneirin, describes the Battle of Cartreath (Catterick), in which he claims he was the only Celtic survivor[116]. Numerous clashes in the late sixth century are also mentioned in the Anglo-Saxon chronicles.

By about 650, the Saxon take-over of England was virtually complete, except for a few mountainous regions and some areas of marginal land, and over the next four centuries, England evolved from a series of small petty kingdoms, with shifting power relationships, into a single kingdom.

The takeover was so effective, that if the English language is examined today, some 1,400 years after these events, over a

---

116   The battle is thought to have been fought between the dates of 570 and 600 AD and is described in the epic poem *"Y Gododdin"* written in Old Welsh. The Gododdin are thought to be the Celtic tribe referred to by the Romans as the Votadini whose capital town was Din Eidyn (Edinburgh). Aneirin describes a year-long feast for three hundred warriors before they attacked a numerically superior Saxon army. Only a single copy of the poem survived. It is thought to have been written by two scribes, sometime during the ninth or tenth centuries, and based on earlier oral tradition. One stanza mentions Arthur, although it is not certain whether this was inserted at a later date. Din Eidyn was captured by the Saxons in 638 and incorporated into the Saxon kingdom of Northumbria.

third of English words come from a Germanic rootstock, and so does virtually all the syntax of the English language. The words that come from a Germanic origin are also the most basic and widely used words in English, words such as why, what, who, where, when, which, while and how[117]. A few place names incorporating Celtic roots survive such as Sherburn in Elmet in Yorkshire and Pen-y-ghent, but very few words of Celtic origin are found in English, and those that are, such as "eisteddfod", have been imported in the last hundred years or so. This would strongly suggest that the Celts were totally dispossessed and not assimilated into Saxon society.

The effects of these epidemics were not felt in Northern Germany and Scandinavia to anything like the same extent, and it was presumably population pressures that had led to the Saxon immigration into England in the fifth and sixth centuries. Similarly, a large increase in the Scandinavian population precipitated the Viking raids of the eighth, ninth and tenth centuries, eventually leading to the Norse settlement of much of Western Europe. The archaeology of grave-sites suggests that the Vikings of this period were considerably more robust physically than people from much of the rest of Europe. The Viking period reached its zenith with the establishment of the Empire of the Northern Seas under Knut (Canute) in the eleventh century.

Similar effects were seen in Ireland. There were severe crop failures and famine from the mid 530s, and a series of major epidemics in the decade 545-555 AD. The Annals of Ulster mention a *"Failure of Bread"* in 539 and *"The first mortality called Bléfed"* in 544 AD. There are further references to a great mortality in the year 549 and again in 556. Many Irish records mention the Yellow Plague, and massive population

---

117   As Kipling put it;

"I have six honest serving men,
They taught me all I knew,
Their names are what and why and when
And where and how and who".

crashes occurred, accompanied by power shifts between the various clans following numerous battles. One record states that an epidemic in 545 killed three kings, numerous princes, bishops and abbots, and one saint! It is reasonable to assume that if it killed so many high-ranking individuals, then the effect on the peasantry would have been devastating. Given the date mentioned, it is almost certainly the Plague of Justinian.

Archaeology suggests that there were significant changes in life style during this period, with many communities building defensive fortifications that are not seen during the excavation of earlier sites. Following the epidemics, a series of great monastic houses were founded, such as the one at Clonfert in 563 AD, presumably in the hope of divine intervention. These became important centres of Celtic culture and art, giving rise to masterpieces such as the Book of Kells[118]. As a result of these monastic foundations, Ireland became an important centre of learning and Christianity in Western Europe during the Dark Ages.

It is possible that the severe outbreak of disease which reached Scotland around 544, facilitated the task of missionaries such as St Columba, who came from a noble Irish family. He arrived in Iona in 560 AD, to convert the pagans to Christianity, as the old gods were seen as powerless to halt the wave of epidemics and associated deaths. The Abbot of Iona (The Holy Island) wrote of *"a great mortality which has ravaged the world twice in our time"*.

Many historians assume that the Plague of Justinian was bubonic plague, but there is no definite evidence to prove that it was. At this time, the tropical black rat and its associated fleas, the main vectors for bubonic plague, would not have been present in Northern Europe as it was an exceptionally cold period, and evidence for epidemics of bubonic plague in Northern Europe is weak. The assumption that the Plague of

---

118   There is some evidence that the Book of Kells may have been written in Iona, and sent to Ireland for safety when the Viking raids started on the west coast and islands of Scotland.

Justinian was bubonic plague is based on its similarity to the Black Death, but this makes the assumption that the Black Death was also bubonic plague, an assertion that is being increasingly challenged.

The disease also travelled to India, China and Persia, reaching China in 610 AD where reoccurring epidemics lasted for 200 years. Contemporary Chinese writers refer to it as being common in Canton and the surrounding area, but rare in the interior provinces leading to the supposition that it travelled to China by sea, which fits in with the known epidemiology of the disease in Europe. No estimates of the number of dead in China are available, but contemporary literature suggests they were extremely large with over half the population of some provinces dying in a series of epidemics beginning in 762 AD. This outbreak, which occurred during a major army revolt that began in 755 AD, reduced the manpower in the coastal provinces that remained loyal to the emperor so severely, that he was forced to rely on nomadic mercenaries from the steppes to deal with the revolt. This theme reoccurs at regular intervals in Chinese history.

A major epidemic started in Japan in 808 AD killing over half the population. No description of the disease is given in contemporary literature, but given the date, the proximity of Japan to China and the severity of the epidemic, it was presumably the same epidemic that attacked China and Europe.

The epidemic disappeared in the eighth century in Europe. The last mention of it in Byzantine literature is 767 AD, but the same or a very similar disease reappeared as the Great Pestilence in the mid-fourteenth century.

Some authors have attempted to link significant climatic changes of the mid-sixth century with the Plague of Justinian. Dendrochronology (the study of tree rings) and ice cores from both Greenland and the Antarctic, show that the Earth underwent a series of very cold summers during the period 536-540, and the few contemporary documents available in

Europe record widespread crop failures and frosts with snow in mid-summer.

Two theories have been suggested to explain this cold period. One of them suggests the cause is the explosion of a large comet or asteroid in the Earth's upper atmosphere whose debris blotted out the heat of the sun. Procopius mentions a comet seen for more than forty days in the year 539 AD, and the Celtic mythology of the period frequently mentions comets and fiery dragons flying through the sky. Other authors, especially Keys, have attempted to link the outbreak of the Plague of Justinian with a huge volcanic explosion (probably Krakatoa) that occurred in the East Indies in 536 AD[119]. Procopius wrote of an entire year (536/7) when *"the sun gave forth light without brightness"*, a statement reminiscent of the year 1816 (known as the *"year without a summer"*), after the volcano Tambura in Indonesia exploded. Keys however, makes the assumption that the Plague of Justinian was bubonic plague, and that the climatic changes caused by this event were responsible for the mass migration of rodents in East Africa, where they formed the focal point of the pandemic.

THE BLACK DEATH

The third great epidemic, usually associated with bubonic plague, was the Black Death. From contemporary fourteenth and fifteenth century accounts, it was obviously seen as a catastrophic event. Many historians from the eighteenth century however, regarded it as a minor event, but by the mid-nineteenth century, most writers regarded it as being of major importance. One author in 1844 described it as *"a convulsion of the human race, unequalled in violence and extent"*, whilst others have called it *"the crucible of the modern world"*. Shrewsbury, writing in 1970 (*"History of Bubonic Plague in the British Isles"*), claimed that the effect had been greatly over-rated, but McNeill writing a few years later did not agree, considering

---

119   The eruption was even more violent than the 1883 eruption of Krakatoa, one of the largest of recent times. It is thought to have blown what was previously one large island into the two modern islands of Java and Sumatra.

it a major epidemic. Gottfried called it, *"the greatest biological environmental event in human history"*. This is perhaps phrasing it too strongly when one considers the effects of the Plague of Justinian. Although there has been controversy over the effect of the Black Death, it is obvious a society cannot lose one-third of its population in a period of about thirty months without some drastic consequences.

Interestingly, most authors recognise that there are a number of major anomalies between the behaviour of the Black Death and modern day bubonic plague, but do not consider the possibility that the Black Death may not have been bubonic plague.

The involvement of bubonic plague in the Black Death, the Great Plague of London, and numerous other epidemics between the fourteenth and seventeenth centuries, was first suggested by the German epidemiologist, August Hirsch, in the nineteenth century, and has been accepted by most people since the early 1900s. This suggestion was based on the one fact that a few contemporary accounts of the Black Death mention buboes. A careful examination of this hypothesis suggests that many historians and scientists have adapted the other facts to fit this suggestion, rather than building a theory to fit the all known facts. In some cases, the people involved have recognised that the available evidence is not compatible with bubonic plague as the cause of these epidemics, but, rather than challenge perceived wisdom, they have introduced various extraneous features and special pleadings to paper over the cracks.

The name, Black Death, only came into common usage in the nineteenth century, in medieval, Tudor and Stuart times it was known as *pestis magna* (great pestilence) or *pestis atra* (terrible pestilence)[120]. The disease was assumed to be bubonic plague solely on the basis of the appearance of the victims. There are, however, a number of diseases that present with very similar clinical symptoms, and, as mentioned earlier,

120   It is still known as "la peste" in France.

contemporary accounts of the appearance of the victims are by no means consistent.

At the beginning of the twelfth century, the population of Europe and the Mediterranean region began to grow. Political stability increased and a middle class started to appear. There were improvements in agriculture with the introduction of windmills and waterwheels. Horses started to replace oxen for ploughing, allowing greater areas to be ploughed as horses are faster and the horse collar plough came into use, allowing the ploughing of much heavier land. Many major epidemic diseases had subsided to childhood infections indicating that the population was acquiring "herd resistance" as it became more disease experienced. Much of the belligerency of Western Europe was siphoned off to the Near East by the Crusades, and no major new diseases appeared after these expeditions, suggesting that the disease pools of the Near East had merged with those of Western Europe. The populations of France and Germany grew and reached population densities not seen again until the nineteenth century.

There were problems, much of the farming in Western Europe was based on a small number of cereal crops with a yield-to-input ratio as low as 2-3 to 1. Obviously, crop yields as poor as this leave very little margin for survival if anything goes wrong. Starting in 1290, there were three and a half decades of poor summers and cold winters causing crop failures and widespread famine. In 1300 AD, the Little Ice Age started in Europe[124], which would have had a major impact on the yields of wheat. In 1315-6, there was a terrible famine referred to as the Great Famine, and the weather of 1346-1348 was

---

121   The dates for the Little Ice Age are controversial. It is generally accepted that it ended in the mid-nineteenth century, however the dates suggested for its start vary widely. In 1250, the glaciers of Northern Europe started to advance as did the pack ice in the north Atlantic. About 1300, the summer weather in Europe became less dependable leading to very poor harvests. A very cold period occurred around 1500 and all these dates are quoted by various authors as the start date. The Little Ice Age reached its peak during the mid-seventeenth century.

extremely bad with a succession of very cold, wet summers. Contemporary sources claim that the harvest of 1346 was the worst for a quarter of a century and the one of 1347 was not much better, leading to large rises in the price of food, especially cereal crops. There were also serious epidemics (murrains) amongst livestock leading to substantial losses. This is of course remarkably similar in climatic terms to the weather preceding the Plague of Justinian, and the widespread crop failures would have meant people were poorly nourished when the Black Death arrived. The poor harvests also meant less paid work for labourers, which meant less money to pay for what little food was available and poor families slipped even closer to the margin of survival.

These problems were compounded by a series of small wars in Europe, a typical example being the Hundred Years War that broke out in 1337, when King Edward III of England laid claim to the throne of France. Whilst several major battles were fought over this period, Crecy, Poitiers and Agincourt being the main ones, the war mainly degenerated into widespread raiding and looting, causing general havoc over a wide area of France. There were also problems in the north of England and an invading Scots army was defeated at Neville's Cross in 1346.

A much more serious problem was the development of the Mongol Empire. This empire started in the early thirteenth century when the Mongol leader, Genghis Khan (1162-1227 AD), conquered the warring tribes of the Gobi desert and welded them into a single force. Under his grandson Kublai Khan (1215-1294), a huge empire developed covering China, most of the Middle East and much of Russia. Communications throughout the empire were carried by relays of horsemen who frequently covered great distances in very short periods of time. This allowed a much more rapid transmission of disease than was possible by slow camel caravans using trade routes such as the Silk Road. Although the Silk Road between

China and the Middle East had existed for centuries, the Mongols also made extensive use of more northerly routes over the steppes. It is possible that this network of messengers or caravans allowed bubonic plague to infiltrate the steppes and their rodent population, and become established permanently in this area. Some authors have suggested that the epidemic of the fourteenth century may have started in the steppes of Central Asia, although there have also been suggestions that it started when the Mongol armies attempted to penetrate into South East Asia, specifically Burma.

By the 1330s, a major epidemic was spreading across the Asian landmass, being compounded in China by a series of earthquakes, droughts, floods, and famines. The ethnic Chinese were also revolting against their Mongol overlords, further exacerbating problems, and by 1340 Arab historians were referring to widespread plague in the East.

It has been proposed that the loss of manpower was a major factor in the sudden collapse of the Mongol Empire in the second half of the fourteenth century, a theory supported by the patterns of migration in the western steppes. Before the massive population losses of the fourteenth century, the nomadic populations of the western steppes were always moving into the agricultural regions of Western Europe adjacent to the steppes. Early examples are the Scythians, Magyars, Avars and Huns, and ultimately the Ottomans. By the sixteenth century however, this migration had reversed and farmers were moving into the western steppes, especially on the Russian borders.

Many authors consider that the European outbreak of plague started in 1346 at Caffa [Kaffa] (modern Feodosia) in the Crimea. Recent work however suggests that this may be merely coincidental. Caffa, a Genoese colony and port central to the Genoese trading empire on the Black Sea, was besieged by the Tartars (part of the Mongol army known as the Golden Horde). When disease broke out in the Tartar army, forcing their retreat, their Khan, Janibeg, ordered diseased corpses to be hurled into the city using catapults, an early example of germ warfare. de Mussis claimed *"what seemed like mountains of dead were thrown into the city"*. The Genoese dumped the corpses into the sea as fast as they came over the walls, but in a besieged city the result was almost inevitable. The Genoese fled from the city and were alleged to have carried the disease to Sicily and Genoa by ship and by 1347 it was widespread in Southern Europe. From the Mediterranean it rapidly spread to most of the rest of Europe reaching England in 1348 and Norway in 1349.

The Muslim writer Ibn-al-Wardi, who lived in the caravan city of Aleppo claimed that plague started in the Land of Darkness and spread from there to China, then India and Islam, whilst a Christian enquiry also stated that it came from China. In 1352, Boccaccio claimed in the *"Decameron"* that, *"It came from the East"*, whilst Gabriel de Mussis, a lawyer of Piacenza, wrote the *"History of the Great Mortality"* and is frequently quoted as describing how the Genoese galleys brought plague from the Crimea to Messina in Sicily. At one time, it was thought that de Mussis had been in Caffa when it was besieged and had travelled to Sicily with the galleys. However, the evidence available suggests that de Mussis never left Piacenza, which is in northern Italy (over five hundred miles north of Sicily), and it appears that the account was written nearly a decade later, presumably using hearsay evidence. He claimed that plague appeared in the city two days after the galleys had docked, that the citizens then expelled them and they went from Messina up the Italian coast to Genoa, carrying the plague with them

Another account by a Franciscan, Michael of Piazza, written twelve years later also claims that the galleys brought the infection with them. It is difficult to know where the facts stop and fiction takes over in this case. Michael writes that the Archbishop blessed Messina with holy water, and a black dog carrying a drawn sword in its paws appeared and attacked the altar scattering the holy vessels.

Several sources hint that no infection was obvious in the galleys when they arrived. It is also reasonable to suppose that if there had been a large number of sick and dying people on the galleys when they docked, the authorities at Messina would not have allowed them to stay for two days, but would have expelled them immediately. If the disease had been on the galleys and had been bubonic plague, there would have been large numbers of very sick people on board.

Guy de Chauliac, physician to the Papal Court at Avignon, gave the advice, "*Fuge cito, vade longe, rede tarde*" frequently abbreviated to "*Cito, longe, tarde*". This translates as flee quickly, go far, return slowly. Unfortunately, such advice if followed only spreads the epidemic more efficiently. de Chauliac also wrote, "*it was so contagious......father did not visit his son, nor the son the father. Charity was dead and hope crushed*". de Chauliac is one writer who mentions buboes but also admits that there were numerous other symptoms and that these did not appear in every case.

The best records for the plague are found in Italy and England. Whilst there is a considerable amount of contemporary information from Italian sources, unfortunately much of this is subject to considerable embellishment and hyperbole, and in many cases it is difficult to distinguish between fact and fiction. The spread of the disease was erratic, and some areas were virtually completely spared. Milan and Parma both remained plague-free by refusing to allow travellers to enter. In Pisa, however, contemporary accounts suggest that 70% of the inhabitants died and in Siena 80,000 people died in seven months. Florence was devastated with over 100,000 dead in five months out of a population estimated at 130,000. In the majority of cases, there is no objective evidence for the numbers of dead given, and all we can deduce is that a very large number of people died. The problems are seen when the figures for Venice are examined. The population is variously given as 120-150,000 and the number of dead as 72-90,000, so if the best-case scenario is taken, then about 48% of the population died. If the worst case is taken, then the figure is 75%, a rather wide discrepancy.

The chronicles of the time claim that the population of many villages was totally destroyed and numerous towns were reduced to only a handful of individuals. As the epidemic spread, infected families were nailed up in houses and left to starve in vain attempts to stop it spreading. Contemporary accounts, by a number of authors including the *"Decameron"* by Giovanni Boccaccio (1313-1375), make terrifying reading. Boccaccio wrote, *"many fell dead in the streets, both by day and by night, whilst a great many others died in their own houses, and drew their neighbours attention more by the smell of their rotting corpses than any other means ......bodies were here, there and everywhere"*, whilst Petrarch commented on the dreadful silence over the whole countryside.

Italy and England were two very different types of states in the fourteenth century. Italy comprised of a number of city-states with relatively small populations, where bureaucratic control of the city was relatively easy to implement compared with a large state such as England. There were also numerous petty wars occurring in Italy, whereas England was a unified state under Edward III.

Various Italian states distinguished between plague and non-plague deaths at an early stage, and required those dying of plague to be buried outside the city walls. This required trained doctors to make the necessary distinction, although the doctors frequently did not agree because of pressure from the civil authorities who would have to implement the necessary control measures. In one case, as late as 1630, the doctor confirming the presence of plague was shot dead. Many families also concealed plague victims because of the repressive actions of the authorities imposing controls such as quarantine.

Quarantine was developed in the Italian states and their satellite towns during this period. This was a period of forty days seclusion during which travellers and ships were isolated, although initially the period involved was trentino (thirty days). The first attempt at quarantine is thought to have been in Ragusa (modern day Dubrovnik) on the Adriatic Sea. The period of forty days was eventually decided as it was the time that the Bible stated Christ spent in the wilderness. Quarantine was difficult to enforce, as traders were obviously losing considerable sums of money during this period of enforced inactivity of their ships and crews and impoundment of their trading goods. Bribery of the guards to turn a blind eye to infringements was frequent[122]. There were also other forms of resistance to plague regulations. Cases are known of bodies placed in mass graves being dug up and reburied in churchyards (it was widely believed that the closer to a church one was buried, the greater the aura of sanctity and the better your chances of a favourable result on Judgement Day).

In Italy, passports and certificates of health were introduced and were required for travel between city-states and this obviously required literate customs and immigration officers. It also required a certain level of trust between states even in time of war, and the development of state bureaucracy, a civil service and diplomatic representation was one of the main results of plague in Italy. The state had to provide doctors who could diagnose and treat plague victims and as a result health boards developed. These instituted Bills of Mortality to track the disease. The health boards were also responsible for running the plague or pest houses, some of which were massive. The

---

122   The most impressive *cordon sanitaire* was the one that ran for hundreds of miles from the north of the Danube down into the Balkans, between the Ottoman and Hapsburg Empires in the eighteenth century. This consisted of a series of customs posts and quarantine stations, supported by troops and militia, that was intended to stop plague entering Europe from the Ottoman Empire.

Lazaretto di San Gregorio in Milan, built in 1488, housed over sixteen thousand patients in the outbreak of 1630.

The organisational and financial control required to run this sort of civil administration was very centralised, and making it function occasionally required persuasion. In Palermo in 1576, the official line was gold, fire and gallows; gold to pay the expenses needed to control the disease and minister to the victims, fire to destroy any infected chattels and the gallows for those who did not co-operate. The tax burden fell increasingly heavily on those still able to work, and many states were forced to negotiate loans so that they could maintain the economic and social cohesion of society. This was not always a straightforward situation as a number of major Italian banking houses had gone bankrupt in the early 1330s.

There are many contemporary accounts of the plague in Italy. Boccaccio comments on the social effects of the epidemic. These included changes in moral behaviour, people refusing to work and enjoying themselves (the *"eat, drink and be merry, for tomorrow we die"* syndrome). This is reminiscent of the comments made by Thucydides during the Plague of Athens (430 BC). High inflation occurred because of the difficulty in obtaining goods and produce. There were huge losses in the labour force and surviving serfs left the land, causing a shortage of agricultural produce and resulting in starvation in urban areas.

Other contemporary authors include Angelo di Tura, a merchant of Siena, who made a chronicle of events. He wrote that *"father abandoned child, wife abandoned husband, and brother his brother. So many died that all believed that it was the end of the world and no one wept for any death"*. His diary ends as a personal tragedy and he writes of *"carrying my five children to the mass grave, and burying them with my own hands as no-one could be found to bury them for friendship or money"*.

He also writes of wolves and dogs running around the towns carrying limbs.

One author mentions "*mass graves containing layers of bodies with a thin layer of earth between them like lasagne layered with cheese*", and comments on grave diggers charging extortionate fees, priests becoming rich from conducting burials, and inflationary prices, especially of food. The church estimated there was a minimum of twenty-five million dead in Europe alone, whilst in Avignon, the Pope (Clement VI) blessed the river Rhône so that corpses could be thrown into consecrated "ground", and sat between two large fires to protect himself. Whilst the Pope might have protected himself, over twenty per cent of the Papal Curia died. Many of the numbers quoted for the victims by the Church, and in countries such as Italy, are mainly symbolic and are not supported by any evidence.

England, however, has the best archival material in Europe. There are several reasons for this, the first being the existence of a database, the Domesday Book. The second reason is that the legal process of England is, to a large extent, based on precedent, and therefore decisions were written down and the third is that England has not been conquered since 1066, and these records are more or less intact. The records include ecclesiastical rolls[123] listing appointments to benefices or livings in the church, and also secular rolls listing land holdings, rents and the heriot (inheritance tax) paid when a feudal landlord died, and his heir inherited the estate. From these rolls, it is possible to calculate how many priests or landlords died during a normal period and compare this figure with how many died during the plague.

Examination of the ecclesiastical rolls, in a number of dioceses across England, shows that approximately forty-five per cent of priests appointed to benefices died between the arrival of plague in England in August 1348 and the end of 1350. In the diocese of Bath and Wells, nine priests were

---

123   The records were written on sheets of parchment that were stitched together then rolled up for storage, hence the name.

appointed to benefices in November 1348 before the plague took hold in that area, and in June 1349, after it had peaked and started to wane, the figure was seven. However, between December 1348 and May 1349, the total figure was two hundred and nineteen. In January 1349, the Bishop wrote to all the parishes in his diocese to inform that them if no priest was available, then the dying could make confession to a layman or *"or if no man is available, even to a woman"*[124]. To allow a layman, or worse still a woman, to hear confession was a public admission that church routine could not deal with the situation. A similar figure for monks dying is found if the monastic rolls are examined. These high figures are presumably due to the fact that priests and monks would have come into frequent contact with the sick, dead and dying

Examination of the manorial rolls across England show that although there were variations across the country, the average suggests that approximately one third of tenants died between September 1348 and the end of 1350. A similar figure was found in Bristol amongst senior merchants and guild members. It has to be remembered that these figures refer to land-holding tenants and wealthy merchants, the death rate would have probably been considerably higher amongst the poor, living in slums, but no one recorded them. The estimates for the population of England in 1347, immediately before the Black Death, suggest a figure of between four and five million, whilst the Poll Tax of 1377 indicates a population of three

---

124   In 1215, the Fourth Lateran Council required the sick to seek spiritual healing before any physical remedy was applied as it was thought that medicine would be more effective once spiritual harmony had been restored. Medieval paintings frequently show the death of an individual accompanied by demons waiting to snatch the soul of the dying person and drag it off to hell, unless there was suitable intercession by a priest. This would have taken the form of repentance and confession followed by administration of the last sacraments. In the absence of the priest, there was nothing between the dying person and hell. In many cases of sickness, the physician was kept waiting outside the bedchamber until the priest had finished, and by the time the doctor was admitted, the patient had expired, albeit in a state of grace.

million. These figures obviously correlate with the deaths of approximately one third of the population.

The rolls suggest that the plague travelled across England as a wave, lasting about seven months in each area. The peak in many areas was during the winter months, the opposite of genuine bubonic plague that tends to be a disease of warmer months.

Although there was obviously severe social disruption in England, the general fabric of society held together, and there is only one record of rioting, in Durham. Many towns had recovered their pre-plague numbers by the mid 1350s, presumably by hiring labour from the surrounding farms and manors. Many of these however had still not recovered fifty years later, although the records show a wide variance. If the manor was owned by a large and rich landowner or the Church, it seems to have fared a lot better than one owned by a small landowner. Many small manors had disappeared or were struggling to survive. The rent returns for the county of Hertfordshire show that over sixty villages disappeared, and William of Dene, a monk of Rochester, wrote *"there was so great a deficiency of labourers and workers of every kind that more than a third of the land in the whole realm was left idle"*. One entry in the Bishop of Durham's rolls states, *"No tenant came from West Thickley because they are all dead"*. When compared with some of the accounts from other parts of Europe, it is obvious that the English were a laconic race even in those days.

One problem was that skilled workers who died could not be replaced easily and the cost of manufactured goods rose as a result. This effect is seen in many of the great cathedrals and churches of England, where there is a marked deterioration in the quality of the stonework of the 1350s compared with earlier dates, reflecting the loss of skilled craftsmen. The Black Death also marks a change in church architecture from the highly ornate Decorated style to the much simpler Perpendicular style. Although this move had started before the Black Death, it accelerated greatly in the decade after.

The fall in the numbers of skilled and agricultural workers led to complaints that the peasants were victimising the nobility by demanding new conditions of employment. In England, The Statute of Labourers passed in 1351 was meant to hold wages to the 1346 level. As there had been a severe depression in 1346, any attempt to have kept wages at this level would have resulted in mass starvation. The shortage of labour meant that the labour force was upwardly mobile, with many labourers renting farms that had become vacant and becoming in effect the ancestors of the land-holding yeomanry of later centuries. The labour shortage also enhanced the movement to sheep farming as fewer men are needed to maintain flocks of sheep than are needed to tend land and grow crops. Dairy farming was not widespread at this time due to the difficulty of keeping cattle over winter.

Before the Black Death there were very few popular peasant movements in Europe, but from 1355 onwards, a number start to appear. There were numerous peasant revolts in France known as Jaqueries and in England the Peasants' Revolt occurred in 1381. The peasants marched on London and several unpopular officials were killed, including the Archbishop of Canterbury. The revolt was only contained when their leader, Wat Tyler, was killed and the king, Richard II, made various promises and concessions. The rebels dispersed, the promises were not honoured and the rebel army was later destroyed by troops loyal to the king.

A movement which had greater long-term effects was the rise of the Lollards who propagated the ideas of John Wycliffe during the 1370s. Wycliffe (1330-1384) who was Master of Balliol College, Oxford, preached against the wealth of the Catholic Church, demanded the translation of the Bible into the vernacular, attacked the sale of pardons, the right of sanctuary and the worship of relics. One of his main attacks however, was on trans-substantiation, the belief that bread and wine were converted into the body and blood of Christ during mass. This anticipated the rise of Protestantism in Europe in the sixteenth century and many of the Lollard ideas became mainstream Protestant doctrine. They also preached social change and one of their preachers, John Ball, is credited with the lines, *"When Adam delved and Eve span, who then was the gentleman"?* Ball later became involved in the Peasants' Revolt and was hanged, drawn and quartered for treason in 1381. Wycliffe and the Lollards were initially protected for political reasons by John of Gaunt, Duke of Lancaster, who acted as regent during the minority of King Richard II. The movement was later destroyed by King Henry IV on charges of heresy in the early fifteenth century. It went underground, but reappeared in the sixteenth century when it was incorporated into the mainstream Protestant movements.

Wycliffe influenced many of the ideas of the reformer John (Jan) Huss (1370-1415) of Bohemia who was burned at the stake, as a heretic, after being given a safe conduct by the Catholic Church. The writings of Huss later played a role in influencing the thinking of Martin Luther (1483-1546), who initiated the Protestant Reformation in much of Northern Europe.

The mortality figures for the rest of Europe between 1347-50 probably averaged out similarly to those of England, with figures for the Mediterranean area being higher, and those for parts of Northern Europe being somewhat lower. In the Islamic world, up to fifty per cent of the population died, and in China, between the census of 1200 and the census of 1400, the population was virtually halved from an estimated one hundred and twenty million to sixty-five million. This figure is almost certainly an underestimate because many people would have attempted to avoid the census as it was used for tax purposes. Some authors consider that the Mongols were responsible for the huge loss of life in China, but even the renowned ferocity of the Mongols is unlikely to account for losses on this scale.

There are several claims as to where plague first appeared in England. The most reliable seems to be that of the fourteenth century chronicle of the Grey Friars of Lynn that reads, "*In this year of our Lord 1348 in Melcombe* [Weymouth] *in the county of Dorset a little before the feast of St John the Baptist* [24th June] *came two ships. One of the sailors had brought with him from Gascony the seeds of a terrible pestilence and through him the men of this town of Melcombe were the first in England to be infected*".

Examination of the records of 1348 show that the graveyards in London's churches were all full within weeks, and mass graves were prepared. The archaeological examination of one, near Tower Bridge, shows that it was one hundred yards long with eight hundred bodies, buried five deep, which had been dumped unceremoniously. The population of London at this time is thought to have been approaching one hundred thousand, and deaths were occurring at the rate of three hundred a day. The records suggest that up to fifty per cent of the population of London may have died within a matter of months, and archaeological evidence shows that in some cases the bodies were incomplete, suggesting that they were not buried until some time after death. This is supported by contemporary authors in Italy, who wrote that dogs and wolves were seen in the streets carrying limbs. The treatment of bodies can be compared with burials dated to before the Black Death, where bodies are laid out in single graves, facing east ready for the resurrection.

One contemporary account by the Frenchman, John of Bassigny, did postulate that a positive effect of plague would be that the Irish and Scots would invade England and "*destroy the sons of Brutus*". This refers to the legend that London was founded by Brutus, a descendant of the Trojan warrior, Aeneas[125].

---

125   The story created by Geoffrey of Monmouth in the twelfth century.

A number of waves of the disease occurred in England between 1348-1665. The second epidemic in 1361 became known as the Children's Plague, because of the large numbers of children who died. These were presumably the ones born after the first outbreak who had little or no immunity. There were also military consequences, in 1399 the northern counties of England petitioned King Henry IV for assistance, as a sequence of epidemics had left them with insufficient men to defend their territories against Scottish raids.

In England, the crowded cities and towns were affected worst, but numerous villages also suffered. In the epidemic of 1531, Henry VIII paid compensation to the poor, and then expelled them from the area as a precaution, when he took up residence in the Palace of Greenwich. Parish records also start around the middle of the sixteenth century, with priests being required to record any plague deaths. The authorities obviously realised that crowding was important because, in the epidemic of 1593 (the last of the sixteenth century), the Lord Mayor of London banned all plays, bear baiting, bowling, bullfights, sports and assemblies within his jurisdiction. It is estimated that during this particular episode over seventeen thousand died with a mortality rate of those infected being near 65%. Similarly, the Universities of Oxford and Cambridge frequently curtailed terms, closed colleges and even moved the location of the two universities when a major outbreak occurred. Other attempts to halt the disease in 1665 included the destruction of all dogs and cats (no mention of rats), and burning tar barrels at the street corners to fumigate the air.

In 1625, a severe outbreak of plague in London killed over forty-three thousand and caused Parliament to move to Oxford. A cartoon of the period shows citizens attempting to leave London with the caption "*we fly*" whilst behind them is a skeleton wielding thunderbolts and standing on coffins crying "*I follow*". The fleeing citizens are being repelled from entering another town by a group of men armed with pikes crying "*Keepe out*" (*sic*). On this particular occasion the Puritans blamed the Queen, Henrietta Maria, a French princess who was a Catholic, for the outbreak, claiming that it was God's vengeance for deviating from the Protestant faith. The reception by a group of men armed with pikes was fairly mild by the standards of the time, it was not unusual for refugees fleeing the plague to be fired upon.

The last of these epidemics in 1665, the Great Plague of London, killed a recorded sixty-eight thousand people in a year, at a rate of three thousand per day at its height. This figure is almost certainly an underestimate as the deaths of Jews, Quakers and Nonconformists would not have been included in the parish records. Modern estimates suggest that the true figure was nearer one hundred thousand out of an estimated population of half a million. The figure would certainly have been higher if a large number of the wealthier members of the population had not fled to the countryside.

This raises another unusual point about this particular disease. Normally one would expect a series of epidemics to become less dangerous as time proceeded. The population would become more disease-experienced and the disease would be downgraded to endemic status. Plague in England however, did not go out into the night quietly, the final epidemic was one of the most deadly; plague went out with a very loud roar.

Although it was known as The Great Plague of London, the epidemic of 1665 was widespread with a number of cities, such as Norwich and Colchester, suffering from a higher percentage of casualties than London, and the epidemic continued well into 1666 outside London. Many other cities such as Exeter and Bristol mounted armed guards on the gates to stop Londoners entering, whilst troops were sent to Portsmouth to reinforce the quarantine restrictions after riots.

The authorities had plenty of warning that it was coming. Plague had been reported in the Ottoman Empire in 1661 and had moved west through Europe reaching Holland with whom England was at war in 1664. Many blamed Dutch prisoners of war for introducing the epidemic into England. In June 1665, the Mayor of London ordered all inns to be closed to lodgers, all theatres were closed and so were schools. Stray dogs and cats were killed and industries such as tanneries that created foul smells were ordered to close (the miasma theory again). The Privy Council recommended the use of fumigants based on brimstone (sulphur) and saltpetre, whilst barrels of tar were burnt at regular intervals on the streets. Tobacco was thought to be a preventative and Pepys records purchasing a roll of tobacco to chew, whilst a schoolboy at Eton College was flogged for not smoking.

There were also political ramifications. The Bishop of London threatened to sack any priest who left his parish as he was afraid that Nonconformist ministers would take over and undermine the King who had only been restored to power five years earlier. The appearance of plague was seen as an Act of God; the question was, why had God sent such a terrible epidemic at this time? This was a simple question to answer in England in the aftermath of the Civil War and Commonwealth. The obvious establishment answer was to punish the population for resistance to authority. This resistance took the form of republicanism and Nonconformity. The Quakers were identified as a major source of the problem and many of them were imprisoned and many more fled to the Americas.

The population in England reached a low point in the mid-fifteenth century taking approximately five to six generations to stabilise after the introduction of this new disease. This closely parallels the experience of Pacific Islanders exposed to new diseases and also rabbit populations exposed to myxomatosis. Similar figures of five to six host generations are seen in other host/pathogen relationships, suggesting that the effects of a major epidemic will be limited over a period of time.

Taxes were raised to help relieve those towns affected by the plague, with weekly payments ranging from a few shillings for a small village to £50 for a large, rich, wool town. During periods of plague, circulars offering advice were issued to villages and towns, one of which entitled *"Advise of ye Colledge of Phisitians"* offered a series of rules to be followed. These included:

- Care to be taken that neither men nor goods come from any suspected place without certificate of health, else to be sent suddenly away or put into the pest house for 40 days (quarantine) till certainty appears.
- Statutes to be executed against beggars and alehouses.
- Persons infected not to be removed without approval of overseers, and caution not to wander till sound.
- Houses infected, though none be dead, must be shut and watched 40 days (quarantine again).

Further rules required that nobody who had died of plague could be removed from their home until a grave was ready for them, and the beadle was required to precede the coffin in order to warn people to avoid it. Houses containing infected people were marked by a red cross and the words, *"Lord have mercy on us"* were painted on the door, whilst any parish official who came into contact with the sick was required to carry a four foot long white stick so that people could identify and avoid him.

Some of the suggested cures make bizarre reading in the present day and numerous herbal remedies were used to little or no avail. The drinking and sprinkling of Holy Water was commonplace. One remedy suggests plucking a live pigeon or chicken around the vent and using it to suck the poison out of any skin eruptions. When the birds stopping dying, the patient was cured. A slightly different version consists of using a freshly decapitated chicken or pigeon as a poultice to draw out the poison. One remedy, published in 1721, suggests that skin eruptions should be poulticed until they suppurate, then cauterised with a red-hot iron. If plague did not kill the patient, then presumably the shock in their weakened state would. After the appearance of syphilis in 1493, it was widely thought that syphilis was a good prophylactic against plague, that is, one poison drove out another.

In 1534, Paracelsus (Ch 2) visited the lazaretto in Sterzing (now Vipiteno) in Italy, and gave people pills of bread treated with a tiny quantity of faeces from a sick patient. He claimed to have learnt of this immunisation technique from the Turks; whether it worked is unknown, but Paracelsus did not succumb to plague.

The only contemporary account of the Black Death in Ireland is by a friar, John Clyn. Clyn presumably had a premonition that he would not survive as he left parchment and writing materials for another to complete his work. The last line of his account, written in a different hand, reads, *"Here it seems the author died"*. Clyn also states that large numbers of people made pilgrimages to various shrines throughout the country; this creates ideal conditions for the spread of disease. The effects in Ireland were severe and a death toll of as high as 60% has been suggested by some historians. Pollen analysis of bogs shows that there was a recovery of the oak forests in the late fourteenth century, suggesting a substantial fall in the population.

Several contemporary accounts in Scotland refer to one third of the population dying and emphasise that the death toll was greater amongst the poor. Several accounts suggest that the Highlands suffered even more with up to 60% of the population succumbing. This again raises the question, if it was bubonic plague, how did a tropical rat and its tropical fleas survive in an area with the most severe weather in the British Isles? It was also the most sparsely populated area in the island of Great Britain, which again raises the question of how it could have spread if it was bubonic plague.

The plague caused major social changes in Europe. The Catholic Church was obviously helpless in the face of repeated outbreaks[126]. This raised serious doubts about the effectiveness of the Church and probably speeded up the movement towards the Reformation and Protestantism. It also encouraged the use of the vernacular instead of Latin in a number of areas of learning. So many scholars died that, after the Black Death, there were a number of contemporary complaints about the quality of Latin used in several walks of life. There were also complaints about the quality of French amongst schoolchildren due to the lack of scholars capable of teaching it.

Many history books claim that plague ended the feudal system in England due to the number of serfs dying or running away to the towns. The evidence shows however that the feudal system had started to disintegrate several decades earlier and plague just hastened the end, rather than initiating the process. The Black Death in England may have speeded up the transition between a barter-based economy and a cash-based one and this would have also accelerated the destruction of the feudal system.

A further effect was to shift of the European centre of power from the Mediterranean to Northern Europe. The effect of the epidemic was worse in the Mediterranean with its warmer climate, more densely populated cities and numerous seaports with links through trade routes to exotic destinations.

In Spain, the disease killed Alfonso XI, King of Castile, and destroyed his army in the period 1349-1350. Alfonso was engaged in defeating the Moorish kingdoms of Spain at the time and his death removed the pressure on the last of the Moorish kingdoms, Granada, which as a result survived until 1492. A further four epidemics, which have variously have been claimed as plague or possibly influenza in Spain between 1596-1682 are estimated to have killed over one million people.

---

126   The first known version of the poem "Piers Plowman" (*ca* 1360) contains the line, *"Prayers have no power this pestilence to halt"*.

This may have been an important factor in Spain's decline as a world power that started during this period.

Numerous reasons for the spread of plague were proposed at the time, these included astrological reasons, terrestrial reasons and divine retribution. The astrologers and physicians of Philip VI of France stated that the astrological reason was the conjunction of Saturn, Jupiter and Mars under the sign of Aquarius in March 1345, which followed a solar eclipse. Aristotle had originally suggested that the conjunction of Saturn and Jupiter would cause disaster. Terrestrial reasons were given as earthquakes releasing noxious odours (the miasma theory). The Church claimed it was divine retribution for the greed and corruption of men (and women). One source claimed, *"The pestilence that threatens us is a punishment for the scandalous behaviour of ladies; their behaviour at tournaments and fornication with knights and champions"* whilst another stated, *"God was also offended by the extravagant dress of courtiers and nobility"*. In terms of divine retribution, numerous people pointed out that in the Bible there are various prophecies of doom; *"There shall be famines and pestilences and earthquakes in diverse places"* (Matthew 24, 7) and if this was not enough, *"Before him went pestilence and burning coals went forth at his feet"* (Habakkuk 3,5). Others saw it as the manifestation of the Four Horsemen of the Apocalypse as described in the Bible in the Book of Revelation[127]. This was powerful prose at a time of great superstition when no rational explanation for the epidemic was known. Whilst some of these ideas may seem rather strange in the modern day, they are not so far removed from some of the recent suggestions about the origin of the virus causing AIDS (Ch 18), including the suggestion that it came from outer space!

The divine retribution theory led to the rise of the Flagellant sect who traversed Europe, whipping themselves

---

127 *"I looked and beheld a pale horse: and his name that sat on him was Death, and Hell followed with him: And power was unto them over the fourth part of the earth, to kill with the sword and with hunger and with death"*. Revelation 6, 8.

to near frenzy and, in some cases, death. They travelled to England but only managed one flagellation session before being expelled back to the continent. The sect was finally destroyed after its behaviour became too outrageous for the authorities to tolerate any further.

The Jews were frequently blamed for the spread of plague, as also were *"prideful women"* and the poor. Lepers were frequently accused of poisoning wells and in parts of France were burned at the stake. Pogroms were started against the Jews in numerous cities; in 1348 they were massacred in Carcassonne in France and in Chillon were tortured until they *"confessed"*. In Mainz, twelve thousand Jews were killed, and in Strasbourg, an estimated sixteen thousand. The Flagellants accused the Jews of being instruments of the Anti-Christ and incited the total destruction of the Jewish quarter of Frankfurt. These measures caused a major exodus of Jews from Europe to Russia to escape the attacks. From the point of view of the local population, killing the Jews made sense as numerous countries barred Jews from a variety of professions, and many of them became moneylenders and bankers. The logic is obvious, if the local banker or moneylender was killed and his records destroyed, then one no longer owed the money. The Pope realised that the effect of the epidemic was the same for all ethnic groups and forbade the killing of Jews, excommunicating those who caused pogroms. One valid point made was that there were no Jews in England as Edward I had expelled them all, but the population of England was suffering as severely as everyone else.

In Florence, the population in the mid-fifteenth century stabilised at about one third of the pre-plague figure. Homosexuals and prostitutes were frequently blamed for outbreaks of plague. Both were seen as sinful practices and if they were driven out of the city, the city was more likely to survive the wrath of God (and the next visitation of plague). Both were seen as unnatural acts that did not produce children, and following the plague replacing the population became a subject of state importance.

Plague also caused major changes in the books of the period and surviving sermons in both England and Italy become extremely apocalyptic compared with earlier ones. Funeral accoutrements become more stark. Vivid illustrations of the Danse Macabre, the Dance of Death, become more frequent, most of them showing dancing skeletons teasing the living, the living usually being the high and mighty. One of the more common themes is three nobles meeting three skeletons whilst hunting. The skeletons tell the nobles, *"as you are, so were we, as we are, so you will be"*. A late fifteenth century stained glass window in Saint Andrew's church in Norwich shows a bishop playing draughts with the devil, illustrating that even the princes of the church were not immune. Skeletons and decomposed cadavers start to appear on graves, especially in northern Europe, and memorial plaques are frequently surrounded with skull and crossbones motifs with the motto *"Memento mori"* (remember you will die). Another theme found is the double-decker memorial, showing a noble or bishop in all his glory on the top deck, whilst the bottom deck shows a skeleton or rotting cadaver.

Plague has been cited as the cause of the destruction of the Greenland settlements of the Vikings, although the Little Ice Age occurred in the same period, probably causing severe famine in a climate that was always marginal for human existence. Recent research has suggested that the Christian Church was extremely rich and powerful in Greenland and when the climate became colder, the Church refused to allow the local population to adopt the Inuit methods of hunting and survival as these were considered pagan. The weather became so bad that the population was unable to survive by subsistence farming, and archaeological work has suggested that the remnants of the population were reduced to slaughtering their dogs for food.

By the time of the Great Plague of London in 1665, the disease had moderated considerably. For example, in 1348, the whole of England had been affected by the epidemic, but by 1665 only towns were attacked, and it was possible to avoid the disease to a large extent by fleeing to the country, a practice frequently resorted to by the English court. Both Daniel Defoe in his fictional account, *"Journal of the Plague Year"*, and Samuel Pepys, who wrote his diary between 1660 and 1669, gave graphic details of the Great Plague, but neither of them mentions dead rats. In his diary, Pepys records purchasing a new wig, and ponders whether the hair might have come from a plague corpse, and if so, whether he would become infected. Although Defoe was writing nearly six decades later (1722), he presumably would have heard first hand accounts from survivors.

The end of the plague in London more or less coincided with the Great Fire of London in 1666. This is often given as the reason for the end of the plague in many history books with the claim that it destroyed the habitat of the rats. Whilst the Great Fire may have contributed to the end of the plague in London, it was certainly not the only factor, as the behaviour of the disease had undergone significant modification prior to 1665. Also of course, this reason did not apply to towns other than London, which also saw huge reductions in the number of cases.

The death rate from plague fell rapidly after the Great Fire. There were tens of thousands of deaths in London in 1665, a few dozen in 1667, and then a few cases each year till 1679, when plague vanished from England and has not been seen since. A similar effect was seen in continental Europe. There was a final epidemic in Marseilles during 1720 imported by ship from Lebanon. This was probably an authentic outbreak of bubonic plague as contemporary reports mention large numbers of dead rats, over ten thousand being counted in the harbour alone, a claim not made in any of the previous accounts of plague in

Western Europe. A number of the crew and passengers were sick or dead on arrival on this occasion. There was the usual disagreement between doctors and city officials whether or not it was plague and a number of diagnoses were suppressed for commercial reasons. The city was finally placed under martial law and the quarantine enforced was so effective that food ran out and there were bread riots. After it was over, one city official was executed for fraud and maladministration. The last major epidemic of plague in Europe was in Hungary from 1739-42, but the causes for the disappearance from Europe are not understood.

Further epidemics categorised as bubonic plague occurred in North Africa, especially Egypt, which had numerous outbreaks. Egypt was ruled by the Mamelukes from 1250 until 1798, when they were defeated by Napoleon. The Mamelukes recruited troops from the Caucasus region where plague was endemic, and new troops arriving in Egypt appear to have been a constant source of re-infection. After the Mameluke defeat, plague in Egypt decreased rapidly once these links with the source of the disease were broken.

However, bubonic plague has not vanished on a worldwide basis; there was a major outbreak in the late nineteenth and early twentieth centuries in China that became widespread, and in India, an estimated six million died of bubonic plague in the first decade of the twentieth century, 1.3 million dying in 1907 alone.

Discovery of the Bacterium causing Bubonic Plague

By the time of the outbreak in China, the bacteriological schools of Pasteur and Koch were well established, and both groups attempted to discover the causal organism. Shibasaburo Kitisato (1852-1931), a Japanese microbiologist, who had worked with Koch's group on tuberculosis and anthrax, arrived in Hong Kong in 1894, where there was a major outbreak, with a team of doctors and technicians. Alexandre Yersin (1863-1943), a Swiss microbiologist, who had worked with Pasteur, and after whom the causative organism is now named, arrived a few days later from Vietnam where he worked with the French colonial service.

Kitisato's team were given a great deal of support by the British, whilst Yersin was given little or none. Within a few days, Kitasato was claiming that he had found the bacterium causing plague in blood samples taken from cadavers, and reported the same to *"The Lancet"*. These claims were later shown to be incorrect.

Yersin however, was being blocked at every step and the medical authorities refused to co-operate with his investigations. He eventually bribed attendants to let him into the morgue where he excised buboes from corpses and found the bacteria in virtually pure culture, each bubo being a bacterial paste of the bubonic plague organism[128]. The Chinese were strongly opposed to autopsies on religious grounds and if Yersin had been caught, it is probable that he would have been thrown out of the colony. The paste of bacteria was used to prepare cultures that were injected into mice, and he noted the progress of the disease which killed them within about twenty-four hours. Yersin also realised that large numbers of rats were dying of plague, claimed they were initiating the human epidemic and recommended a campaign to kill and control them. He wrote, *"they* [rats] *are the principal progenitors of the epidemic"*, but he was not, however, able to show how they were involved. The bacterium was named *Pasteurella* in honour of Pasteur in 1923, but renamed *Yersinia* in 1954, although this name was not adopted internationally for another quarter of a century.

The mode of transmission was discovered in Bombay (Mumbai) by Paul-Louis Simond (1853-1947), another scientist who had worked with Pasteur, and independently by Ogata Masanori (1853-1919) who was working in Formosa (Taiwan). By 1898 when bubonic plague reached India, the correlation between rat and human mortality was known and

---

128   Yersin later claimed that the Japanese had purchased all the cadavers of those who had died of plague.

dead and dying rats were very widespread in plague areas in both China and India. Simond noticed fleabites on the wrists and ankles of human victims and when he removed the fluid from these bites it contained the plague bacterium. Dissection of the stomachs of rat fleas showed the same organism. He caught diseased rats, removed the fleas and used them to infect healthy rats (an incredibly dangerous experiment given the laboratory conditions of the time), and he was extremely lucky not to have been bitten and infected. Simond had made the link between fleas, humans and rats, and realised that large numbers of dead rats meant large numbers of dead humans. Typically his work was largely ignored for about ten years.

Plague reached the USA in 1900 when there was an outbreak in Chinatown in San Francisco. Anti-plague regulations forbade any Orientals from using the ferries, trains or trams, the reason being given that Oriental races were thought to be extremely susceptible to plague. It finally disappeared in February 1904 after killing over one hundred people. After its disappearance, the Governor and various other politicians claimed it had never been present and tried to sack the medical boards and doctors who had diagnosed it.

Simond's theories were proved correct when a large outbreak of plague reached San Francisco in 1907, after the great earthquake and fire of 1906 that destroyed the city and displaced the rats. The city paid a bounty for each rat caught, and posters appeared exhorting, *"all citizens to wage a relentless war on the rat"*. By the time plague was brought under control, two million rats had been killed and it was proven beyond any reasonable doubt that rats and their fleas spread the disease.

Plague is now found widely in the USA in the ground squirrel population and has expanded its range every year since 1900, reaching both the Mexican and Canadian borders. Under natural conditions, maturing rodents are expelled from their home burrow and often move several miles to a new colony, taking the disease with them. It is also spread by human agency. Ranchers frequently trap sick animals and carry them hundreds of miles before releasing them into new ground squirrel communities to reduce numbers as they compete with grazing animals, such as sheep, for pasture. The disease is now well established in the USA, and there have been a number of cases of plague in recent years due to campers coming into contact with ground squirrels. One incident in 1983 caused forty cases resulting in the deaths of six people.

It is noteworthy that bubonic plague did not appear in the USA until after the advent of steamships that were able to make a very rapid passage from the Old World. Speed was essential to convey an unbroken chain of infection from port to port. In the days of sail, *Y. pestis* would have run out of susceptible hosts on a long voyage before a new port was reached. This is at odds with the claim that bubonic plague came to Sicily and Europe from the Crimea in 1347, a journey that would probably have taken at least four weeks by galley. The problem of the transmission of plague worldwide has now been greatly exacerbated by the speed of modern transport, and cases can easily be transported by air around the world before the symptoms become obvious.

In Hong Kong in 1896, Yersin became the first person to cure plague when he injected anti-plague serum from horses into a plague victim who recovered within a few days. Yersin had worked with Roux (Ch 7), whilst in Pasteur's laboratories, on the development of anti-diphtheria toxin. He was able to treat about another twenty victims successfully although the quality of the serum was very variable. He also worked on the development of a plague vaccine and was able to show that heat-killed bacteria had some effect in protecting rabbits from the disease.

One interesting outbreak occurred during 1911-2 in Manchuria. Bubonic plague in this area is carried by marmots, which are large rodents, whose skins are sold to the fur trade. The nomadic tribes of Manchuria had strict rules to cover the killing of marmots that allowed them to avoid becoming infected. Marmots could only be shot from horseback and it was not permissible to kill any sick animal or one moving slowly. If the marmot colony became sick, the nomads moved away to avoid bad luck. In 1911, as the Manchu dynasty collapsed due to a series of civil wars, political and military upheaval, so also did the regulations preventing the ethnic Chinese moving into the steppes. The Chinese started trapping both sick and healthy animals; plague broke out and spread along the railway lines back into China. Traditional ways had stopped outbreaks of plague in Manchuria, and it was only when the newcomers failed to observe these "superstitions" that the disease took a hold. There are frequently good reasons for local taboos, no matter how bizarre they may appear to outsiders.

Plague is one of the diseases that has frequently been considered as having considerable potential for biological warfare. Japan carried out extensive biological warfare research from 1931-45 in Manchuria. It was also alleged that the Russians carried out trials in Mongolia in 1941 on plague, in which one prisoner escaped and caused an epidemic killing between three and five thousand local people. The USSR had also developed a major biological warfare programme after World War II, contrary to various international agreements. This involved strains of bubonic plague resistant to antibiotics. The dissolution of USSR has made this very dangerous as financially destitute scientists could easily sell their expertise to the highest bidder. Bubonic plague also appeared amongst American troops in Vietnam on a number of occasions, although it never progressed to a full-scale epidemic.

Plague is still endemic in Africa and Asia, with about two thousand cases per year being reported to the World Health Organisation, and in the 1990s there were reports in India of antibiotic resistant strains of *Y. pestis* appearing. This is extremely worrying as the main method of treating plague is by means of antibiotics. The vaccines currently available are relatively ineffective providing immunity to only about fifty per cent of those immunised. This particular outbreak was also marked by disagreements between politicians who claimed there was no plague, and the doctors who diagnosed it, a theme which frequently re-occurs with this particular disease.

WAS THE BLACK DEATH BUBONIC PLAGUE?

The assumption has been made by most historians for many years that the Black Death, and by extrapolation, the Plague of Justinian were outbreaks of bubonic plague. A number of authors have recognised that the epidemiology of the Black Death did not fit the known epidemiology of authentic bubonic plague, but have not made the conclusion that the Black Death was not bubonic plague. Instead numerous special factors have been suggested, such as the disease being spread by dogs. A thorough examination of the evidence for, and against, this theory was made by Scott and Duncan in 2001.

The Victorians decided that the Black Death was bubonic plague solely on the basis of contemporary descriptions of the victims of the disease although these descriptions are very variable. A few accounts mention a high fever followed by the appearance of buboes and death a few days later. Many fourteenth century accounts give a different picture of symptoms mentioning pustules and haemorrhages breaking out all over the body, which is not characteristic of authentic bubonic plague. Numerous contemporary reports mention the victim vomiting blood and all accounts make it clear that once this occurred the patient died. There are numerous diseases recognised today which produce similar, although not identical symptoms, especially diseases caused by a number of haemorrhagic viruses, the most notorious being Yellow Fever and Ebola.

What is the evidence against the Black Death being bubonic plague?

Firstly, how did the Plague of Justinian or the Black Death spread through England and many of the other countries of

Western Europe? There was no resistant rodent host in England or Western Europe, so no reservoir of the disease could have been established enabling it to survive over winter. There were also no brown rats in England until the eighteenth century (i.e. one hundred years after plague disappeared from England). The number of black rats was limited and found only in ports. In addition, the black rat is a tropical species that would have had difficulty surviving a British winter, especially as Europe was entering the Little Ice Age at the time of the Black Death, and a very cold period at the time of the Plague of Justinian. There is also no mention anywhere in contemporary literature in Britain or Western Europe of dead rats being associated with either epidemic. There were two severe epidemics of plague in Iceland in 1402 and 1494, but there is no evidence of rats being in Iceland at this time. The date of 1494 also coincides with one of the coldest periods of the Little Ice Age, again raising the question of how a tropical rat and its tropical fleas could survive in a country suffering from very severe cold weather. In addition, Marchionne, writing in 1348 about the city of Florence (where the plague was particularly bad), states, *"even animals such as dogs, cats, hens, oxen, donkeys and sheep died of the same disease"*. He does not mention rats.

The only major outbreak of bubonic plague that has been authenticated, using modern bacteriological techniques, was that occurring in China and India at the end of the nineteenth and beginning of the twentieth centuries. Accounts of this epidemic mention large numbers of dead rats and make it plain that the deaths of rats preceded the deaths of humans. Secondly, in India, it attacked and killed approximately three to four per cent of the human population. This contrasts very markedly with the Plague of Justinian which is thought to have killed half of the population of Western Europe, and the Black Death which is known to have killed between one third and one half of the population of the same area, well over half of the population of some of the Italian cities it attacked and approximately half the population of China.

There is also the question of how the Black Death became established in England. Bubonic plague was imported into the UK through a number of seaports (Cardiff, Glasgow and Liverpool) on several occasions in the early twentieth century. Although each introduction caused a small number of cases and a few deaths, it failed to become established on every occasion, in spite of the facts that both the rat and human populations were significantly higher, and the climate considerably milder than during the fourteenth century[129]. These importations of bubonic plague include several that occurred pre-antibiotics, so antibiotics did not play any role in limiting the spread of the disease. Generally, the conditions determining the initiation of an epidemic of bubonic plague are considerably more stringent than the conditions required for the initiation of many other epidemic diseases.

There are also several serious problems relating to the spread of the Black Death. The incubation period of bubonic plague in humans is two to three days with death usually occurring within six days of infection and in rats the period is even shorter. Contemporary fourteenth century accounts alleged that the epidemic was imported into Europe through Sicily by means of galleys coming from the Black Sea. Most historians consider it started in central Asia in the 1330s, reached the Crimea in 1346, and Europe in 1347. Although the general consensus of opinion is that it came from the Crimea, there have also been suggestions that it may have come from North Africa, the same source as the Plague of Justinian.

If the most popular theory is considered, it would have taken several weeks for a galley to travel from the Black Sea to Sicily, which would have allowed a number of cycles of bubonic plague to occur. Any infected rats would have died, and the crew would have been greatly depleted and sick on

---

129   The average temperature of England in the early twentieth century was approximately 3°C higher than that in the middle of the fourteenth century.

arrival. Several contemporary accounts however, suggest that the crews were in good health when the galleys arrived, and that plague broke out a few days after their arrival. A long voyage of an apparently healthy crew and passengers, followed by an outbreak of an epidemic two days after they landed, does not fit the known epidemiology of bubonic plague. The arrival of the galleys may, therefore, have been coincidental with a disease which had arrived in Sicily earlier and was being already being incubated on the island.

The problem of bubonic plague reaching Sicily is also mirrored by the problems of this disease reaching Iceland and Greenland, both of which would require a long period of travel in a sub-arctic climate. These problems should be considered alongside the fact that authentic bubonic plague did not reach the New World until the advent of steamships able to make a fast passage.

There are further problems relating to the spread of the Black Death. Authenticated outbreaks of bubonic plague move slowly, in many cases only travelling a few miles from the epicentre of the outbreak over several years. This behaviour has been observed during outbreaks in both India and South Africa. In one outbreak in South Africa the epicentre of the disease took a decade to move twenty or thirty miles. The Black Death moved from Sicily to Norway in less than three years, frequently jumping twenty or thirty miles between one known outbreak and the next. This included crossing mountain ranges and moving substantial distances during cold, wet European winters. This again does not equate with a disease spread by a tropical and sub-tropical rodent and a flea that needs an ambient temperature of at least 18°C (65°F) to breed.

The spread of plague more closely resembles the spread of measles, another viral disease spread by droplet infection. Measles typically jumps from one urban centre to another, then retraces its steps infilling the rural areas between the urban ones. Those authors invoking the bubonic plague theory frequently argue that this pattern of spread of the disease could have been achieved by human victims suffering from pneumonic plague. This, however, ignores the fact that pneumonic plague is the terminal stage of the disease. It kills all its victims within a couple of days and no one suffering from the pneumonic version of plague could travel any sort of distance, at a time when one either walked or rode. In addition, it ignores the fact that pneumonic plague requires an outbreak of bubonic plague to initiate it, and any outbreak of pneumonic plague is so deadly that it dies out rapidly, as the susceptible victims are eliminated, unless there is a focus of bubonic plague to restart it.

Penrith and Eyam

Scott and Duncan have examined two outbreaks of plague in England in some detail, one in Penrith which started in 1597, and one in Eyam starting in 1665, both showing similar behaviour. By this time, priests were required by law to fill in parish registers showing the number of deaths in their parish, and mark those occurring from plague with the letter P. It is a reasonable assumption that the priests were sufficiently familiar with plague to recognise it when they saw it; indeed, an outbreak in Stratford in 1546 is noted in the parish register with the laconic statement, *"Hic incipiet pestis"* (Here will start the pestilence).

The case study on the outbreak of plague at Penrith in 1597-8 traced the path of the epidemic on a family-by-family basis using the parish register. In the past, several authors had assumed this epidemic to be an outbreak of bubonic plague. Entries in the parish register show that 606 people died out of an estimated population of 1,350 giving a death toll of 45%. This is probably a slight underestimate as the register was not filled in for ten days, following the death of the vicar's wife who acted as parish clerk. This figure is very much higher than any morbidity or mortality rate produced by bubonic plague.

The first victim was a visitor to the community (Andrew Hodson), presumably a travelling packman, who was staying in the town and who died on the 22nd September 1597. Given the subsequent behaviour of the epidemic, it is probable that he became infected sometime during August, at some location remote from Penrith. There were no further deaths until the 14th October 1597, that is, twenty-two days later. This again does not equate with bubonic plague, which has an incubation time of two or three days, and kills within six days from the point of infection. The epidemic peaked in June/July, 1598 and the last victim was buried on 6th January 1599. It never reappeared in the town again, in spite of the fact that there were a number of epidemics in England during the first half of the seventeenth century. This suggests that the surviving population had developed a high level of herd immunity.

The analysis carried out by Scott and Duncan does not correlate totally, but the minor deviations that occur can be explained by the presence of immune individuals, who did not develop the disease in spite of coming into contact with it, and infected individuals who recovered and therefore do not appear in the parish register of burials.

Mathematical modelling and analysis of the first 130 days of the epidemic in Penrith suggest a disease with the following parameters. It was spread by droplet infection or possibly fomites; bubonic plague is spread by vectors. The latent period was 10-12 days, followed by a very long infectious period of 20-22 days, before the symptoms (which lasted for five days) appeared and were followed by death or recovery. The total infectious period was therefore 25-27 days, and the time from the point of infection to death was approximately 37 days. This is a very long infectious period compared with many other diseases and is in complete contrast to bubonic plague.

The long infectious period would explain how individuals, showing no symptoms, could have been travelling around spreading the disease and explains why it frequently jumped thirty miles between outbreaks in Europe. It would also explain how the epidemic spread to places such as Iceland and Greenland. If it had been bubonic plague, then nobody showing symptoms would have embarked on such a voyage and survived long enough to spread the disease. As already mentioned, it is inconceivable that infected tropical rats could have survived such long sea journeys along the southern edge of the pack ice. It should also be pointed out that in the case of the Penrith epidemic, the winter would have been too cold and wet for a tropical species of rat and its fleas to survive in a mountainous area in the north of England at a time approaching the coldest period of the Little Ice Age.

The disease also appears to have spread between families. After an outbreak in one house, the next house infected would belong to a family member such as a brother or cousin, even although they lived some distance away. It was therefore spreading through family members socialising, whereas, if it had been spread by vectors such as rats and fleas, one would expect it to have spread from one house to the ones on either side in the same street. This spread through family members living at some distance from each other is not typical of a disease spread by a vector.

One interesting point about the Penrith analysis is that it shows that the first death in a house was usually a young person, and the disease appears to have been spread from house to house by teenagers who were presumably courting or socialising. Nothing changes!

Scott and Duncan also examined the epidemic in Eyam in Derbyshire in 1665. This shows some remarkable similarities to that in Penrith. The first person to die in Eyam on 7th September was George Vicars[130], a journeyman tailor, who was also a visitor to the village and was lodging with the Cooper family. The traditional story in the village is that Vicars was sent a box of cloth from London, and removed the cloth to dry it in front of the fire. An infected flea is alleged to

---

130   Also spelt Viccars depending on the source.

have jumped out and bitten him[131]. The second person to die was Edward Cooper on the 22nd September some fifteen days later. Assuming this story is correct, it immediately raises the question of why a hungry flea, that was unable to feed properly because its gut was blocked with bacteria, should wait fifteen days before biting a second person in the same house.

The third person to die was Peter Hawksworth on the 23rd September, but his fourteen month old son, Humphrey, living in the same house, did not die until 17th October, a twenty-four day interval. Using the same argument, it seems inconceivable that a hungry flea would wait twenty-four days after biting the father before biting the child. Neither the Vicars/Cooper deaths nor the Hawksworth deaths fit the known epidemiology of bubonic plague.

Eyam is in the Peak District of England, another rural high altitude area, where the movement and survival of a tropical rat through the winter months is most unlikely. Eyam was also unusual for the self-imposed quarantine. The vicar, William Mompesson, who took control of the situation in June 1666, was twenty-eight, and had only been vicar for two years. It was a difficult position politically. The post had been held by Shoreland Adams who had been appointed in 1630. He had been evicted from his office by the Puritans in 1644, and replaced by Thomas Stanley who was evicted in turn in 1660 after the Restoration, when Adams was reinstated. Adams appears to have been unpopular and when he died, Stanley returned to the village and when the epidemic started, Stanley and Mompesson agreed to work together.

Several decisions were made, the first was that there would be no organised funerals and burials in the churchyard. This avoided villagers congregating and families buried their dead in gardens and orchards, which also allowed bodies to be disposed

---

131   Given that the involvement of fleas in the transmission of plague was only discovered at the end of the nineteenth century and not generally accepted until the first decade of the twentieth century, this story must have originated at least two hundred and thirty years after the event.

of quickly. The second decision was that church services would be held outdoors and a natural amphitheatre was used, which again avoided people crowding together in enclosed places. It has to be remembered that the miasma theory was widely believed at this time, so these were reasonable precautions to take.

The third decision was the imposition of a *cordon sanitaire* to avoid spreading the disease to surrounding villages and towns. The village was not totally self-sufficient, and items that were purchased were paid for by placing money in a local stream, which it was thought would wash away any contagion. Alternatively, holes were drilled into parish boundary stones; money was placed in these and covered with vinegar.

The epidemic peaked in July and August 1666, and the last burial took place on 1st November. The Hearth Tax of 1664 indicates that there were one hundred and sixty households in Eyam, which if an average of five individuals per household is taken gives a population of about eight hundred. There is a slight discrepancy over the number who died; Mompesson claimed that it was two hundred and fifty-nine, whilst Joseph Hunt who became vicar in 1683 and transcribed the records, claimed it was two hundred and sixty. These figures suggest that about thirty-two per cent of the population died, a figure very close to that given for the Black Death in England between 1348 and 1350.

Interestingly, the dead were not spread evenly across the village, all of those who died were from seventy-six households. Mompesson wrote, *"Here hath been 76 Families visited within my Parish out of which have died 259"*. On the basis of five individuals per household, the death rate amongst these families was over sixty-eight per cent. The other eighty-four families were virtually untouched. It is impossible to believe that in a small village they did not come into contact with those infected, which would strongly suggest that members of these eighty-four families had some genetically based resistance to the disease.

Several cottages from the seventeenth century are still in present day Eyam. The effect of families living in some of these cottages was devastating. Mary Hadfield, formerly Cooper, lived in Plague Cottage with her two sons, and her new husband, Alexander Hadfield. George Vicars, the first person to die, was staying there. They all died except Mary, but she lost nineteen relatives living throughout the village. Nine members of the Thorpe family lived in Rose Cottage in the same street, they all died.

The suggestion has been made on several occasions that the disease might have been anthrax. This is most unlikely as anthrax is an animal disease, humans do not catch it easily, and during the plague at Eyam numerous farmers wrote wills, leaving their livestock to various family members, with no mention of any of the stock being sick.

Examination of the DNA of modern day residents of Eyam, who can trace their ancestry back to seventeenth century families living in the village, shows that a significant percentage of them possess a genetic mutation known as CCR5Δ32 (CCR5 *delta* 32). Sampling across the UK and Europe shows that this gene is carried by about 10% of the white ethnic population of the UK, rising to about 15% in Sweden. This mutation is virtually unknown amongst Asian and African populations where genuine bubonic plague has been present for hundreds if not thousands of years.

The gene CCR5 codes for a protein receptor on the surface of the macrophages. Certain viruses must bind to this receptor before they can enter and infect a cell. The Δ32 means that a piece of DNA, thirty-two base pairs long, has been deleted from this gene rendering it ineffective. The result is that the protein receptor is missing and therefore the virus cannot bind to the host cell and enter it. Anyone possessing two copies of the gene CCR5Δ32 (i.e. homozygous for the gene) is completely resistant to any virus requiring that receptor to enter the cell. Any person having one copy of the gene (i.e. heterozygous) would have a reduced amount of the receptor protein. This would produce a high level of resistance to the virus, slowing down the infectious process and giving their immune system time to counter the viral attack.

It is speculated that the mutation only occurred once. New mutations have a mathematical probability of disappearing within a few generations if they are neutral, that is, if they do not confer a selective advantage on the individuals possessing them. Statistically, it is highly unlikely that the mutant gene CCR5Δ32 increased to its present frequency by random genetic drift, and therefore there must have been some event(s) that gave individuals possessing this gene a considerable selective advantage over the rest of the population.

Several variations of the CCR5Δ32 gene have developed since its first appearance. These are further mutations of the original mutation. Mathematical examination of these variations suggests that the original mutation occurred three to four thousand years ago in North Western Europe. It was then subjected to some strong selective event(s) that occurred between about eighteen hundred and three hundred years ago. This strong selective event was an epidemic caused by some pathogen with a high mortality rate that used the CCR5 membrane receptor protein to gain entry into the cell. Those individuals possessing the mutant gene were resistant to this epidemic. Both the Plague of Justinian and the Black Death fit this time frame, which suggests that at least one and possibly both were caused by a pathogen that entered the cell via the CCR5 membrane protein.

One interesting feature of the Black Death is its relationship to HIV. This virus docks with the susceptible cell by binding simultaneously to two membrane proteins, one of which is the CCR5 protein. Individuals homozygous for the Δ32 mutation are totally resistant to infection by HIV and in heterozygous individuals there is a much longer delay before the onset of AIDS (Ch 18).

The differences between authentic bubonic plague and the Black Death are shown in table 9.1.

Table 9.1. Comparison of Bubonic Plague and the Black Death

Bubonic Plague	Black Death
Considered to be tropical or sub-tropical disease	Widespread throughout Europe during winter months
Needs reservoir of resistant rodents to initiate epidemic	No resistant rodents present in Western Europe
Needs rats	No brown rats in Western Europe until the mid-18th century. Black rat is a tropical species, rare in Europe in the 14th century.
Human flea is very inefficient vector. Oriental rat flea needs temperature of $18.3°C$ ($65°F$) to reproduce.	Very cold period, Little Ice Age just starting. Winter temperatures in Eyam and Penrith well below $18.3°C$.
Typically kills 2-5% of the population	Killed 30-35% of the population.
Epicentre typically moves 2-3 miles per year	Moved from Sicily to Norway and Iceland in three years. Frequently jumped 20-30 miles per day.
Kills large numbers of rats	Dead rats not mentioned in contemporary literature.
Kills within six days	Epidemiological studies in Penrith and Eyam show that time of infection to death was thirty-seven days.
Spreads as vector spreads, i.e. from one house to next-door neighbour	Frequently jumped a quarter of a mile from one house to house of relative in Penrith. Suggests droplet infection
Bacterial disease	Selected and concentrated CCR5Δ32 mutation giving immunity to HIV. Suggests Black Death caused by virus entering cell in the same way as HIV.
Introduced to UK several times in 20th century prior to antibiotics. A small number of people were killed.	Never took hold even though conditions more favourable than 14th century. Warmer, more rats, more people.

When a theory is proposed, the theory should explain all the known facts. If one fact does not fit, then the theory needs tweaking, if none of the facts fit, the theory is wrong and needs to be completely rethought. When all the facts in the table are considered, it becomes obvious that the case for the Black Death being bubonic plague is extremely weak, and the case for it being some other pathogen such as a haemorrhagic virus is very strong.

Perhaps the most frightening aspect of the Plague of Justinian and the Black Death is this thought. If they were not bubonic plague, then there is some unknown pathogen that causes major pandemics with a very high mortality rate, which has appeared at least twice with an interval of seven to eight hundred years. It is now nearly seven hundred years since it last appeared in Western Europe, and if there is an, as yet, unknown pathogen capable of causing death on this scale of magnitude, we need to know about it.

Whatever this disease was, it is obvious from this chapter that it had a massive and profound influence on the history of the Old World, especially Europe and the Near East, an effect whose consequences are still with us today.

Chapter 10

Smallpox

"The most terrible of all the ministers of death".
Lord Macauley (1800-1859).

Introduction

Smallpox is caused by a double-stranded DNA virus, known as *Variola,* belonging to the pox group of viruses, which include cowpox, monkeypox, camelpox and myxomatosis. The pox group are amongst the largest viruses known in terms of size and are a very stable group genetically. Unlike many viruses they have their own enzymes for transcription and replication (Ch 4), and are therefore able to replicate in the cytoplasm of the host cell. Most viruses must multiply in the nucleus so that they can access the host cell enzymes for nucleic acid synthesis.

The smallpox virus occurs in two forms, *Variola major* and *Variola minor.* The form occurring in most of recorded history is *V. major,* which generally had a mortality rate of approximately thirty percent, although this could rise to as high as ninety per cent in a population that had not experienced the disease previously. *V. minor,* which was fatal in less than one percent of cases, did not appear until 1896 in the USA, although it had been described in the Caribbean about thirty years earlier[132]. It is also possible that Jenner may have recognised it. In his "Inquiry" (see later) he mentions, *"a species of smallpox of so mild a nature, that a fatal instance was scarcely ever heard of"* found in Gloucestershire. *V. minor* caused much less scarring but still gave immunity to *V. major.* The appearance of *V. minor* was

---

132   This mild form is occasionally referred to as alastrim.

possibly a response to the increasing use of vaccination at the end of the eighteenth century, or it may have been due to the virus moderating its behaviour after the very severe epidemics of the seventeenth and eighteenth centuries. Whilst most virologists only recognise the two strains mentioned above, a few claim that there were also a number of intermediate types. A comparison of *V. minor* strains from a number of countries shows considerable variation between them that may account for these reports.

Some of the pox viruses are specific to one host. Smallpox is only found in humans and camelpox in camels, whereas others such as cowpox can live in a number of species including humans, cattle and rats, whilst monkeypox can live in most primates and a variety of rodents.

Smallpox is transmitted by airborne infection, the victim breathes in droplets containing infected material that have been coughed out by a person already suffering from the disease. The virus can also survive on dry fomites, such as the bedding or clothes of a victim, for considerable periods of time and dust from these was a regular source of infection. It has been claimed that there is a theoretical risk of contracting smallpox from human remains, especially if the bodies of smallpox victims were buried in permafrost and there are a number of anecdotal stories suggesting that this may have happened on a few occasions.

About ten to twelve days after infection, the victim develops headaches, severe pains in the muscles and joints and a high fever followed by a rash appearing about forty-eight hours later. Over the next ten days or so, the pustules become raised and hard, and have been described as being similar to, *"lead shot embedded under the skin"*. The pustules fill with a clear fluid that changes to pus and if the victim has survived this far, these pustules slowly dry up and the fever abates. When the scabs fall off they leave deep scars frequently described as pitted. The pock-marks are found over the whole body, but are especially bad on the face and in many cases the victim is blinded. They may also destroy the pigmentation of the skin creating a mottled appearance.

If the pustules remained separate, the attack was known as discrete and usually had a death toll of about thirty percent. If the pustules fused, it was called confluent smallpox, and was frequently followed by a secondary infection of *Streptococcus*, a bacterium commonly found on the skin. In this case the death toll was of the order of sixty percent. In rare cases, the victim developed severe internal bleeding of the lungs and other organs to give haemorrhagic smallpox, which usually killed the victim from haemorrhaging and toxaemia before the characteristic rash appeared. The survival rate from haemorrhagic smallpox was extremely low and victims frequently died before it was realised they had smallpox.

There are only two outcomes from an infection of smallpox, death or life-long immunity, and in many societies parents were exhorted not to count their children until they had experienced, and survived, smallpox. Although the death toll from smallpox has been immense[133] and it has played an extremely important role in history, it is the only human disease to date that it has been possible to eliminate completely. The reasons for this are discussed later.

HISTORY

One interesting question is the origin of the *Variola* virus. The only known hosts are humans and there is no animal reservoir. The infected human is only infectious for a few weeks and if victims survive they are immune for life. Under these conditions, the virus could only survive in large human communities with a constant supply of new susceptible individuals (children), and therefore could not have appeared earlier than about six or seven thousand years ago when urban society started to evolve.

---

133   It is estimated to have killed 300 million in the twentieth century alone.

The virus must have originated in some animal host then jumped to humans, where it mutated, and lost the ability to survive in the original animal host. The origin was probably not monkeypox, because although this can attack humans and cause a fatal infection, it does not spread easily from human to human. In addition, DNA sequencing shows that smallpox and monkeypox are very different to each other and it is highly unlikely that one could have evolved into the other.

Arab tradition claims that smallpox came from domestic camels although camelpox very rarely attacks humans. However, the DNA sequence of camelpox is closer to *Variola* than any other known poxvirus. It is also known that if camels are inoculated with *Variola,* they only develop a local reaction and are protected from a future infection of camelpox. Close proximity of humans to camels in desert regions would have given the virus the opportunity to jump the species barrier. Alternatively, the two diseases may have evolved from a common viral ancestor that has now vanished.

SMALLPOX IN THE OLD WORLD

Smallpox was frequently confused with measles as these two diseases regularly occurred more or less simultaneously, or in close succession to each other and when dealing with contemporary historical accounts it is very difficult to separate them. In addition, measles was also confused with scarlet fever, and smallpox with chickenpox.

The first person to distinguish between smallpox and measles was Abu Baka Muhammad ibn Zakariyya ar-Razi, known as Rhazes (Ch 2) in Western Europe (and considered by some to be the greatest Islamic physician of all time). Rhazes wrote a *"Treatise on the Small Pox and Measles"* around 910 AD, giving a very detailed description of smallpox. He noted that it usually occurred in spring, and that it mainly attacked children. He stated that smallpox was very common throughout the Islamic Caliphate, and both Rhazes and Avicenna (Ch 2) implied that smallpox and measles were relatively mild childhood infections at that time. Even after his descriptions, considerable confusion was still found until well into the seventeenth century, with many doctors considering the two to be the same disease, measles occurring in children and smallpox in adults. It was thought there was a single cause, and the differences were due to the variation between adult and children's blood. There are considerable similarities, both smallpox and measles are virus diseases spread by droplet infection, both can produce high death rates especially in young, non-immunised children and antibiotics are ineffective against either of them.

There are numerous theories about the source of smallpox and how long it has afflicted the human race. The sixth plague of Egypt (boils) was described by Philo of Alexandria, in the first century AD, in terms that suggest it could have been smallpox. There are also claims that it appeared in China during the first millennium BC. India has been suggested as the source about 2,000 years ago, on the basis of descriptions in various texts, but some of these suggest that it was not a serious disease. Indian sources do not describe a deadly disease with all the characteristics of smallpox until the seventh century AD.

Marc Ruffer, a pupil of Pasteur, who became Professor of Bacteriology at Cairo School of Medicine, claimed to have found smallpox vesicles on mummies of the eighteenth dynasty (*ca* 1539-1295 BC) and also the twentieth dynasty (*ca* 1186-1069 BC). The most convincing of these is the pharaoh, Rameses V, who died around 1143 BC. There is however, no description in any known Egyptian papyrus of a disease resembling smallpox.

Some authors, including Zinsser, consider the Plague of Athens was possibly smallpox. However, smallpox is not mentioned recognisably in early Hebrew texts or by Hippocrates, who was writing a number of years after the Plague of Athens. The symptoms of smallpox are so obvious to even the untrained observer, that if the disease had been endemic or epidemic at the time, it is certain that Hippocrates would have mentioned it. It is known however, that some of the writings of the *Hippocratic corpus* have been lost and it is possible that these include ones mentioning smallpox.

A description of a disease that may have smallpox is given by the doctor Ko Hung, who described an epidemic occurring in China in 49 AD. Chinese literature describes a great epidemic in 162 AD that killed forty per cent of the population of the north-western provinces. This date would tally with the suggested appearance of smallpox in Europe three years later. Other Chinese sources describe an epidemic that may have been smallpox in 310 AD, following a plague of locusts and famine. This is claimed to have killed over ninety per cent of the population in the north-western provinces and thirty per cent nationwide. There are also sources suggesting that it appeared in China during wars with the barbarians in Northern China around 495 AD.

The nineteenth century German epidemiologist, August Hirsch, suggested that the first recognisable attack in Western Europe of a disease that was probably smallpox, was the epidemic known as the Antonine Plague or the Plague of Galen. This started in 165 AD, and caused an epidemic lasting fifteen years that killed an estimated twenty-five to thirty percent of the population of the Roman Empire, although some authors claim it killed as many as fifty per cent. The total number of dead has been estimated at up to seven million throughout the Roman Empire and it is claimed that two thousand a day were dying in Rome itself. Whilst these figures might seem excessive, they are not outrageous for a disease of the severity of smallpox attacking an immunologically naïve population. One of the people killed was the emperor, Marcus Aurelius Antonius in 180 AD. His *"Meditations"* claimed that the epidemic was not as deadly as the lies and treachery around him.

Legend claims that the epidemic began when the Roman legions attacked Mesopotamia during the Parthian Wars, and a legionary forced open a sealed casket in the Temple of Apollo (the God of Medicine), whilst Seleucia was being sacked. This was Pandora's box with a vengeance as out came smallpox that ravaged the world for the next eighteen hundred years.

Galen left Rome in 166 AD to return to his home in Asia Minor and some authors have accused him of fleeing from the epidemic as he could nothing to stop it. It has also been claimed that the loss of manpower from this epidemic was one of the reasons for the Romans being unable to contain the Germanic tribes threatening the Roman Empire's northern border on the Rhine.

It is difficult to match epidemics of this period to a specific disease, as descriptions of the symptoms of many diseases are very similar in the early stages. Frequently there are only one or two primary sources describing the epidemic, and usually these have not been written by trained doctors. There is the possibility that the disease has altered its behaviour over a period of two thousand years, and it is also very probable that more than one epidemic was raging at any one time, and that these have become confused in the minds of contemporary writers, especially if they were writing some time after the event. Major epidemics that may have been smallpox were reported in Cyprus in 251-66 AD (the Plague of Cyprian[134]), Japan 552, Mecca 569-71, and Europe generally from about 4-800 AD (a ninth century manuscript in the British Museum is an Anglo-Saxon prayer against smallpox).

One epidemic thought to be smallpox stopped the Huns led by Attila in the middle of the fifth century. They retreated from the gates of Rome because of the threat from disease. Nicaise, Bishop of Rheims, who was decapitated by the Huns on his cathedral steps, had recovered from smallpox the

---

134   This was named after Saint Cyprian, Bishop of Carthage, who, when asked to pray for the victims of the disease, is reported to have said, *"let them all die, God will decide the righteous".* He was obviously an early advocate of Malthusian theory.

previous year. He became the patron saint of smallpox victims, and is always pictured carrying his head, as legend claimed that after being beheaded, he walked through the cathedral carrying it and did not fall dead until he reached the altar.

An epidemic in Saudi Arabia in 569 AD that may have been smallpox occurred during the War of the White Elephant. Mecca was besieged by Christian Ethiopians based in Yemen, led by Prince Abraha who rode a white elephant into battle. The besieging army was destroyed by the epidemic, and Mecca was not conquered until 630 AD, when Mohammed and his supporters launched an attack from Medina. This epidemic is mentioned in the Koran and several authors, including Keys, suggest that it was not smallpox but an outbreak of bubonic plague.

In 573 AD, the Bishop of Avenches described an epidemic and appears to have been the first to use the word *variola,* derived from the Latin word *varius,* meaning spotted or mottled. In 580, Geoffrey of Tours gave a very accurate account of smallpox when he described the disease occurring in much of Europe at that time.

Smallpox is thought to have arrived in Japan in the middle of the sixth century with an embassy from Korea, which was attempting to introduce Buddhism. The disease was reintroduced on several occasions over the next hundred years or so by embassies from both Korea and China. There were a series of epidemics from about 700-1050, the worst being from 735-7 AD which killed many members of the ruling Fujiwara clan, destabilising Japan politically.

Smallpox would certainly have been spread by the expansion of Islam in the seventh to ninth centuries, but so also were a number of other diseases such as the Plague of Justinian. Whether these epidemics helped Islam to spread, by causing huge movements of people and depopulating numerous countries in the paths of their conquests is debatable (see the Plague of Justinian, Ch. 9).

The disease appears to have become a lot more virulent in the mid-sixteenth, seventeenth, and eighteenth centuries. In Italy, it killed an estimated thirty per cent of the population in epidemic years in the eighteenth century, and in eighteenth-century London, smallpox was virtually continuous, causing some ten to fifteen per cent of the annual deaths, with eighty per cent of those being children under the age of ten. One estimate suggests that it killed sixty million people worldwide during the eighteenth century. In 1668, Pepys complained it had been the worst season for smallpox for many years, and John Evelyn (1694) wrote, *"the smallpox increased exceedingly and was very mortal"*.

After 1665, it replaced plague as one of the main causes of death in Europe. The reason for this increase in incidence and mortality is not known, although it has been suggested that the Black Death may have masked the smallpox death toll in the fourteenth and fifteenth centuries. The effects on small or isolated populations could be devastating. In 1707 it appeared in Iceland for the first time in generations and killed an estimated eighteen thousand out of a population of fifty thousand. In percentage terms, it was even worse when it broke out on the island of Foula off the coast of Scotland in 1720 when it killed one hundred and eighty out of a population of two hundred. Perhaps the most poignant outbreak in 1727 was on St. Kilda, which is forty miles west of Uist and the most isolated island in the British Isles. Three men and eight boys were taken to Boreray, an island four miles from St. Kilda, to catch gannets, which were a staple part of the diet. The boat left promising to return a few days later. However, in the interim, there was an outbreak of smallpox on St Kilda that killed most of the islanders, only nineteen surviving out of approximately one hundred and eighty. Most of the survivors were children and there were too few adults to man the boat. The result was that the eleven on Boreray were marooned within sight of their home for nine months and were not rescued until a boat called at St. Kilda.

The political consequences could also be considerable. In England, it killed Queen Mary II (the wife of William of Orange) in 1694, leaving her husband as sole monarch, and in 1700, it killed William, Duke of Gloucester, the eleven-year-old son of her sister (who later became Queen Anne), thus ending the Stuart dynasty. The consequence of this death was "The Act of Settlement" of 1701, in which the throne of England passed to Sophia, Electress of Hanover, or her heirs on the death of Princess Anne. Anne became queen in 1702 after the death of William of Orange. The House of Hanover descended from James I through his daughter, Elizabeth.

Mary II and Anne were daughters of James II by his first wife and had been brought up as Protestants at the insistence of their uncle, King Charles II. Mary and her husband, William of Orange, had become joint monarchs after James II fled from England in 1688 during The Glorious Revolution. James II had made his Catholic tendencies obvious over a period of years, but the trigger for this revolution was the birth of a son, James Edward to James II and his second, Catholic wife, Mary of Modena. This son (who later became known as the Old Pretender and led the Jacobite rising of 1715) would have taken precedence over his half-sisters, Mary and Anne. He was recognised as James III of England by the French king Louis XIV, after the death of his father in 1701 at the French court where he had taken refuge.

The Young Pretender, Charles Edward Stuart (Bonnie Prince Charlie) was son of the Old Pretender, and led the Jacobite rising of 1745 that culminated in the Battle of Culloden in 1746. This battle finally destroyed the clan system of Highland Scotland (the last tribal society of Western Europe).

In addition to the inheritance problems of Great Britain, smallpox also caused major problems in continental Europe when it killed Prince Joseph Ferdinand of Bavaria in 1699.

The Spanish king, Charles II (last of the Spanish Hapsburgs) was childless and England, France and the Dutch Republic agreed the "First Treaty of Partition", in 1698, in which Joseph Ferdinand would have inherited a major portion of the Spanish Empire. When he died, a second treaty was agreed in which the portion he would have received went to the Archduke Charles, second son of the Holy Roman Emperor, Leopold I. Leopold refused to ratify the treaty unless his son received all the Spanish Empire intact. The inheritance was further complicated when Charles II was persuaded to write a will, a few weeks before he died, leaving the whole empire to Philip, Duke of Anjou, the grandson of Louis XIV of France. The whole balance of power in Europe would have been upset by this arrangement and three weeks after the death of Charles, the French invaded the Spanish Netherlands. Britain, the Dutch Republic and the Holy Roman Empire formed an immediate alliance against France, and were later joined by the Prussians and various other Protestant German states. The War of Spanish Succession (1701-1716) had started and several major victories at Blenheim and Ramillies led to the elevation of the English general, John Churchill (ancestor of Winston Churchill) to become the First Duke of Marlborough.

There was major confusion in England over numerous diseases until Thomas Sydenham, in 1670, described measles, which was confused not only with smallpox, but also with scarlet fever and to some extent diphtheria, in spite of the fact that Rhazes had distinguished smallpox and measles in the tenth century. However, even as late as 1857, some doctors were still confusing smallpox and chickenpox. In addition, Sydenham distinguished between the discrete and confluent stages of smallpox and recommended that if it were discrete, the physician should do nothing, a novel suggestion coming from a physician of that time.

One of the most widespread treatments for smallpox was the so-called red treatment, thought to have started in tenth century Japan, which lasted until the early twentieth century. It was suggested that a red cloth hanging in the room would help cure the patient, and this theory reached Europe in the twelfth century. The explanation given was that red bedclothes had a warming property, and would help expel undesirable humours. It was considered that bad humours were the cause of the pustules and heating the patient would cause sweating and the evil humours would be expelled.

The red treatment became widespread throughout Europe, and was given a pseudo-scientific explanation by the late nineteenth century. Niels Finson, who won the Nobel Prize for treating patients suffering from *Lupus vulgaris* (the common wolf, i.e. skin TB) using UV light, suggested that red curtains or glass would exclude short wave length light from the sick room. This would supposedly stop the pustules suppurating and the patient would be cured with no scarring. The method was discredited and its use died out in the early twentieth century.

The Role of Smallpox and Measles in Colonisation

The first European colonisation expeditions were to the Atlantic islands of the Azores, Madeira and the Canaries. The Azores and Madeira were uninhabited and were colonised by the Portuguese. Sugar cane was introduced, which needs intensive labour, so the Canaries were raided for slaves. The indigenous stone-age inhabitants known as Guanches, who were related to the Berbers of North Africa, had an estimated population of one hundred thousand, but vanished in less than a hundred years, leaving only a few artefacts such as stone tools and a small number of mummies. Two major epidemic diseases were involved, measles and smallpox.

Smallpox and various other diseases also played a major role in the European colonisation of the Americas and other countries. The colonisation of the Americas by the Amerindians is described in Chapter 5. The dates for these migrations are controversial, but whenever they happened, migrations would have taken place long before crowd diseases evolved in the Old World. The migrating bands scattered, and developed into a number of different cultures ranging from hunter-gathers to advanced Neolithic. In some areas, large urban populations such as the Aztec in Mexico and the Inca in the Andes appeared, the communities involved being significantly larger than those required to support epidemics in the Old World.

At the beginning of the twentieth century, the number of Amerindians in pre-Columbian America was thought to have been relatively low, but these numbers have been revised upwards at regular intervals. Many authorities now consider that there were between one hundred and one hundred and twenty million Amerindians immediately pre-Columbus.

A report, written in 1857 by Britain's first medical officer of health, estimates the pre-Columbian population of Santa Domingo at one million, but more recently the figure has been put as high as four million in 1513. Estimates of the mortality rate from smallpox in Santa Domingo also vary widely; whilst some reports claim a third of the population died, others state that only 1,000 survived by 1548. Figures from another Caribbean island, Puerto Rico, claimed it killed over half of the population, whilst in Cuba, smallpox is estimated to have killed half the indigenous population in 1518 and the measles epidemic, which followed in 1529, killed two thirds of the survivors. The Caribs have now effectively disappeared from the islands of the Caribbean and been replaced by a population mainly of African descent.

It is difficult for us to comprehend epidemics on this scale, but a contemporary account from the nineteenth century illustrates the situation. In 1837, the Mandans, a group of Plains Indians, caught smallpox from passengers on a steamboat going up the Missouri from St Louis. The population fell from two thousand individuals to less than forty in a few weeks.

No large animals were domesticated in the New World with the exception of llamas in the Andes and they do not live in large herds. They also were not kept in houses as live-in stock, as was the case in much of Europe. This meant that the human population did not come into contact with the various zoonoses that the human population of the Old World experienced. There was no malaria, yellow fever, smallpox, measles, diphtheria, or influenza, all of which arrived with the Europeans or their African slaves. Smallpox arrived in the second decade of the sixteenth century, measles arrived in the third, typhus is thought to have followed in the 1540s, influenza in the period 1556-60, whilst mumps and diphtheria appeared in the seventeenth century. Falciparum malaria and yellow fever arrived with African slaves, but could not become established until the appropriate mosquito vectors were present.

Archaeology shows that the health of the pre-Columbian Indians ranged from good to very bad, but that life expectancy was generally low and about forty per cent of the population were dead by the age of twenty. In some areas such as the central valley of Mexico, the population had become too large for the available arable land to support. The Aztec codices mention several major crop failures and famines in the years before the Spanish arrived (for example, there was a major famine in 1450), but none of these were accompanied by an epidemic.

By the fifteenth century, diseases were becoming stabilised in the Old World, and, following the Black Death, the European balance of power shifted from Mediterranean states such as Venice and Genoa, to countries on the Atlantic seaboard such as England, Spain, Portugal and Holland. Major advances in areas such as ship-building and navigation were made, and a wave of expansion started. In Europe, by this time, many epidemic diseases had become common childhood diseases with relatively low death rates and a high level of herd immunity, and by the time most children were about five years old, they were either immune to them or had died from them.

The Europeans carried these diseases to the Americas where they killed millions. Many people think that the conquests of the Conquistadors were due to their guns, horses and steel weapons. However, biological warfare (diseases) was the most deadly weapon by far.

Because the Indians had no experience of European crowd diseases, even one person with a mild dose of some disease such as measles could initiate a lethal epidemic. It happened regularly, smallpox being the worst culprit killing millions between 1514 and 1520. It has been suggested that one of the reasons for the massive effect of Old World diseases on the Indian population was that they suffered from a lack of biodiversity. All the Amerindians were descendants of a few very small groups emigrating across Beringia, in relatively recent times in terms of human evolution. There is also the suspicion that numbers may have been reduced to very low levels by some extra-terrestrial event such as an asteroid strike that destroyed the Clovis culture (Ch 5). Their genetic diversity was therefore small, and disease micro-organisms had a good chance of encountering the same, or a very similar immune system, as it moved from host to host. Studies on measles show that it becomes more virulent as it passes from relative to relative and sibling to sibling, and the mortality rate in closely related families is significantly higher than similar sized groups of non-related people. The virus, in effect, becomes a bespoke killer for extended human families.

The effect of this on the Amerindians was catastrophic. Their populations fell to an estimated five per cent of their original numbers and only started to recover in the twentieth century.

A few examples illustrate the problems the Indians faced. Hernán Cortés landed in the New World at Vera Cruz in 1519, and when his small army attacked the Aztec capital

Tenochtitlán in 1521 the population was estimated at 400,000. The first Spanish attack was beaten off, but losses from smallpox stopped the Aztec from following up their success. Cortés was able to rally his men and when they attacked the second time, approximately half the population had died, and many more were sick from smallpox. The Spanish captured the city with a few hundred men. They also captured the Aztec emperor, Montezuma, and after Cortés had exacted a massive ransom for his release, he was murdered. His successor, Cuitláhuac, was killed by smallpox. The social and political infrastructure of the Aztec empire was destroyed and there was a rebellion against the Aztec rulers by various subject tribes, followed by civil war. It is estimated that the population of the Mexico Valley was twenty-five to thirty million when Cortés arrived, but that within less than fifty years (1568), it had fallen to about three million, and by 1618, it was down to approximately 1.6 million.

A similar situation occurred in Peru when smallpox arrived in 1526 and killed the Inca emperor Huayna Capac and his heir Ninan Cuyachi. This was followed by a dynastic civil war between two rival claimants, Atahuallpa and his half brother Huascar. Atahuallpa was victorious, but in 1531, Francisco Pizarro[135] attacked the Incas, and in the Battle of Cajamarca in 1532, less than 200 Spanish, with some local levies opposed to the Inca, defeated an estimated 30,000 Inca, captured the emperor and sacked the Inca capital, Cuzco.

This was again followed by a catastrophic demographic collapse. Census figures compiled by the Spanish show that between 1553-1791, the Inca population fell from eight to three million.

Some of the contemporary accounts make terrifying reading, one author claims, *"more than half the population died...many more died of starvation because they were all sick at once, they could not care for each other"*. Another states, *"the streets, squares and houses were covered with dead bodies; we*

---

135   Pizarro is alleged to have given the Inca smallpox infected blankets.

could not avoid treading on them". In 1541, a Spanish priest wrote that, *"so many died it was impossible to bury the dead and their houses were pulled down on top of them"*.

The Aztec account of "the Great Rash", quoted by Wood, shows how devastating an attack on a non-immune population could be. *"Sores broke out on our faces, our breasts, our stomachs, we were covered with painful sores from head to toe. The sick were so helpless that they could only lie on their beds like the dead, unable to move their limbs or heads. They could not move their bodies, if they did they screamed in pain"*.

One of the major effects of the defeats of the Aztec and Inca Empires was that vast amounts of gold and silver flooded into Spain, and it was this treasure that funded the fleet that defeated the Ottoman fleet at Lepanto in the Mediterranean in 1571, the Spanish armies in the Low Countries and the Spanish Armada that attacked England in 1588.

By 1530, smallpox had spread from the Canadian border to Argentina. It attacked the Mound Builders of the Mississippi valley in 1539, destroying their civilisation. When Hernando de Soto advanced through the Mississippi Valley in 1540, all the Indian towns had been abandoned as most of their inhabitants had died of disease in various epidemics. When French settlers arrived in the late 1600s, the towns themselves had vanished.

In 1620, the Pilgrim Fathers found the area around Plymouth, Massachusetts, depopulated. An epidemic several years earlier, which had spread from the French in Nova Scotia, had killed about ninety per cent of the Indians along the coast. In 1634 John Winthrop (1588-1649), the Governor of Massachusetts, wrote that, *"the natives they are all neere dead of the Small Poxe, so as the Lord hathe cleared our title to what we possess"*. One Puritan preacher wrote of disputes with the Indians over land but concluded by writing, *"God ended the controversy by sending the smallpox amongst the Indians"*.

All the colonists, Spanish, French, English and Americans, were accused at one time or another of deliberately infecting the Indians, usually by giving them blankets that had been used by previous smallpox victims.

Demographic changes of these magnitudes cause massive consequences in terms of the psychology, culture and politics for the societies involved. Faith and belief in the established political order and religion are destroyed frequently triggering revolutions or civil war. The skills and knowledge required to farm the land and maintain irrigation systems that have built up over generations disappear, labour shortages and economic problems appear and the population flow is reversed from cities back to rural areas.

Throughout these massive epidemics, the Europeans were virtually untouched, whilst the Indians, who had no experience of epidemic diseases, attributed this to the power of the European god, and the supernatural belief that, *"their god is stronger than our gods"*. The massive death rate and near-total destruction of the indigenous culture and infra-structure made it easy for the Europeans to penetrate the countries politically and militarily, and impose their religions and cultures on what had effectively become a power vacuum.

Initially, the biggest problem for the Europeans in the Americas was the shortage of labour. The Indians who were used first died of disease, then convicts were used, but there were insufficient numbers. Black slaves were then imported from West Africa and these brought a whole new range of diseases with them including yellow fever and malaria, both of which became epidemic in the Americas and are considered elsewhere. Slave ships also brought the mosquito vectors necessary to carry these diseases. The first record of African slaves in the New World is on the island of Santa Domingo in 1503.

The white population also died as they became isolated from European crowd diseases. Until well into the eighteenth century, most white Americans lived on farms and in villages, and the towns and communities were too small to support crowd diseases. There are many reports of settlers dying in the seventeenth and eighteenth centuries from smallpox, malaria and yellow fever in addition to various other diseases and malnutrition. Many of these diseases were reintroduced at regular intervals into the ports, with yellow fever being a serious problem until the early twentieth century. Some of the diseases that became established permanently evolved into local strains that developed different characteristics to the parent strains in the Old World. It was not until the nineteenth century that the urban population of the USA grew sufficiently large to enable crowd diseases to become endemic and start behaving as typical childhood diseases.

The epidemic diseases of the Americas were repeated as Europeans penetrated the Pacific and Siberia. Measles killed twenty per cent of the population in Hawaii in 1853 and a similar percentage in Fiji in 1874/5. Tuberculosis and sexually transmitted diseases were widespread in Polynesia and the Maoris suffered severely from smallpox, measles, whooping cough and influenza in the mid-nineteenth century, their numbers falling from one hundred thousand to forty thousand. It was a similar story in Australia amongst the aboriginal population, although in this case the Europeans were probably not responsible for introducing smallpox. Smallpox is thought to have arrived in Australia in 1789, probably from Indonesian fisherman who made annual trips to harvest sea slugs. They are also thought to have caused further smallpox epidemics in 1830 and 1860 which killed large numbers of aborigines. Smallpox was probably brought to Indonesia from China as it was already there when the Portuguese arrived in the sixteenth century.

Variolation

Smallpox was the first disease against which an effective immunisation system was developed. This was introduced into

Western Europe in 1721 by Lady Mary Wortley Montagu (1689-1762), the wife of the British Ambassador to the Ottoman Empire, using a process she observed in Istanbul known as variolation. It is thought that the tradition of using the variolation process to inoculate against smallpox in Turkey went back at least several hundred years before 1720. Lady Mary was a famous beauty in her youth but an attack of smallpox had scarred her severely.

In 1717, Lady Mary wrote to one of her friends as follows, "*The smallpox, so fatal and general amongst us, is here entirely harmless by the invention of engrafting* (variolation)". There had been a number of previous reports on variolation to the Royal Society, from 1700 onwards, from Turkey and Greece and also one from America by Cotton Mather, a minister who observed a variolation scar on one of his African slaves in 1706.

The first variolation in England was carried out by Charles Maitland, a doctor from the embassy in Istanbul, on the three year old daughter of Lady Montague. Maitland insisted on having two other doctors present as witnesses, and a report on the procedure was written by Sir Hans Sloane, President of the Royal Society, and published in a Royal Society journal.

Variolation consists of taking living material from the pustules of a victim suffering from a mild case of smallpox and using it to scratch the skin of a susceptible person. The material used causes a pustule at the site of the scratch and confers a long-lasting immunity against a subsequent infection by the smallpox virus. The mildness of the infection caused is usually attributed to the abnormal route of inoculation, the more usual route being through the lungs by droplet infection. Variolation had a significant risk as a number of people did develop smallpox, and about one per cent died from the process. This however was considerably less than the death toll from "natural" smallpox during an epidemic. The major problem with variolation was that the person variolated was infectious and could initiate an epidemic of smallpox amongst non-immune contacts. Numerous epidemics are known to have started in this manner.

In China and India an alternative method of variolation was practised. A piece of cotton, infected with material from the pustules of a smallpox victim, was placed into the nostrils. This is theoretically considerably more dangerous as it is the normal route of infection, however, material was only taken from very mild cases and was dried at body temperature for a month to reduce its pathogenicity (basically an attenuated culture was used). As an alternative in China, the doctor would blow infective material up the nostrils of a child using a tube, right nostril for a boy and left for a girl. The powder used would have produced larger particles than the virus containing aerosol from an infected person, and when inhaled would have been filtered out in the upper respiratory tract, and not penetrated very far into the lungs. As mentioned in Chapter 3, the particle size of inhaled bio-warfare agents is critical.

The Chinese and Indians probably practised nasal inoculation at an earlier stage than the Turks used engrafting. Officials of the Honourable East India Company mentioned inoculation in India in the eighteenth century, and commented that it had been common for at least 150 years, whilst there were some claims that the practice went back hundreds of years earlier. There were also claims that variolation had been practised in China from the mid-sixteenth century.

Following the variolation of Lady Montague's child, the Princess of Wales, Caroline of Brandenburg Ansbach, with the agreement of King George II, arranged for six condemned prisoners who had not had smallpox to be variolated. All the prisoners recovered and were freed. Sir Hans Sloane paid one prisoner to nurse smallpox victims and the prisoner did not catch smallpox. The princess then arranged for six foundling charity children to be variolated and when they all survived she had her own children inoculated. Large numbers of the upper classes followed the example of the princess and had themselves, their children and servants variolated. These were followed by the middle classes, including people such as Josiah Wedgwood, the founder of the Wedgwood factory and grandfather of Charles Darwin. Maitland did have some problems in families when children, who had been variolated, infected other members of the family and servants with smallpox. A number of upper and middle class families would not employ servants unless they had survived an attack of smallpox and had the scars to prove it.

There was initially strong vocal opposition to variolation in England from many of the clergy. In 1722, Sir Edmond Massey claimed in a sermon that Satan inflicted boils on Job, therefore Satan was the first inoculator and it therefore followed that variolation was a diabolical practice. It was also thought that smallpox was one of the punishments God used to chastise sinners and fear of it kept men on the straight and narrow.

By 1758, variolation by physicians in England had evolved into something complicated and mystical. Lady Mary had reported that variolation in Istanbul was carried out with no preparation, a small scratch producing a minor skin abrasion was made, and a minimal amount of infectious material inserted into it. In England however, on the principle that more must be better, several deep cuts were inflicted and a large amount of material was rubbed into the wounds. These frequently produced blood poisoning or gangrene. In addition, the prospective patient was frequently dosed for a number of weeks prior to variolation, with drugs such as mercury and antimony, and subjected to regimes of dieting, purging and bleeding. Jenner himself was variolated at the age of eight and went through six weeks of preparation that was later described as, *"human veterinary practice"*.

Eventually there was a reaction against such barbaric treatments, initiated by variolators in the Sutton family. They cut out the preparatory period, and used minimal incisions as used by Islamic doctors. They also used infectious material taken from the pustules of a smallpox victim on the fourth day of development, whilst they were still immature, and the material in them was still clear. Earlier variolators had used pus from mature pustules. The Sutton method produced a much milder reaction using these techniques.

By this time the need for quarantine to avoid the variolated person spreading smallpox was widely realised, although there were still dissidents. One member of the family, Daniel Sutton, set up isolation clinics where he charged rich patients for variolation, making substantial profits, but treated the poor free of charge. By 1768, there were numerous authorised partnerships using the Sutton methods of variolation in the British Isles, Europe and the American colonies. Jenner trained using the Sutton methods, and adapted their idea of taking immature material for his own vaccination methods.

In 1743, variolation was made compulsory for orphans at a hospital in England and, in 1746 the first smallpox hospital in England was opened. The hospital was split with one part for quarantining those who had been variolated, and the other half for naturally occurring cases of smallpox.

In 1768, an English doctor, Thomas Dinsdale, travelled to Russia and successfully variolated the Empress, Catherine the Great, and most of her court. Dinsdale also helped to establish inoculation hospitals in Russia and trained Russian doctors. The process became very popular, it is estimated that two million Russians were variolated and Dinsdale was rewarded very handsomely by Catherine. He also realised the importance of quarantining the variolated person, and strongly advocated variolating whole families, villages and districts simultaneously, rather than variolating isolated individuals.

Not everyone agreed with Dinsdale about the importance of isolating those variolated. The influential Quaker doctor, John Lettsom, was worried that only the rich could afford variolation followed by isolation. He advocated free clinics available to everyone and also initially did not believe in the necessity for isolation. The satirical poem written about him was a bit unfair, it probably applied to most of the doctors of the day:

> *"When any sick to me apply,*
> *I physics, bleeds and sweats 'em*
> *If after that they choose to die,*
> *Why verily, I Lettsom".*

By the time Jenner started to vaccinate people, Lettsom's views had modified, and he had realised the dangers of not isolating freshly variolated patients.

Variolation was not popular in France, even although it suffered from severe epidemics of smallpox, an estimated twenty thousand dying in Paris alone in 1723. Variolation was opposed by both the Church (it interfered with God's will) and the Sorbonne (it was not French), and by 1769, although over 200,000 had been variolated in England, only 15,000 had been treated in France. Although some members of the French royal family had decided to have their children variolated in 1756, it was not until 1774, when Louis XV died from smallpox, that resistance to variolation ceased.

At the beginning of the nineteenth century, it was thought that 45,000 were dying annually in the UK from smallpox, but in France the figure was of the order of 150,000 per annum. The mathematician, Daniel Bernoulli, claimed, in the middle of the eighteenth century, that six hundred thousand were dying of the disease in Europe every year which was probably a conservative estimate.

The drive to variolate and vaccinate was led to a large extent by the military. The Prussians began variolating their troops in 1775, the Duke of York ordered that the whole of the British army and navy should be vaccinated in 1800, and Napoleon enforced it in France in 1805 and again in 1811. France abandoned immunisation after Napoleon was defeated and suffered very badly from smallpox in the mid-nineteenth century as a result.

Smallpox was also a serious problem in America during the eighteenth century War of Independence, and George Washington had all his troops variolated. It was carried out in great secrecy so the British could not take advantage of the fact that the soldiers were incapacitated whilst they recovered. Many of the general public were also variolated at the same time. Washington had had smallpox himself in 1751, and in 1777 he wrote to a friend stating that, *"it is more destructive to an army than the sword"*. After the worst epidemic in Canadian history from 1775-7, John Adams, the future president of the USA, wrote that, *"Our misfortunes in Canada are enough to melt the heart of stone. The smallpox is ten times more terrible than the British, Canadians and Indians together. This was the cause of our precipitate retreat from Quebec"*.

In the United States, variolation was practised widely, although there was considerable controversy about its effectiveness. Massachusetts passed a smallpox act in 1701 allowing houses to be commandeered for the isolation of victims, and Boston had a smallpox quarantine hospital in 1717, whilst quarantine stations had been set up to check ships for smallpox. A large epidemic occurred in Boston in 1721 which killed a considerable number of people. Variolation was used to bring it under control and only one of those variolated died, although some doctors objected to the process, claiming that it helped spread the epidemic. Some American states went as far as banning variolation because of the risk of spreading the disease. Benjamin Franklin, writing in 1736, stated that one of his sons aged four had died of smallpox and he greatly regretted not having him variolated.

By 1755, the College of Surgeons in England were writing that they judged variolation *"to be a Practice of the utmost benefit to Mankind"*. During the last decade of the eighteenth century, both doctors and the clergy in England were advocating variolation, and it was widely known that the main problems were incomplete variolation of the population and inadequate quarantine of those who had been treated during the period they were infectious. A number of towns had variolation hospitals, where variolated patients were isolated to reduce the risk of them causing an epidemic but these were frequently too small for the numbers involved.

Several doctors recommended compulsory variolation of everyone, and one, John Hoggarth, claimed in 1793, that although it was an *"invasion of personal liberty"*, if his ideas were followed, smallpox could be eliminated from Britain within a few weeks.

James Jurin, the Secretary of the Royal Society, suggested that a profit/loss from variolation should be prepared, and collected figures of those variolated, which suggested a death rate from the process in the region of one per cent. He also studied the Bills of Mortality and was able to show that the average death rate due to smallpox was over seven per cent. His figures were somewhat suspect, as it was difficult to make the appropriate allowance for those who had contracted smallpox from people who had been variolated. His opinion was that the risk to the individual variolated was worth taking, but that the risk to society needed to be minimised by quarantining those who had been variolated until they were no longer infectious.

A similar exercise had been carried out by Charles-Marie de la Condamine in 1754, when he published *"Mémoire sur l'Inoculation"*. He calculated that ten per cent of deaths in France were from smallpox and considered that it destroyed, maimed or disfigured a quarter of the population. He also made the novel suggestion, for the time, that the lives saved would increase the wealth of the state, a statement echoed in the attempts to control HIV and AIDS in Africa today.

VACCINATION

"Among those whom in the country I was frequently called upon to inoculate, many resisted every effort to give them the smallpox. These patients I found had undergone a disease they

called the cowpox, contracted by milking cows affected with a peculiar eruption on their teats". Edward Jenner, 1801.

The process of vaccination was discovered by Edward Jenner (1749-1823), an English country doctor, who published his results in 1798. Jenner was a Fellow of the Royal Society who elected him for his work as a naturalist, specialising in cuckoos. Some of his observations regarding cuckoos were not confirmed until the twentieth century, when they were validated by techniques such as time-lapse photography. He was also a life-long fossil hunter who realised that fossils were an extinct form of life.

Jenner trained in the Sutton method of variolation, but by the end of his apprenticeship around 1769, he became aware of the disease cowpox, and the fact that it appeared to prevent smallpox. He realised that a number of his patients had acquired cowpox from milking diseased cows and that it was impossible to carry out a successful variolation on these people. The observation that milkmaids never caught smallpox is the origin of the song, *"Where are you going to my pretty maid?"* to which the answer is, *"I'm going a-milking"* followed by, *"What is your fortune my pretty maid?"* with the response, *"My face is my fortune"*.

There had been a tradition in folk medicine in a number of counties of using cowpox to vaccinate against smallpox before Jenner. It has been suggested that he got the idea from a Dorset farmer, Benjamin Jesty, who vaccinated his wife and two children in 1774, over twenty years before Jenner's work[136]. The difference between Jenner and Jesty however, was that Jesty did not challenge the people he had vaccinated with

---

136   Jesty is buried in the churchyard at Worth Matravers in Dorset; his gravestone was cleaned and re-dedicated in 2008. It reads, Sacred to the Memory of Benj^m Jesty (of Downshay) who departed this life April 16th 1816 aged 79 years. He was born at Yetminster in this *County*, and was an upright honest *Man;* particularly *noted* for having been the first Person (known) that *introduced* the *Cow Pox* by *Inoculation*, and who from his *great strength of mind made the Experiment from* the *Cow* on his Wife and two Sons in the year 1774.

variolation (smallpox), Jenner did. Jenner also vaccinated a number of individuals, carried out a scientific investigation of the process and then published his results[137].

Technically, one can only vaccinate against smallpox, as the name is derived from the Latin word *vacca* for cow. Immunisation against every other disease is done by inoculation, Pasteur however, recommended that all immunisations should be called vaccinations in honour of Jenner. The terms vaccination, inoculation and immunisation are now used virtually synonymously.

Jenner wrote a report on his work in 1798 entitled, *"An Inquiry into the Causes and Effects of the Variolae Vaccinae"*. In his "Inquiry" he stated that in July 1796, he had inoculated an eight year old boy, James Phipps, with material from a pustule on the hand of a milkmaid, Sarah Nelmes, who was suffering from cowpox. He commented that he was surprised at the close resemblance of the pustules to those of smallpox. He then challenged James Phipps by attempting to variolate him with smallpox six weeks later, but was unable do it successfully. Jenner gave details of twelve patients in his inquiry who had had cowpox, all of them were resistant to variolation and smallpox. It is an unusual situation that infection with one virus, *Vaccinia* or cowpox, can confer immunity to a disease caused by a second virus, *Variola* or smallpox.

Jenner also stated, *"What renders the Cow-Pox virus so extremely singular is that the person who has been thus affected is for ever after secure from infection of the Small-Pox"*. He actually got that wrong, infection with cowpox does not provide life-long immunity against smallpox, although it is long-term. This distinction between life-long and long-term caused considerable confusion and controversy during the nineteenth century, when the subject of re-vaccination was

---

137   It is worth pointing out that a modern medical ethical committee of the British Medical Association would have struck Jenner and numerous other medical practitioners off the register. The methods they used to develop a smallpox vaccine would certainly not be tolerated today.

hotly debated. Jenner probably had not appreciated that people working with cattle came into contact with cowpox at regular intervals throughout their life. This would have produced a much higher level of immunity than an adult who had only been vaccinated once as a child. They would have effectively re-vaccinated themselves every time they came into contact with cowpox, and boosted their immunity to smallpox on each exposure to the cowpox virus.

It is also interesting to note in the previous paragraphs, that Jenner used the word *"virus"* approximately one hundred years before viruses were discovered or their existence inferred. He would have been using it in the Latin meaning of the word, i.e. poison.

Jenner speculated that diseases in humans might have been caught from domestic animals, stating, *"There is a disease to which the Horse, from his state of domestication is frequently subject. The Farriers have termed it the Grease. It is an inflammation and swelling in the heel, from which issues "matter" possessing properties of a very peculiar kind which seems capable of generating a disease in the Human Body which bears so strong a resemblance to Smallpox, that I think it highly probable it may be the source of that disease".* He thought that people coming into contact with an infected horse, then milking a cow could pass the infective agent onto the cow where it manifested itself as cowpox. This could in turn be passed onto other humans during the milking process. Again he was considerably in advance of his time, and by speculating that smallpox may have made the species jump from animals to man, he was articulating an idea that only really became accepted in the twentieth century.

Jenner showed that it was possible to transfer cowpox from the arm of one child to the arm of another through a sequence of five children, and wrote, *"they proved that the matter in passing from one human subject to another through five generations, lost none of its original properties".* This became extremely important in practical terms as it was used as the source of an active vaccine in the absence of refrigeration or storage methods.

He also pointed out that *Vaccinia,* unlike *Variola,* was not infectious, and did not initiate an epidemic of smallpox, and even realised that children with eczema or other skin problems such as herpes should not be vaccinated due to the possibility of a generalised skin reaction.

Henry Cline, one of Jenner's friends, wrote to him in 1798 saying, *"I think the substituting of the Cow-Pox poison for the smallpox promises to be one of the greatest improvements that has ever been made in medicine".* In 1806, Thomas Jefferson, the President of the USA, wrote stating that, *"Medicine has never before produced any single improvement of such utility".* He was even praised by Napoleon; Jenner wrote to him requesting the release of certain prisoners during the Napoleonic Wars, and Napoleon is reported to have said, *" Jenner, I can refuse him nothing".*

By 1801, Jenner was predicting the end of smallpox by means of vaccination, but there were numerous practical problems to be overcome before this dream could be realised.

Not all doctors agreed with Jenner about the advantages of vaccination and some continued to offer patients the choice of variolation or vaccination for many years. There were numerous problems with doctors attempting to vaccinate people using material from lesions on cattle that had not been caused by cowpox. When these people were challenged with variolation or came into contact with smallpox, they developed the disease, and as a result it was frequently claimed that vaccination was ineffective.

There were also problems over the purity of the cowpox material, and Jenner considered that in some cases, cowpox had become contaminated with smallpox as a result of careless practice by certain vaccinators. This could initiate an epidemic of smallpox as the person, who was thought to have been vaccinated, had in fact been variolated. As far as Jenner was concerned, one William Woodville at the London Smallpox and Inoculation Hospital was the main culprit, but it is impossible to sort out the facts amidst all the accusations and counter-accusations, many of which would certainly be considered libellous today and finish up in court.

The *Variola, Vaccinia* and cowpox viruses produce markedly different reactions when grown on fertile hens' eggs, and analysis of their DNA sequences shows that although there are many similarities, they are three distinct viruses. The question therefore arises, what was the origin of the Vaccinia virus used in vaccination? The answer is that nobody knows for certain. Cows were not the only source of the material used for vaccination, both Jenner and other doctors used material from lesions in horses as Jenner had problems of obtaining sufficient cowpox virus. The genetic makeup of horsepox cannot be checked as the disease appears to have disappeared from Europe during the twentieth century.

Cowpox is uncommon in cattle, but one sample of the virus found in Pennsylvania in 1882 was used to found the vaccine-producing laboratory that eventually became Wyeth Laboratories. One of Jenner's original theories was that cows only developed cowpox when handled by people who had handled horses with *"grease"*. The immunity patterns led Jenner to suggest that *"grease"* had to pass through cattle before it became very effective. The theory was difficult to prove and Jenner eventually dropped the idea. Several other doctors tried to inoculate people using *"grease"* and claimed to have been successful. One went as far as to suggest that the immunising material should be called equine instead of vaccine, after the Latin word "equus" meaning horse.

Some priests condemned Jenner's work as interfering with God's design for keeping the population under control, and one Dr Birch suggested that smallpox was a, *"merciful provision on the part of providence to lessen the burden of a poor man's family*". The Church also complained about introducing an animal disease into humans, a complaint reminiscent of some of the comments made in the present day about the uses of genetic engineering. Gilray ridiculed the hysteria over vaccination with his famous satirical cartoon of 1802, showing cows erupting on various parts of peoples' anatomy after they had been vaccinated by Jenner.

Thomas Malthus (Ch 5) also became embroiled in the argument, and wrote that smallpox was, *"one of the channels and a very broad one, which nature has opened for the last thousand years to keep down the population to a level of the means of subsistence"*. As late as 1826, he described doctors advocating vaccination as, *"those benevolent but much mistaken men"*.

In 1832 Thomas Hood wrote the satirical poem, "Ode to Malthus".

> *"Oh Mr Malthus, I agree*
> *In everything I read with thee,*
> *The world's too full, there is no doubt*
> *And wants a deal of thinning out.*
> *Why should we let precautions so absorb us*
> *Or trouble shipping with a quarantine,*
> *When if I understand the thing you mean,*
> *We ought to import the cholera morbus"!*

He is admittedly talking about cholera rather than smallpox, but presumably could not get smallpox to scan, and as cholera had just reached the shores of the British Isles for the first time, it would have been a highly topical subject.

Even Charles Darwin became involved in the discussion. In the *"Descent of Man"* (1871) he wrote, *"There is reason to believe that vaccination has preserved thousands, who from a weak constitution would formerly have succumbed to smallpox. Thus the weak members of civilised societies propagate their kind. No one who has attended to the breeding of domestic animals will doubt that this must be highly injurious to the race of man. It is surprising how soon a want of care, or care wrongly directed,*

*leads to the degradation of a domestic race; but except in the case
of man himself, hardly anyone is so ignorant as to allow his worst
animals to breed".*

Thomas McKeown (1912-88) suggested that improvement
in mortality rates and the rise in population was due not
to improved medicine and vaccination, but rather due to
improved nutrition and sanitation. Most experts do not agree
with this suggestion. Population increases were not influenced
by improved sanitation before about 1870, and most authors
think that the introduction of smallpox vaccine had a major
impact on population demographics.

One early success of vaccination was in 1800, when a
case of smallpox appeared in Westmoreland. The local doctor,
Robert Thornton, vaccinated all the contacts in the village
(about 400), ring-fencing the epidemic and stopping it in its
tracks. This later became the standard method of dealing
with outbreaks of smallpox. It works because smallpox has an
incubation time of 10-12 days whilst vaccination is effective
within 3-5 days. Therefore if people are vaccinated sufficiently
quickly after coming into contact with smallpox, the epidemic
can be ring-fenced and contained. Erasmus Darwin, the
grandfather of Charles and a physician, suggested that all
children should be vaccinated when they were christened.

By 1801, an estimated one hundred thousand people had been
vaccinated in England, and Jenner's work had been published in
Latin, with translations into a number of European languages.
In 1802, Jenner was rewarded by Parliament who voted him the
sum of £10,000 for his work and a further £20,000 in 1806.
These were enormous sums at that time, when one could live
reasonably comfortably on an income of £100 per year.

Jenner was also capable of self-promotion; he acted as the
patron of the poet, Robert Bloomfield, who wrote a number
of poems praising Jenner and advocating vaccination. One of
these pieces "The Farmer's Boy" included the lines,

> *"or dreamt that in the blood of kine there ran*
> *Blessings beyond the sustenance of Man".*

At this point there was no method of storing vaccine, so when it was sent any great distance it was done as an arm-to-arm transfer. A number of "volunteers" were sent on a ship, the first being vaccinated before leaving and the others were vaccinated at intervals during the voyage to keep an active vaccine going until the voyage ended. In 1803, the Spanish sent 22 foundling boys to South America, who were vaccinated in pairs at intervals and the last pair provided material for the start of a vaccination programme in South America. More children were "recruited" in South America, and the vaccine was sent using the same method to China, the Philippines and Mexico. Portugal also used this technique to take vaccine to its South American colonies.

Although this method was successful, there were numerous problems. It was necessary to have a constant supply of suitable children, and there was a possibility of transmitting syphilis or some skin disease such as erysipelas. As a result, Jenner suggested it would be better to use material taken directly from a pustule, rather than the arm-to-arm method, and advocated the use of cotton threads impregnated with material from cowpox pustules and dried. These could then be applied to the scratches to introduce the material into the body. The main problem with this approach was one of reliability and the efficacy was variable.

Because of the problems of using virus from children, a number of doctors and scientists started to use calves. Two methods were used, the first of which was to inoculate calves with smallpox in an attempt to induce cowpox. A number of people claimed to have done this successfully, but twentieth-century opinion considers that the smallpox used was almost certainly contaminated with cowpox.

In the second method, calves were inoculated with cowpox from the arm of a person who had been recently vaccinated.

This was attempted as early as 1805, and in 1843, Pietro Negri in Italy carried out inoculations from calf-to-calf, then dragged a calf through the town inoculating people calf-to-arm in roadside clinics. The process spread widely across Europe, Russia and the USA. In England, calf-to-arm vaccination clinics were established, one of which in London later became the Lister Institute.

The vaccine from calves became known as lymph and before its use became widespread it was necessary to store it safely without it losing its efficacy. Negri used glycerine (glycerol) as a stabilising agent, which had the additional advantage of killing contaminating bacteria. Lymph treated with glycerol became widely used, and arm-to-arm vaccination was banned in England in 1898. Even when treated with glycerol, calf lymph only retained its efficacy for about six weeks; this could be improved by refrigeration although it was not always possible in the tropics.

During World War I, the Pasteur Institute developed a method of treating the lymph with glycerol and then freeze-drying it. This is a process in which the material is frozen rapidly and all the moisture is removed by the application of a high vacuum. Once the freeze-dried material was vacuum packed, the vaccine lasted for months irrespective of storage conditions.

The College of Physicians warned of the dangers of variolation in 1807, and recommended that, *"vaccination should be offered to the poorer classes without expense"*. However, variolation was still causing epidemics of smallpox in Britain as late as 1818/9, when it caused more than 3,000 cases in Norwich, killing over 500. Only approximately fifteen percent of the population of the city had been vaccinated which is well below the level needed to establish herd immunity.

Variolation caused problems for much of the first half of the nineteenth century. In Britain, the Vaccination Act of 1840 offered free vaccination to all young children, and also at the insistence of many doctors, banned variolation. The British banned variolation in India in 1870 but it was still being used in China as late as 1965. By the 1840s, vaccination was widespread throughout Europe, and is credited with playing a major role in the reduction of the death rate of children during the nineteenth century.

A new Bill in 1853 proposed that all children should be vaccinated by the age of four months, with parents who refused being fined or imprisoned. In many other countries vaccination was made compulsory for children before they were allowed to attend school, and vaccination certificates had to be produced to claim poor relief, become an apprentice or get married. As late as 1856, anyone was allowed to carry out vaccination, including clergyman and midwives.

In 1896, the British Medical Journal stated, *"Primary vaccination vastly reduces the mortality from smallpox, but it also shifts the incidence of this mortality from childhood to adult life".* They pointed out that a single vaccination as a child does not give permanent protection, it lapses with age and is not as effective as the immunity created by surviving smallpox. The article finishes by stating, *"More adults now die of smallpox than in the early days of vaccination".* Because vaccination was not life-long, if a person who had been vaccinated some years previously came into contact with the disease, it was possible for them to acquire a sub-clinical infection. Such a person would become a carrier, and could pass the disease onto susceptible individuals, without it being realised that they were the focal point of the infection. Generally however, the person vaccinated in the distant past usually presented as a very mild case of smallpox. During the nineteenth century, many countries introduced re-vaccination and made it compulsory for army recruits and other state jobs.

There was some danger associated with vaccination. It killed about one individual in every fourteen thousand vaccinated, caused encephalitis in a few isolated cases, and could cause a generalised outbreak of pustules in individuals with eczema and herpes. There were also cases of erysipelas caused by careless vaccination that could be fatal before the discovery of antibiotics. Arm-to-arm vaccination caused a few cases of syphilis, probably due to material being taken from the arm of a child suffering from an unrecognised case of congenital syphilis. These problems were however trivial when compared with those of a major epidemic of smallpox.

Smallpox was not a problem for the British in the Crimean War of 1853-6, but it was very serious during the American Civil War from 1861-5. It was much worse in the South than in the North and amongst black soldiers rather than white ones. It also caused a very high death toll in prisoner-of-war camps.

In Canada, there were major riots in Montreal when vaccination was enforced during a serious epidemic, due to the fear that it would spread syphilis, and troops were needed to restore order. Many people were not vaccinated and the final death toll was over three thousand.

These worries led to the rise of the English Anti-Vaccination League established after the 1853 Act (the first attempt to make vaccination compulsory). One review at the end of the nineteenth century pointed out that the majority of leaders of the AVL had had no contact with smallpox, the implication being that if they had, they would support vaccination. Jurin had stated earlier that, *"people do not easily come into a practice in which they apprehend any hazard unless they are frightened into it by a greater danger"*. By this time, the death rate from smallpox was so low that it did not seem to be the greater danger. When smallpox was finally eliminated, vaccination risks were very low at 1-2 deaths per million, with about fifty individuals per million suffering from adverse side-effects.

There was considerable opposition in England to vaccination throughout much of the nineteenth century. Much of this opposition was generated by educated men such as the

Victorian reformer, Edward Chadwick (see Ch 12). He thought most diseases were due to miasmas, filthy conditions and poor sanitation. He included smallpox with other diseases such as typhus, typhoid and cholera, which could be dealt with by improving conditions. In addition, well-known people such as George Bernard Shaw referred to vaccination as, "*a particularly filthy piece of witchcraft*". Shaw had no medical knowledge and regarded Pasteur and Lister as scientific charlatans. Vaccination was also opposed by the naturalist, Alfred Russel Wallace, whom one would have expected to know better. He was of the opinion that, "*vaccination is quite powerless either to prevent or to mitigate smallpox*", and stated that the statistics produced in support of vaccination were useless.

Shaw was opposed by the writer, Sir Henry Rider Haggard (author of the novel, "*King Solomon's Mines*"), who had experienced a severe epidemic of smallpox in Africa. In 1898, Rider Haggard wrote a novel, "*Doctor Therne*", extolling the advantages of vaccination.

The advantages of vaccination and re-vaccination were demonstrated by two outbreaks in England in the last two decades of the nineteenth century. The first was in Sheffield in 1887. Ninety-five per cent of the population had been vaccinated, and when the epidemic started nearly three hundred died in the unvaccinated five per cent of the population and only two hundred in the vaccinated ninety-five per cent. There were no deaths amongst those who had been revaccinated.

In 1895 however, in Gloucestershire, there was a strong opposition to vaccination and a large number of children had not been immunised. An outbreak infected a significant part of the population and killed over four hundred, including many children. Compulsory vaccination and revaccination eventually brought the epidemic to an end.

One major epidemic in Europe in 1870 coincided with the outbreak of the Franco-Prussian War. It was spread across Europe by French refugees and prisoners of war, and is estimated to have killed over half a million people. It killed approximately 23,000 French troops but less than five hundred in the Prussian army, where compulsory vaccination and re-vaccination were enforced with Prussian thoroughness.

The effectiveness of these types of measures was seen on several occasions in the twentieth century. In 1947, a visitor from Mexico died of smallpox in New York, and infected a number of other individuals. Two people died, but the outbreak was controlled by vaccinating six million people in a few weeks. A similar incident occurred in Moscow in 1960, when one case infected forty-six people and over six million were vaccinated in one week.

Because of strong opposition, the 1898 Vaccination Act in Britain allowed parents to refuse to vaccinate their children, that is, to become conscientious objectors. A cartoon of the time shows a cloaked skeleton, crowned with a laurel wreath, holding a scythe in one hand; around its feet are symbols of death such as an hourglass and a snake. The skeleton is triumphantly waving aloft a scroll with the title, *"Anti-vaccination Bill"*. The cartoon is labelled, *"Triumph of De-Jenner-ation"*, an interesting play on words.

By the end of the nineteenth century, the effectiveness of vaccination throughout Europe was obvious. In those countries where vaccination and re-vaccination were compulsory and enforced, the number of deaths due to smallpox had fallen to virtually zero. By the twentieth century, *V. major* had more or less disappeared from the UK, Europe and North America except for isolated epidemics caused by infected immigrants, although there were serious outbreaks caused by returning troops after World War I. Vaccination was mandatory in the UK until the late 1940s, although it was never 100% successful because of conscientious objectors.

A statue of Jenner was placed on one of the plinths in Trafalgar Square. It only stayed there for four years before being moved in 1858 to Kensington Gardens to make room for some obscure general. As usual, Punch made the appropriate satirical comment that says it all:

> *"I saved you many million spots*
> *And now you grudge one spot for me".*

Routine vaccination against smallpox in the UK ended in 1971, and stopped worldwide in 1980. After this time the only vaccinations carried out were in emergencies.

<u>THE ERADICATION OF SMALLPOX</u>

Although the process of vaccination was well known and widely practised in Western Europe and North America, from the early nineteenth century onwards, its use in other areas of the world was sporadic, and as late as the early 1960s, smallpox was still estimated to be killing two million people each year.

Smallpox was finally eliminated from the human population in 1977, the last few cases occurring in Somalia. It was a relatively easy disease to defeat for a number of technical reasons, and to date, it is the only human disease we have managed to eliminate. There are a number of reasons for this, and although many people regard smallpox eradication as an example of how to deal with other diseases, many epidemiologists would regard the elimination of smallpox as a lucky aberration, not an ideal model for the elimination of other diseases. The reasons for the effectiveness of smallpox eradication are as follows;

- People were frightened of smallpox in a way that they were not frightened of other diseases. This meant that most people are prepared to undergo the discomfort of vaccination, when they would not undergo immunisation against many other diseases.

- There is a single, very effective vaccine against all types of smallpox which is simple to store and can be administered by personnel with only a minimum of training. In addition, as the vaccination site usually produces an easily recognisable scar, it is possible to distinguish between those who have, and those who have not, been vaccinated in a population. The vaccine can also be given as a single application with no booster necessary in the short term, this single application producing a long-term immunity of ten years or more in most individuals.

- The disease is simple to diagnose even for an untrained layman due to the massive pustules. These produce serious permanent scarring, so it is easy to determine who has had disease and therefore has a high level of natural immunity.

- Smallpox is a human virus only; there are no animal reservoirs and no vectors. Therefore once it has been eliminated in humans, the disease has been beaten.

- The progress of the disease is rapid. Once a person is infected the symptoms appear within about ten days and people are only infectious for a short period. This makes the process of tracing contacts relatively simple. In addition, the victims are so weak that they are effectively immobilised and access to them can be controlled, thus reducing the possibility of them infecting large numbers of other people.

The main problems of dealing with smallpox were that cases were not reported for a variety of reasons. In many parts of the world, it was regarded as a fact of life, and local authorities did not report it, and in a number of countries, cases were concealed or vaccination was refused by various religious groups. In addition, in a number of colonial administrations, houses were burnt to control the spread of the disease, obviously leading to a marked reluctance to report cases. Finally, smallpox was widespread in rural areas and frequently the authorities did not hear of an outbreak for some time. Between 1901-60,

Ghana was an example of these problems. There were six major epidemics of smallpox, with a death rate of about fifty per cent of those infected, but in no year were more than 2,000 cases reported to the authorities.

In 1955, the WHO, which had been founded in 1948, agreed that eradication of malaria should be a world-wide policy, and this should be done before mosquitoes became resistant to insecticides such as DDT. There was a massive attempt at eradication over the next ten years, but by 1969, it was obvious that this was ineffective in spite of the huge sums of money spent, and the programme was ended in 1973.

This delayed the start of the smallpox eradication programme that had originally been proposed to the WHO in 1959, although Jenner had suggested this was a possibility one hundred and fifty years earlier. In 1966, the WHO agreed a programme aimed at eliminating smallpox worldwide within ten years. Millions of doses of vaccine were donated by the USSR and Cuba and the programme started in 1969. The programme emphasised detection and containment, that is, detecting cases, and ring-fencing them, with a vaccination programme in areas where smallpox was endemic, and mass vaccination in areas where the disease was epidemic. A major part of programme was the education of the public.

In India, smallpox was causing over one million deaths/year in the 1950s, and there were still large numbers of cases as late as 1967 in spite of claims that eighty per cent of the population had been vaccinated, a figure that had almost certainly been falsified. There were a series of bad outbreaks from 1972-4, the last case in India occurring in May 1975, and in Bangladesh in November 1975. There were also problems in Afghanistan, when an epidemic in 1970 spread to Iran, Iraq and Syria. This was finally stopped in late 1971.

In 1973, a major famine in Ethiopia led to mass migration into Somalia, and in 1974 a revolution deposed Haile Selassie, the Emperor of Ethiopia, this being followed by a bloody civil war in 1975. The last outbreak in Ethiopia was in 1975, but in 1976, there were reports of over 500 cases in Somalia by the end of the year. By May 1977, over 600 cases had been reported from Southern Somalia. The WHO saturated the area with medical teams and the epidemic peaked in June with 1,300 cases. By September ninety per cent of the population had been vaccinated and the last case occurred in October 1977. There were considerable problems in dealing with the last few cases in Sudan/Somalia which was effectively a war zone. In addition, the population are Muslim and the Hajj (the annual pilgrimage of Muslims to Mecca) was close. It would have only needed one infectious case, amongst several million pilgrims, to spread the disease world wide again.

Serious problems occurred in many countries where the reporting of cases was ineffective and there were also problems of vaccination records being falsified to meet projected targets. Several methods of improving the situation were used including replacing inefficient staff and cash rewards for anyone informing about cases.

No cases were reported from 1977 to 1979, with the exception of two cases, one of them fatal, in England in 1978, whose source was a laboratory accident in Birmingham University. In 1979, the world was officially declared free of smallpox.

The total cost of the eradication programme was estimated by the World Health Organisation to be $300 million.

Routine smallpox vaccination has now been discontinued, and by the mid-1980s a number of countries had destroyed their smallpox stocks. The virus is now officially kept in only two laboratories throughout the world, one in the Center for Disease Control in Atlanta, USA, and one in the Institute of Virology in Moscow ready to make the vaccine should it ever again be necessary, whilst the UK keeps a library of fragments for the identification of any future outbreak.

Military personnel were vaccinated against smallpox during the second Gulf War in 2003, and it was also used in the summer of 2003 when monkeypox was introduced to the USA by a wildlife importer. This caused over seventy human cases of monkeypox, but smallpox vaccination is reasonably effective at immunizing against this disease.

SMALLPOX AS A WEAPON OF BIOLOGICAL WARFARE

The USSR saw eradication of smallpox as an opportunity; eradication of a disease makes it very tempting for use as a biological weapon. In 1987, the Russian scientist, Ken Alibekov, started supervision of a new smallpox weapon ordered by President Gorbachev. Factory production of *Variola* was begun with the intention of producing 80-100 tons of *Variola* per year that could be delivered either by aircraft or missile. In the late 1980s and early 90s, several Russian scientists including Alibekov defected. When debriefed, some of Alibekov's claims shocked western scientists about Russian progress. These included manipulating *Variola* genetically to make it resistant to existing vaccines, and also inserting new material into *Variola* to create a novel virus capable of causing two lethal diseases simultaneously. Following the disintegration of the USSR, Russian scientists have gone to numerous countries, and there is now the suspicion that *Variola* may be circulating in a number of countries usually regarded as terrorist states.

There is also the problem that the complete nucleic acid sequences of several strains of *Variola* are known and have been published, which raises the possibility of it being synthesised in a laboratory. Whilst this is not possible at present as the genome is too big, polio was synthesised several years ago and it is probably only a matter of time before *Variola* is synthesised successfully.

Leprosy and Tuberculosis

Leprosy and tuberculosis are both diseases caused by Gram-positive bacteria from the genus *Mycobacterium.* They are closely related, and are therefore considered in the same chapter.

Leprosy

Leprosy is also known as Hansen's disease, after the Norwegian doctor, Gerhard Hansen (1841-1912), who discovered the causative organism in 1873. It is caused by the bacterium, *Mycobacterium leprae,* and probably infected humans from soil thousands of years ago. *M. leprae* only causes disease in humans, although bizarrely it is possible to infect armadillos in the laboratory. Much of the research work on it was carried out on mice, which can be infected on the pads of their feet, although it is not possible to pass it from mouse to mouse, thus limiting the value of these animals for laboratory study of the disease. Scientific work on leprosy is very difficult, as it is one of a small number of pathogenic bacteria that cannot be grown on artificial media. Hansen found it impossible to either grow the bacterium or to establish the chain of infection in humans. The incubation period of the disease is extremely long and contrary to widely held public opinion, it is one of the least contagious diseases known and person-to-person transmission may take many years. It is therefore very difficult to demonstrate cause and effect in its passage between victims. It is assumed that it enters the body either through skin lesions or through the respiratory route and there is still controversy over the method of transmission.

Leprosy occurs as a continuous spectrum of symptoms between two extreme forms, the tubercular and lepromatous forms, the difference between the two types appearing to depend to some extent on the intensity of the victim's immune reaction. In both types however, the progress of the disease is very slow. The lepromatous form, which is the classical manifestation of the disease, involves infection by large numbers of bacteria and appears to be a more serious problem in light-skinned races. The bacterium forms nodules especially on the face, these attack the membranes of the nose and mouth and also the peripheral nervous system (that is the nerves outside the brain and spinal cord). The disease is characterised by swellings on the face, skin ulcers and the paralysis of nerve endings in the fingers and toes. This typically causes the loss of digits as the victim does not feel pain, does not realise when the fingers and toes are being damaged and therefore does not take evasive action. The upper lip and nose are destroyed progressively producing severe disfigurement and the bacteria invade the nerves of the vocal chords causing a harsh voice and in a few cases vision may become impaired. Although further progress of the disease can usually be halted using modern drugs, the damage already caused is permanent and cannot be reversed.

The tubercular form of the disease is generally less severe, and involves a relatively small number of bacteria, typically patches are formed on the skin and all feeling is lost in these areas. The victims have a good chance of making a more or less complete recovery if the disease is diagnosed and treated in the early stages.

Although there are now effective drugs against Hansen's disease, it is still a common problem in much of the tropics. As with tuberculosis, it is frequently necessary to continue treatment for a prolonged period, occasionally as much as two years.

Leprosy is now regarded as a curable disease, and in the 1990s the WHO launched a campaign to eliminate it worldwide by 2000. This failed due to the large numbers of infected people including many living in war zones, the exceptionally long incubation time of the disease and the fact that the epidemiology is still not fully understood.

HISTORY OF LEPROSY

The main problem when discussing the history of leprosy is to reconcile the modern description of the disease with ancient descriptions such as that found in the Bible. The incidence rate of leprosy in antiquity has always been controversial. Several authors have suggested it was widespread in Persia by 2,000 BC and Egypt and India by 1,000 BC, but others consider that the number of authentic cases of Hansen's disease has always been low. Biblical descriptions of leprosy do not closely resemble any disease recognised today. The Book of Leviticus that was probably written about 1,000 BC describes leprosy as a *"disease of one's dwelling place"* (Leviticus 14, 33-38). Much of this controversy is due to problems of translation of the Bible from early Hebrew. The word for leprosy used in the Bible is Tsara'ath, this implies a ritual impurity and in Jewish law, lepers were people forced to live outside society. The rabbi would diagnose leprosy, and the infected person or house would be isolated until the blemish was removed. Once this had been done, an individual could present him or herself to the rabbi who would certify that he or she had been cured. This *"cure"* would suggest that there were a number of cases that were not true leprosy or Hansen's disease, as the effects of this are irreversible.

Confusion arose when the Bible was translated into Greek, then Latin and various Arab sources. The Greek word *lepra,* from which leprosy is derived, was used by Hippocrates. This means any disease producing a scaly skin or thickening of the skin such as the localized keratoses found in older people and discoloured patches of skin. These could include problems such as eczema, scabies, ringworm and psoriasis, all of which may be curable or self-limiting.

A number of other cultures beside the Jews describe diseases that may be leprosy; these include the Ebers papyrus from Egypt, but this is controversial and depends on the translation of several unknown words. There is a Chinese reference from the first millennium BC, and early Indian texts (500 BC) describe diseases of discoloured skin with flaking, which may have been leprosy, psoriasis or one of several other diseases. It was also frequently confused with various venereal diseases in antiquity. The lepromatous form of the disease was known as leontiasis in Roman times from the lion-like features, especially during the early stages of the disease. Sources such as Galen and Celsus refer to elephantiasis that is thought to be the tubercular form of leprosy and describe it as incurable and Avicenna described leprosy very accurately in his "*Canon of Medicine*" in the tenth century AD.

There are several traditional beliefs explaining its appearance in Western Europe. One is that the army of Alexander the Great brought it with them on their return from Asia in the fourth century BC, and that it spread from Greece to the rest of Europe. There are suggestions that Roman soldiers in the army of Pompey the Great carried the disease from Africa to Italy in the first century BC, and that Roman legionaries later spread it all over the empire. Other groups were also blamed for spreading it throughout Europe in addition to the two above. These include the Persian armies attacking Greece, the Phoenicians around 1,000 BC via their trading empire and the Jews driven out of Jerusalem after its destruction by the Romans in 70 AD. By the Dark Ages, the disease was widespread throughout Europe, the Near East and North Africa. It appears to have spread along trade routes in Europe, especially during the twelfth and thirteenth centuries, probably as a result of the Crusades and pilgrims visiting the

Holy Land. Prominent victims were Baldwin IV, the *"leper king"* of Jerusalem, and Robert the Bruce, King of Scotland.

Leprosy spread rapidly throughout Europe, and a number of skeletons from the late Roman period with the lesions of leprosy have been found in England. In 583, the Edict of Lyons limited the movement of lepers in France, although in Anglo-Saxon England lepers do not appear to have been isolated and their bodies are found in cemeteries with those of uninfected people. By the time of the Normans however, hospices known as lazar houses (St Lazarus is the patron saint of lepers), were being established as places of refuge. Many of them were associated with monasteries and the word Lazars is still found in village names in England, an example being Burton Lazars in Leicestershire. Approximately two hundred lazar houses were thought to be present in England, a significantly larger number in France, and most Italian towns and cities had a lazar house outside the walls. Many of them were later used as pest-houses for the confinement of plague victims.

By the end of the twelfth century, the Christian Church was following various ecclesiastical ordinances based on Leviticus, and the Third Lateran Council of 1179 required priests to exclude lepers from the community to avoid them infecting others. Papal decree declared they were dead in civil law and their heirs inherited any property they possessed. Special masses were said with the victim being present in which they were declared to be *"dead amongst the living"*[138]. In some cases they were required to stand symbolically in a grave, dressed in clothes with a yellow cross on them whilst the funeral service was read over them. They could not marry, were excluded from their family if they were married and could only associate with other lepers until physically dead. The French king, Philip V, decided in 1321, that lepers were conspiring with the Sultan of Babylon and the

---

138   *"Be thou dead unto the world, but alive unto God".*

Moorish Kingdom of Granada to poison wells in France, and ordered that all lepers should be burnt at the stake.

The Fourth Lateran Council (1215) required lepers and Jews to wear identifying badges (the Jews were thought to be particularly prone to leprosy because of their alleged lecherous tendencies). Victims of the disease were required to carry bells or clappers to give warning of their coming and allow people time to get out of their way. They were also forced to wear distinctive clothing with a yellow cross and carry a long staff to enable them to reach food and alms without going near uninfected people. Most countries exempted them from the anti-begging laws.

The horror with which the medieval population must have regarded leprosy is described graphically by Robert Louis Stevenson in his novel, *"The Black Arrow"* published in 1883. *"Upon this path, stepping forth from the margin of the wood, a white figure now appeared. It paused a little and seemed to look about; and then, at a slow pace, and bent almost double, it began to draw near across the heath. At every step the bell clanked. Face, it had none; a white hood, not even pierced with eyeholes, veiled the head; and as the creature moved, it seemed to feel its way with the tapping of a stick. Fear fell upon the lads, as cold as death. "A leper" said Dick hoarsely. "His touch is death" said Matcham. "Let us run"".*

The Church believed leprosy was a divine punishment for debauchery and decreed separate burial places for lepers on the basis that if it was a divine punishment, then lepers could not be buried in holy ground. In spite of this, most Christian communities, especially the monasteries, provided charity for lepers in the form of food, clothes, shelter, medical and religious services. Although they had been banned from the community, there are contemporary accounts of lepers banding together to extort money and food from villages. The horror and fear of the disease was such that these blackmail attempts were frequently successful.

The medieval concept that leprosy was a punishment for sin, especially excessive and debauched sex (many early physicians were of the opinion that leprosy was spread by sexual contact), and suggestions that leprosy may have had some venereal characteristics have led certain authors to consider that it may have been a pre-sixteenth century form of syphilis.

Leprosy was also widespread in the Arab world where it was thought to be both contagious and hereditary. It was considered to be a divine punishment for immorality, and therefore lepers had their legal rights limited, giving them the same rights as slaves and the insane. Similar attitudes were found in the Far East. It was also considered a divine punishment in Japan, and lepers were regarded as untouchable.

Medieval treatment for leprosy was limited to salves for the skin, many of them containing the mediaeval cure-all, mercury, although both the Jews and Arabs believed in the efficacy of hot sulphur springs in treating the disease. Even today, chemotherapy for leprosy is limited to a very small number of drugs that frequently have to be taken for periods exceeding a year.

The disease reached its zenith in Europe in the twelfth and thirteenth centuries when some authorities consider it may have infected as many as ten per cent of the population. After reaching a peak around the year 1300 in Western Europe, it then more or less disappeared from this area, although it continued to flourish elsewhere. The one part of Europe where it persisted until the early twentieth century were rural areas of Norway, where Hansen carried out a great deal of his work. It has been estimated that as many as two to three per cent of some communities in Norway were infected but the reasons for its persistence in these isolated areas are not known.

Leprosy was first studied in Norway by Daniel Danielssen and Carl Boeck in Bergen who published a book, *"Om Spedalskhed"* (On Leprosy) in 1847. They were convinced however that it was a hereditary disease rather than an infectious one. Danielssen attempted to infect himself and several associates with material taken from the nodules of a patient in 1856. None of them developed leprosy which reinforced the opinion that it was a hereditary disease. This study was continued by Hansen who was Danielssen's son-in-law. Hansen later lost his medical position for inoculating a patient suffering from the milder form of leprosy with the more dangerous form, to determine whether the mild form conferred immunity. This was essentially very similar to the variolation process carried out with smallpox in the eighteenth century, but times had changed.

The reasons for the decline of leprosy in Western Europe are controversial. Some authors argue that the number of victims fell because lepers were killed by the Black Death, which reached Europe in 1347, and suggest that numbers fell to a point where there were insufficient to continue spreading a disease transmitted so slowly. This is not correct as contemporary accounts make it obvious that the incidence rate of leprosy in Europe had fallen significantly, approximately fifty years before the Black Death appeared. The disappearance of leprosy may be due to the spread of tuberculosis caused by *Mycobacterium tuberculosis,* which is a far more efficient human pathogen than *M. leprae.* There is a considerable cross-immunity between the two diseases, and people carrying *M. tuberculosis* have significant resistance to leprosy, although the converse is not true.

It has also been suggested that the fall in the number of lepers around 1300 may have been due to improved diagnosis. The Papal physician, Guy de Chauliac (1300-1368), writing *"Le Grande Chirurgie",* in the mid-fourteenth century, defined the medical symptoms of leprosy accurately. This would fit in with the fact that before the fourteenth century, leprosy was diagnosed mainly by priests, after this date it was usually diagnosed by physicians. The fall in numbers also coincided with the beginning of the Little Ice Age in Europe and it is possible that the lower temperatures may have influenced the spread of a disease that generally had a higher prevalence in the tropics and sub-tropics.

There are relatively few drugs available for the treatment of leprosy for reasons similar to the problems found in treating tuberculosis (see later). One treatment used since 1,500 BC in India and China was chaulmoogra oil, derived from the seeds of a tropical evergreen. The efficacy was debatable and its use was stopped when the sulpha drugs became available. The first effective drug used in Western medicine was the sulpha drug, prontosil, which appeared in the mid-1930s. A number of other sulpha drugs followed, the most effective one being dapsone. The sulpha drugs are bacteriostatic, that is they stop the bacterium growing, the first bactericidal drug that actually killed the leprosy bacterium was rifampicin, developed in the 1960s.

Resistance to the drugs used has been described on numerous occasions, and the WHO now recommends that treatment should be the use of multi-drug therapy to stop resistant bacterial strains arising. Killing the bacterium does not restore body tissues that have already been damaged or destroyed, and in spite of the fact that patients have been cured and are no longer infectious, in many cases they have to deal with the social stigma still attached to the disease.

Leprosy was probably brought to the Americas by European colonists and West African slaves. One group who seem to have been more than usually susceptible were the Acadians, a group of French Canadians expelled from Nova Scotia in 1755, who went to Louisiana[139]. It still occurs occasionally in this area in people of Acadian descent. In 1894, a leper colony was created near Carville, Louisiana, which in the early twentieth century became the Hansen's Disease Center and has become a major research centre for the disease.

---

139   Louisiana was still a French colony at this date.

There was a major outbreak of leprosy amongst the native population of Hawaii in the 1860s linked to the immigration of Chinese labourers. All the cases diagnosed were expelled to the island of Molukai where they lived in appalling conditions. In 1873 the Belgian priest, Father Damien, went to Molukai to minister to the sick and died there in 1889 after contracting leprosy.

In the 1960s the WHO recommended the abolition of compulsory isolation, although it was continued in certain countries, such as Japan, until the mid-1990s. The WHO now supplies all the drugs for the treatment of leprosy free of charge, and although it has been eliminated from a number of countries, it still causes approximately 250,000 new cases per year, mostly in sub-Saharan Africa, Latin America and Asia.

TUBERCULOSIS

"The captain of all the men of death that came against him to take him away was the consumption".
John Bunyan, Life and Death of Mr Badman, 1680.

In 1961, the British Medical Association was told, *"The defeat of tuberculosis in our young adult population has probably added hundreds of thousands of working man-years to our productive and economic capacity".* In 1993, the World Health Organisation declared tuberculosis was a *"Global emergency",* the first infectious disease to receive this dubious accolade. The WHO stated that approximately two billion people were infected (i.e. one third of the world's population), making it the most prevalent chronic disease in the world. There were eight to ten million new active cases (see later) each year, two to three million deaths each year, the epidemic was increasing, and the WHO predicted that TB will kill thirty million people over the next decade, most of them in South East Asia and sub-Saharan Africa.

By 2004, the WHO stated that it was gaining ground against TB[140], and a spokesman announced, *"It was thought*

---

140   The initials TB originally stood for *Tubercule Bacillus,* but are now used to mean the disease, tuberculosis.

that …the tuberculosis epidemic could be controlled". The stated goal of the WHO was the detection of 70% of all cases, and curing 85% of those detected by 2005. The charity, Medicins sans Frontieres disagreed; they argued that the current tests were ineffective, especially when a combination of TB and HIV was present, and stated that, *"We are losing the fight against TB"*. Given the past track records of the WHO and MsF, most informed individuals would probably incline towards the MsF point of view and events since then tend to confirm this opinion.

What happened between these statements in 1961, 1993 and 2004?

PATHOLOGY OF TUBERCULOSIS

The pathology of tuberculosis and the relationship between the human host and the bacterium, *Mycobacterium tuberculosis,* is complex, and a number of different forms of the disease can be recognised in humans. Most non-medical personnel tend to think of tuberculosis as a disease of the lungs which is indeed the most common form of the infection. The bacteria can however infect many other organs of the body including the bones, joints, skin and glands and the symptoms are very variable depending on where the disease is located. This can make tuberculosis difficult to diagnose as it frequently mimics the symptoms of other diseases.

Different mycobacteria are found in humans causing tuberculosis type symptoms, and there is some argument about whether they are different varieties of the same species, or different species. *M. tuberculosis* is accepted as the organism that generally causes human tuberculosis, but a second organism, *M. bovis*, which normally causes tuberculosis in cattle, is also found in humans. Tests on the DNA of the two organisms indicate that they are virtually identical and any genetic differences are very small. Tuberculosis is also found in numerous other domesticated animals such as pigs and in wild animals such as badgers. In a small number of cases, the human disease scrofula is caused by a non-tubercular *Mycobacterium* known as *M. scrofulaceum,* and rare cases of an avian variety of *Mycobacterium* causing disease in humans with damaged immune systems are also found.

Tuberculosis can be transmitted in one of two ways. In the case of *M. tuberculosis,* the bacterium is spread by droplet infection from an infected person, and in the case of *M. bovis,* by the ingestion of infected milk. Tuberculosis spread by drinking infected milk tended for obvious reasons to be a disease of young children. In previous centuries, in northern latitudes, farmers frequently lived in the same houses as their cattle, mainly because it would have been warmer in winter, and this may well have increased the general exposure to infection.

The most commonly occurring form of the disease is pulmonary tuberculosis, which is transmitted by droplet infection, and is highly infectious. Droplet infection is more effective in overcrowded conditions and for that reason pulmonary TB is frequently found in families (it can also be spread from mother to child *in utero).* This caused frequent arguments between doctors about whether there was a genetic predisposition towards it or whether it was exacerbated by prevailing social conditions. These arguments complicated an understanding of the disease for many years.

In the nineteenth and early twentieth centuries, virtually everyone in Britain and Europe was exposed to the disease, but it only developed into a clinical form in a portion of the population. There are also widespread differences in morbidity and mortality between different races, and in the past, this has led to considerable disagreement between scientists and doctors as to whether these differences reflected genetic, cultural or social differences between races. It is a disease whose study has been more bedevilled by political correctness than probably any other disease in history until the advent of HIV.

Once the bacteria enter the body, there is a complex interaction between the host and bacteria that is determined by both the virulence of the bacterial strain and the resistance of the host. In a small number of individuals, the macrophage defensive system is strong enough to destroy the bacteria at this point and there is no infection. In the vast majority of cases however, the bacteria survive, and one of several interactions are then possible between host and bacteria.

When bacteria are inhaled they reach the alveoli (tiny air sacs in the lungs), and are attacked by the macrophages. Normally, when most types of bacteria attack the body, they are engulfed by macrophages and become imprisoned inside a sac known as a phagosome. These fuse with bags of bacterial-destroying enzymes known as lysosomes and the bacteria are killed. In *Mycobacterium* however, the cell wall contains waxy materials that protect the bacteria from the lysosomes. Not only do these bacteria survive, they are inside the macrophage that acts as a Trojan Horse, camouflaging them from the other immune reactions of the body.

The initial confrontation between the host and bacteria is known as the primary infection, and results in the formation of tubercles in the lungs. These are aggregates of defensive macrophages around the bacteria, and are characteristic of infections of tuberculosis. These tissues contain large amounts of fat and protein, look like cheese, and are named *caseus necrosis*. The tubercles effectively wall the bacteria off from the host so that in most cases there is no acute infection and the bacteria remain isolated and localised in the lungs. These bacteria are dormant however, not dead. The result is that an estimated ninety to ninety-five per cent of people who are carrying dormant *M. tuberculosis*, do not exhibit any symptoms of TB, and do not realise they are infected. In this state, even although people are carrying the bacterium, they are not infectious.

Tubercles may appear in large numbers in lung tissue resisting attack and they can be very damaging over time. In spite of the fact that they are re-absorbed if the patient's immune system gets the upper hand, they form scar tissue that may calcify thus reducing lung capacity. These calcified areas can be seen using chest X-rays and this constitutes a major diagnostic test for pulmonary tuberculosis.

In some infected people, the immune response is inadequate to stop the progress of the disease at this point and the infection progresses to an acute state, in which there is widespread destruction of lung tissue. If this occurs, the victims start to cough-up blood which is accompanied by sweating, rapid weight loss, and frequently pleurisy. In addition to destroying large areas of lung tissue, the bacteria become disseminated throughout the body, start to multiply in other tissues and finally death occurs. Once active in the lungs, the disease is characterised by blood stained sputum and dried sputum containing *Mycobacterium* can remain infective for months. In this form, tuberculosis is highly contagious by droplet infection, and can be spread by coughing, sneezing and spitting. Mathematical modelling suggests that if it is not treated, each active case of tuberculosis will infect 10-15 other victims during the course of a year.

A more common situation however, is that the disease can be reactivated in those people carrying dormant bacteria to give secondary tuberculosis; this period of dormancy may be many years. This reactivation takes place as a result of the immune system becoming weakened because of factors such as aging, over-indulgence in alcohol, poor diet or starvation, working in a dusty environment, overcrowding, stress, the use of drugs or the presence of another disease such as AIDS damaging the immune system. During secondary tuberculosis, tubercles coalesce to form large areas of *caseous necrosis* that break down to form cavities. These rupture into the blood vessels of the lungs and the patient starts to cough-up blood.

Once in the blood vessels, bacteria spread throughout the lungs producing large numbers of small tubercles. This is known as miliary tuberculosis as it looks like millet seed when lung samples are examined microscopically. This secondary form of tuberculosis is also highly contagious by droplet infection.

Tuberculosis may be found in a glandular form. In naïve populations that have not been exposed to the disease previously, the symptoms are frequently not the same as those found in disease-experienced populations. When tuberculosis first attacked Amerindian tribes in Western Canada in the late nineteenth century, for the first two generations it was a generalised glandular disease and not confined to the lungs, unlike tuberculosis as normally recognised in Europe. It only became the typical pulmonary tuberculosis after several generations and had an extremely high mortality rate amongst the Amerindians. One glandular form of tuberculosis, considered in some detail later, is scrofula, a type of tuberculosis infecting the lymph glands of the neck.

Tuberculosis of the bone and joints also occurs, and provides us with evidence that it is a disease with a long history in humans. This type of TB is usually as a result of infection by *M. bovis* caused by drinking infected milk and it has virtually disappeared from those countries where milk is pasteurised. Some scientists consider that on genetic grounds, it may have jumped from cattle to humans as long as 20,000 years ago. Tuberculosis of the spine (Pott's disease) has been found in Neolithic skeletons and also in Egyptian mummies dating from as early as 3,000 BC. The typical spinal curvature found in this form of TB is depicted in a number of Egyptian wall paintings. The first known case of tuberculosis to whom we can put a name is Nesperehan, a priest of Amon, who suffered from Pott's disease and died around 1,000 BC. It appears to have been a common problem in Egypt by about 600 BC.

Many people do not realise the danger of tuberculosis as it kills its victims relatively slowly and can take several months, even in its most virulent form, compared with other epidemic diseases, such as cholera and smallpox that can kill in a matter of hours or days. The incidence rate is closely related to a number of public health issues. These include overcrowding, nutritional standards, social deprivation and the presence of other debilitating diseases. In the industrialised countries, the incidence rate is considerably higher in the homeless, alcoholics and drug addicts than it is in the general population. Historically, the morbidity rate has been significantly higher in cities than in rural communities because of the greater degree of crowding, poorer sanitation and hygiene. It peaked in Britain in the late nineteenth century, but then started to fall gradually with the improvements in public health, hygiene and improved nutritional standards. This fall occurred before the development of any drugs capable of attacking the bacterium. The trend has been reversed in both the UK and USA in the last two decades for a number of reasons, these include cuts in public health services, increased poverty, the rise in incidence of immune compromised diseases and the huge increases in the number of immigrants from the developing world.

The genus *Mycobacterium* has a cell wall consisting of a very thick coat that contains a number of unusual sugars and waxes (lipids) that are chemically unique to this genus. Antibiotics have great difficulty in penetrating the organism because of this waxy coat and treatment therefore frequently takes 6-12 months or longer[141]. One major problem is that when bacteria are treated with antibiotics for this length of time, there is a very high probability that they will mutate to drug resistance. In an attempt to deal with this situation, multi-drug therapy was started in the 1950s. Victims were given a cocktail of drugs, rather than a single drug, on the

---

141   The first effective antibiotic against tuberculosis was streptomycin discovered by Waksmann in the 1940s. Its use however, has been limited by several major problems; the first is that the bacteria rapidly develop resistance, and the second is that it causes severe deafness in a significant number of patients. It is also relatively expensive.

premise that whilst the bacteria might become resistant to a single drug, they are unlikely to become resistant to three or four drugs administered simultaneously.

A further serious problem is that many victims stop antibiotic treatment before it is complete, as they feel better after a few weeks of treatment that kills the more susceptible bacteria. However, the bacteria remaining are the drug-resistant types and the patient becomes sick again. Dropouts from long-term treatment programmes tend to be the socially deprived, drug addicts, alcoholics and the mentally ill. Frequently they are of no fixed address, are difficult to trace and even when traced they cannot be legally forced to continue their treatment. The result is that these people become a reservoir and focus for the spread of antibiotic resistant tuberculosis, the so-called MDR-TB (Multi-Drug Resistant TB), and the even more dangerous version XDR-TB (Extremely-Drug Resistant TB).[142]

This is extremely important from the point of view of cost as well as drug resistance. Multi-drug therapy usually involves a cocktail of what are known as first line drugs; typical examples are isoniazid, rifampicin, pyrazinamide and ethambutol. All of these are of relatively low toxicity, and all are cheap, costing about £50 for a six-month course. Generally all four drugs are taken for two months, then just one or two for a further four months, and this treatment is effective in about 95% of cases. Although the patient remains infected for several months, they cease to be infectious after a few weeks of treatment. If the bacteria become resistant to the combination of first line drugs, then the drugs that have to be used in the second line cocktail, for example kanamycin and cycloserine, are invariably significantly more expensive and frequently more toxic also. The figures for the difference in cost are startling, to treat

---

142   From a public health point of view, it could be argued that a poorly supervised or incomplete treatment of TB causes more long-term problems than no treatment.

an ordinary case of TB requires drugs that can be taken orally and costs approximately £50 over a six month period. MDR-TB treatment may take as long as a year or more, involve hospitalisation, intravenous drug treatment and cost in excess of £100,000.

XDR-TB was first diagnosed in South Africa in May 2005. The South African government did nothing about it, and by early 2007 there were well over two hundred cases with a mortality rate of 85%, death frequently occurring within a few weeks of the disease being diagnosed. Given the high rates of AIDS in South Africa and the interaction between AIDS and TB, this figure was almost certainly a serious under-estimate. The first case of XDR-TB occurring in the UK was confirmed in late 2007.

The problem of resistance is one that is common to most diseases that can be treated with antibiotics. It also means that a poorly run treatment programme can generate dangerous multi-drug resistant strains faster than they can be eliminated. The scale of the problem can be seen from the following figures. In 1982, six per cent of strains tested resistant to one drug, by 1992 thirty-five per cent tested resistant to one drug, nearly twenty per cent were resistant to two and some isolates were resistant to all the main antibiotics normally used to treat TB[143].

One method of administering the drugs that is being used more frequently in the treatment of TB is the so-called DOTS (Directly Observed Therapy, Short Course) system. This requires a trained observer to stand over the patient whilst they swallow the medication and it is proving to be very effective. In some countries such as the USA, the DOTS programme is linked to social security payments; patients refusing to take their medication do not qualify for payments.

---

143   No new antibiotics for the treatment of tuberculosis have been developed in recent years. Generic first line drugs used to treat TB are so cheap that any new drug would have to be significantly more effective to compete in the marketplace.

Before the discovery of antibiotics, TB was treated by isolating the patient in a sanatorium, frequently at high altitudes with prolonged periods of bed rest, diseased areas of the lungs were removed surgically and the patient was given a high protein diet. Whilst active cases of TB are still isolated and an adequate diet is still part of the treatment, surgical removal of infected tissue is now only carried out rarely.

The unusual cell wall structure of *Mycobacterium* mentioned earlier may prove to be its Achilles heel. The waxy coat contains a number of chemicals unique to this genus, and searches are being made for drugs attacking the synthesis of these unique molecules. Hopefully such drugs will show a high degree of selective toxicity, that is, they will kill the bacterium without side effects on the human host. The genome of the bacterium was published in 1998. Not surprisingly given the waxy coat, a large part of the genome is given over to lipid chemistry and this may facilitate a search for new drugs against a disease that is rapidly increasing in importance.

There are a number of other technical problems in the treatment of TB. Traditional detection methods are slow and unreliable. One of the standard methods of testing for the presence of the disease is the staining of sputum samples using a technique known as Acid-fast, or Ziehl-Neelsen staining. The stained samples are then examined for the presence of *Mycobacterium*. This technique is widely used, but even in the hands of an experienced technician it is probable that thirty per cent of positive cases are missed.

M. tuberculosis is also extremely difficult to grow in the laboratory, and numerous cases of MRD-TB, especially in the developing world where laboratory facilities are poor, are not diagnosed until the patient is dead. The bacterium is very slow growing, and laboratory diagnosis frequently takes 4-6 weeks, with several more weeks being necessary to determine the drug resistance pattern of the organism under consideration. In the highly active form of the disease, death frequently occurs within 10-12 weeks, and by this time, the patient may well have infected a large number of other people, especially family members, with whom they have been in close contact.

Further problems relating to tuberculosis include the fact that unlike many bacteria, one bout of the disease does not give life long protection. Infection can also flare up in an individual and then subside for no obvious reason.

HISTORY OF TUBERCULOSIS

The appearance of TB in Egyptian mummies has already been mentioned. It appears to have been uncommon in sub-Saharan Africa prior to European colonisation, and the pulmonary form at least does not appear to have been present in pre-Columbian America. It was generally thought that tuberculosis was introduced into Britain by the Romans, but the skeleton of a man suffering from advanced TB, dated to about 3,000 BC, has recently been found in Dorset.

Several early accounts of tuberculosis are known. Hippocrates considered it non-contagious, but Galen thought that it was contagious and recognised that it was dangerous to live with active TB cases. Fracastoro, writing in the sixteenth century, also held it to be highly contagious.

A number of names were used for different types of tuberculosis in the UK until the end of the nineteenth century. Tuberculosis of the lymph glands of the neck and face was known as scrofula, a skin infection was referred to as *Lupus vulgaris* (this is translated as the common wolf[144] although the Linnean name for the wolf is *Canis lupus*). Pulmonary TB went under several names; these included phthisis (derived from a Greek word meaning "to decay"), consumption because of the way it consumed the victim, the graveyard cough and the "White Plague" from the bloodless appearance of the victims. The privileged classes of the eighteenth and nineteenth centuries did however not suffer from consumption, they were

---

144   A description of 1590 describes the ulcers of skin tuberculosis as being *"very hungry like unto a woolfe"*.

"*in decline*". Richard Manton, an English doctor first used the word tubercle (derived from a Latin word, *tuberculum*, meaning a lump) to describe the nodules he found in the lungs of people dying of tuberculosis. The word tuberculosis itself did not come into common usage until the 1830s.

In earlier centuries, scrofula was widespread in Western Europe and became known as the King's Evil in thirteenth century France and England. This is a very unsightly form of tuberculosis (the name means "little pig" and is the diminutive of the Latin word, *scrofa* meaning a sow), in which enlarged lymph glands in the neck fill with blood and pus, and drain into the skin of the face, neck and chest. Scrofula, which was rarely fatal, is much less common today and generally responds well to antibiotic treatment.

It was believed that the touch of the monarch, who had been anointed by God, could affect a cure, hence, "*touching for the King's Evil*". The English claimed that this practice went back to the reign of Edward the Confessor, the last but one Saxon King of England from 1042-1066, although there is no record of "*touching*" for at least another hundred years. The French claimed it originated with the Kings of France, the first being Philip I (1052-1108), and there are claims that it started with Clovis, King of the Franks around 490 AD. Edward the Confessor was proclaimed a saint in 1161 and the Plantagenet kings of England, starting with Henry II, tried to link themselves to saintliness by carrying out the same treatment. The practice of "*touching for the King's Evil*" became widely used in England, especially by monarchs who needed to make a political statement or who felt that their grip on the throne was not as firm as it might be. There is a certain amount of natural remission of scrofula, presumably this occurred sufficiently frequently to give some credence to the "*King's touch*", and no doubt the King's physicians would also have chosen victims suffering from less severe forms of the disease on the basis that these were more likely to be *"cured".*

Several doctors of the period were not convinced, Arnold of Villanova, a fourteenth century physician, made no mention of the king's healing power when he described scrofula, whilst Jan Yperman, a doctor of Ypres, claimed that it was unsuccessful.

In England, Henry VII (the first of the Tudors) carried out the practice with great pageantry, and also introduced the gift of a gold angel (a coin worth approximately two thirds of a pound, and so-called as it showed the Archangel Michael killing a dragon on one side) to each applicant. This was a substantial sum of money at the time and would have represented several months wages for a labourer. Henry had won the crown in battle in 1485 at Bosworth Field (the last great battle of the Wars of the Roses) and his legal claim to the throne was extremely dubious. He also had the reputation for being miserly, and his decision to spend both time and money in touching for the King's Evil certainly owed more to politics than charity. The royal touch was also practised by Henry's grand-daughter, Elizabeth I, to prove she still ruled England despite being excommunicated and called a bastard by the Pope.

The next dynasty, the Stuarts were also under threat politically on numerous occasions, and one of the best ways to reinforce the concept of the Divine Right to Rule was to touch for the King's Evil, as this was regarded as a gift from God direct to the monarch. James I (1603-1625), the first of the Stuart kings, had angels specially minted for the healing ceremony. During the reign of his son, Charles I, a proclamation fixed Easter and Michaelmas (feast of St Michael, 29th September) as the dates for touching, and each applicant was required to produce a certificate signed by the clergyman of their parish, confirming that the person had not been touched by the King previously. A further proclamation, in 1638, ordered that every candidate was required to obtain a further certificate from a physician or surgeon, authenticating his or her condition. Confidence tricksters obviously go back a long way. Charles I continued to touch for the King's Evil whilst imprisoned on the Isle of Wight in 1648 in order to reassure his followers.

The Office of *"Touching for the King's Evil"* was included in the English Book of Common Prayer in 1633 (during the reign of Charles I). It stated that the monarch, *"shall lay their hand on the sick and they shall recover"*. It was removed in the mid-eighteenth century by the Hanoverian kings because of the Catholic implications.

Charles II (son of Charles I) also found touching for the King's Evil very expedient politically during his years of exile from 1649 (after the execution of his father) to the Restoration of the Monarchy in 1660. He touched numerous people from England and various other places, whilst he was a refugee in the Low Countries, and in 1660 (immediately after the Restoration), he touched a further 600 individuals according to Pepys's diary. The custom reached its peak under Charles II, with thousands being touched. The event eventually was so successful that numbers had to be limited although this was frequently exceeded, sometimes with disastrous consequences. John Evelyn wrote in his diary for March 1684, *"There was so great a concourse of people with their children to be touched for the Evil, that 6 or 7 were crushed to death by pressing at the chirugeon's doore for tickets"*.

Charles II had no legitimate children and his illegitimate son James, Duke of Monmouth, attempted to assume the throne on the death of his father in 1685, using the rallying call of *"No Popery"*. The Duke touched numerous people in his attempt to establish his claim to the throne but it did him no good. His amateur army of rebels was defeated at Sedgemoor by the professional army of his uncle, James II (brother of Charles), and Monmouth lost his head on Tower Hill. It is reputed to have been the most botched royal execution in English history, the executioner took five blows of the axe and had to finish the job off with a butcher's knife. It was also alleged that the authorities forgot have a portrait of him painted before the execution, as was customary for royal executions, so his head was sewn back on, a cravat was wrapped round his neck and his body propped up in a chair whilst the court painter, Sir Godfrey Kneller, did a quick portrait. One of the charges against Monmouth, at his trial for treason, was that, *"he touched children of the King's Evil"*. The irony is that if the Duke had waited until 1688, James II was deposed anyway because of his Catholic tendencies.

One herbal cure mentioned during this period is by the apothecary, Nicholas Culpepper (Ch 2), who considered that bruised leaves of tobacco would ease the pain and discomfort of the King's Evil.

It was not only English people who sought the royal touch, records exist of patients from France, the Netherlands, Germany, Scotland, Ireland, Wales and also early settlers from Virginia and New Hampshire.

During the reign of William III (William of Orange) and Mary II, the practice was discontinued as William considered it to be a useless superstition. On the few occasions he did touch people, he is reputed to have told them, *"God grant you better health and more sense"*. The tradition was resurrected by Queen Anne (1702-14) as a useful means of asserting the royal authority and she was the last English ruler to do it. One of Queen Anne's patients in 1712 was Dr Samuel Johnson as a child, brought by his mother on the recommendation of Sir John Floyer, a physician of Lichfield. The treatment was unsuccessful, Boswell commented that Johnson's scrofula, *"disfigured a countenance naturally well formed, and hurt his visual nerves so much that he did not see at all with one of his eyes, though its appearance was little different from that of the other."*

Once George I (the first of the Hanoverians) ascended to the English throne in 1714, the practice of touching came to an end. However, James, the Old Pretender (the Catholic son of

James II), continued to touch sufferers during his exile in Paris, presumably to give credence to his claim to the English throne. During his return to Scotland to lead the Jacobite Rising of 1715, James touched the sick at Glamis Castle, in an attempt to derive the maximum political mileage from the practice.

In France, Louis XV touched two thousand people at his coronation in 1722 and *"touching"* was continued by various monarchs until the French Revolution in 1789. There was a brief attempt to revive it when the Bourbons were restored to power after the defeat of Napoleon in 1815 and Charles X, who believed in the Divine Right of Kings, did it for the last time in 1825.

It was not just monarchs who touched for the evil. In 1799, two highwaymen found guilty of robbing the mail were hanged and then hung in irons in Horsham. When the bodies were taken down from the gallows to be placed in irons before being gibbeted, it was reported that, *"two young women of genteel appearance, labouring under scrofulous complaints, presented themselves to have their necks stroked with the hand of one of the dead men"*. It was thought at the time that being touched by the hand of an executed criminal was an infallible cure for numerous ailments. This was an extension of the *"Hand of Glory"*, the belief that if the hand of an executed felon was cut off and dried, when a lighted candle was placed in it, it conferred occult powers on the owner.

Scrofula had become very rare in Western Europe by the second half of the twentieth century, but it has now started to reappear in people who are compromised immunologically.

A second form of tuberculosis is pulmonary TB, a disease generally associated with poor living and social conditions. This was widespread in Greek and Roman cities, and was described accurately by Hippocrates, who described it as a wasting disease and also recognised that a change of climate from urban to rural was beneficial in the treatment. Galen also prescribed the sea air and sent rich patients to the coast near the

Isle of Capri. The Arab physicians, Rhazes and Avicenna, both recognised tuberculosis and prescribed milk with powdered crab shells as a cure, a treatment that would have provided extra calcium.

During the Dark Ages, when much of the population lived in rural conditions and overcrowding was not a serious problem, the incidence rate of TB fell in Europe, apparently allowing leprosy to appear. When cities started growing again, the poor living conditions allowed the resurgence of TB, and the incidence rate of leprosy fell. Whilst many scientists and doctors have suggested this scenario, there have been a number who dissent, but generally the dissenters have not been able to suggest a reasonable alternative hypothesis apart from an improved recognition of leprosy.

In the sixteenth century tuberculosis developed into a major epidemic in Europe that lasted well into the twentieth century. This was caused by urbanisation and overcrowding under poor conditions. The mortality rate increased significantly during the sixteenth century, and by the seventeenth century the Bills of Mortality suggest that approximately twenty per cent of those dying annually in London, during non-plague years, were killed by tuberculosis. Even in 1665, during the Great Plague of London, consumption and phthisis are listed as the third most common form of death after plague and fevers, causing some five thousand deaths, with a further eighty-six caused by the King's Evil. Regulations appeared in Italy in the early eighteenth century regarding consumptives and in 1783, Naples made it compulsory for physicians to report cases to the appropriate authorities, who then took various precautionary measures. Some experts consider that when the epidemic reached its peak, virtually everybody in Western Europe was infected. The worst affected countries were those undergoing industrialisation and urbanisation, and by the nineteenth century, TB was thought to be responsible for twenty-five per cent of all deaths in European and North American cities. By

1900 it was probably killing more people worldwide than any other epidemic disease.

Tuberculosis became a major epidemic disease of the Industrial Revolution when conditions such as malnutrition, overcrowding, damp housing and poor ventilation in dusty industries and mines were widespread. Paracelsus had noted the relationship between mining and pulmonary diseases in the fifteenth century, and in 1799, Thomas Beddoes recorded that stoneworkers were very prone to consumption. Beddoes was unusual in that he thought it important to monitor not only the sick person, but their family as well. He was also notorious for believing that it was possible to cure a wide variety of diseases by inhaling gases such as oxygen and carbon dioxide, and attempted unsuccessfully to cure the daughter of James Watt of tuberculosis by treating her with carbon dioxide. This belief was taken to a ludicrous extent by his conviction that the breath of cattle was beneficial to consumption victims, and he arranged sickrooms next door to cowsheds so that cows could breathe on sufferers. Beddoes also hired Humphrey Davy as his assistant, who successfully synthesised nitrous oxide or laughing gas. Unfortunately the medical potential of this as an anaesthetic was not realised until the 1860s.

By 1815, TB was causing about one quarter of all deaths in Britain and the figure in France was even higher. The rate did start to fall in Britain in the second half of the nineteenth century although autopsies showed that virtually every corpse examined had had the disease at some stage of their lives.

The tragic, pale and listless heroines of many Victorian novels were almost certainly consumptives, the classic symptom in these novels being the racking cough and blood stained handkerchief. It was not just the characters who died of TB, it was also their creators. Many authors, poets, playwrights and composers, such as Anne and Emily Brontë, Keats, Chekov, Chopin, Dostoevsky, Goethe and Robert Louis Stevenson succumbed to TB. Twentieth century novelists were not immune either, it killed George Orwell in 1950, although it was self-inflicted to a large extent. He lived in squalor for a considerable period of time to write, *"Down and Out in Paris and London"*, and moved to a primitive farmhouse on the island of Jura, off the west coast of Scotland in 1948, when he was already showing clinical symptoms of TB, to write the novel, *"1984"*.

During the nineteenth century, opium was frequently used to treat consumptives, and this has led to the suggestion that an opium induced haze may have been responsible for the works of certain authors. Even opera has been based on tuberculosis; *"La Traviata"* written by Verdi in 1852 took its theme from the novel, *"La Dame aux Camélias"*, written by Alexandre Dumas in 1848. The main character was one of Dumas' mistresses, the famous French courtesan, Marie Duplessis, who died of TB at the age of twenty-three.

A major research effort was concentrated on tuberculosis during the last quarter of the nineteenth century and the first half of the twentieth century and in 1882, Robert Koch (Ch 3) isolated the tubercle bacillus using guinea pigs as laboratory hosts. Although he isolated the organism causing the disease, Koch did make several major mistakes during his studies. He claimed that humans could not be infected by the bovine strain of the disease and in 1890 he also claimed that tuberculin, a protein extract he had isolated from the tubercle bacteria, could be used as a cure, although within a year of making this claim Koch was forced to retract it. Tuberculin did however become an important diagnostic reagent in the fight against the disease, being made use of in the Mantoux test. This test consists of injecting a small quantity of tuberculin under.the skin and examining the site of injection several days later for a small rash. Contact with *M. tuberculosis* hypersensitises an individual to the organism, and the Mantoux test measures this hypersensitivity. A positive reaction shows that the person either has tuberculosis or has antibodies to it suggesting that they have been in contact with the disease in the past; this includes anyone injected with the BCG vaccine (see later). People testing positive for no apparent reason can be further checked for TB by chest X-rays, and sputum samples. The test is not completely reliable and occasionally gives false results.

For many years it was thought that there was a genetic predisposition to tuberculosis as it occurred so frequently in families. It is however, a disease of population density, poor social/economic conditions and inadequate public health and it is extremely difficult to separate these factors from the biology of both *Mycobacterium* and their hosts. We now know that the epidemiology of tuberculosis is probably more closely related to poor social conditions than the epidemiology of any other disease.

One of the most common genetic diseases in Europe today is cystic fibrosis caused by a mutation in a gene known as CFTR; this faulty gene causes the secretion of a sticky mucus into the lungs. If both parents are carriers and the child has two copies of the faulty gene, s(he) suffers from severe lung and breathing problems requiring regular physiotherapy and will probably die relatively young from some chest infection. A single copy of the faulty gene, however, produces sufficient mucus to immobilise pathogenic bacteria and provides a significant level of resistance to lung diseases such as TB. It is another example of a Mendelian recessive disease similar to that found in sickle cell anaemia and resistance to malaria (Ch 16). This is also known as a heterozygotic advantage, as although possession of a double copy of the gene (homozygotic) is dangerous, possession of a single copy confers a significant advantage in the presence of a dangerous disease. The faulty gene occurs at a significantly higher level in Caucasian than in African or Asian populations, suggesting that tuberculosis, in the past, has been a more serious problem in the first group.

Tuberculosis can be spread in different ways. Until around 1950, about 25% of the cases found in humans in the UK were bovine in origin, although the percentage was much higher in children below the age of fifteen. These cases were caused by drinking milk infected with *M. bovis* which initiated intestinal infections that frequently spread to other organs. In most developed countries, the problem has been more or less eliminated by the frequent testing of milking herds for TB, followed by the slaughter of cattle testing positive, and the pasteurisation of the vast majority of cows milk. Implementation of these two measures in the first half of the twentieth century led to a significant fall in the incidence rate of TB in the UK, especially in children. Prior to pasteurisation, contaminated milk is thought to have caused 50,000 cases of TB in the UK each year, approximately 2,500 of them being fatal. Not all doctors agreed with pasteurisation. Some claimed that although a few children infected with bovine TB would die, many had little more than a slight fever that they threw off and were then left with resistance to a more severe and dangerous attack later in life.

Several methods have been used for the pasteurisation of milk, all involve heating the milk for a period of time sufficient to kill a variety of pathogenic bacteria. The most popular method is flash pasteurisation or the High Temperature, Short Time (HTST) method in which milk is raised to 72°C for 15 seconds, and then cooled rapidly. Alternatively, milk can be heated to 63°C and kept at this temperature for 30 minutes. The heating should be sufficient to kill *M. tuberculosis,* which is the major objective of the process. It has the additional advantage of killing various other pathogenic bacteria found in milk, such as the *Streptococci* causing tonsillitis and scarlet fever, and *Brucella* species causing undulant fever (brucellosis).

The use of the tuberculin test to identify infected cattle also contributed greatly to the reduction in TB. During the first two decades of the twentieth century, it is thought that as many as a quarter of all cattle were tubercular. Initially in the UK a policy of paying a premium for TT (tuberculin tested) milk was used. This was a premium, paid to farmers, for milk from cattle guaranteed free of tuberculosis but this was then followed by a policy of slaughtering all milking cattle testing positive for the disease. This protection comes at a price, it is estimated that the slaughter policy costs the British taxpayer £100 million per year in compensation. Similar policies in the USA and many developed countries have resulted in the virtual elimination of human infection by the bovine strains of *M. tuberculosis.*

Tuberculosis was virtually eradicated from the British milking herd in the 1970s but has started to reappear on a considerable scale. It has been suggested by farming groups that the rise in incidence appears to be correlated to the rise in the numbers of badgers (*Melus melus),* after the 1973 Badger Protection Act. There is certainly a reservoir of tuberculosis in wildlife, especially badgers, but there has been, and still is, considerable scientific controversy over the role of badgers in spreading the disease.

A report by the Krebs group in 1997 claimed there was, *"compelling evidence that badgers are a significant source of infection",* and in 1998 badgers were culled at a number of trial sites in England to study if there was any effect on the levels of TB in cattle. These trials were due to finish in the year 2003, but were invalidated by a widespread outbreak of foot and mouth disease in 2000. This period coincided with a large increase in TB in the milking herd. By 2004 animals in over 5,500 herds were infected compared with less than 2,000 in the year 2000, and bovine TB had spread from the traditionally infected areas in the West Country to the Welsh Borders, Cumbria, the Midlands and parts of Scotland. However, there is also a serious problem with bovine TB in the Irish Republic, where the levels are twice the UK figure, in areas where badgers have been virtually eliminated, suggesting that there is some additional factor involved.

The problem of accusing badgers of spreading bovine

TB in the UK is that generations of British children have been brought up with Kenneth Grahame's book *"Wind in the Willows"*. The badger is regarded as an irascible but likeable old gentleman, who can be relied on in an emergency, and as far as the public is concerned, separating the facts from the emotional background is not easy.

The National Farmers Union, the Ministry of Agriculture and Fisheries and various big landowners claim that badgers cause 80-90% of the tuberculosis outbreaks in cattle, and that the correlation between the rise in the number of infected badgers and the increase in bovine TB is more than coincidental. These groups insist that thousands of badgers need culling in the most badly affected areas.

The supporters of badgers agree that there is a wildlife reservoir of TB, but claim that cattle could be infecting badgers. They suggest that the reservoir could be deer that are known to carry *M. tuberculosis,* as are cats and the brown rat. They regard the case against badgers as *"not proven"*. The badger supporters do make a number of interesting points. They claim that the tubercular lesions in cattle are initially confined to the pulmonary region suggesting transmission by droplet infection It is difficult to visualise how badgers can pass the bacteria to cattle by droplet infection. Also, in most badgers, the initial tubercular lesions are found in the mandibles, indicating that badgers are taking in bacteria through their food, presumably by eating worms under infected cowpats, which suggests that cattle may be infecting badgers rather than the other way round.

There are other relevant questions; how was TB in cattle virtually eliminated in Great Britain prior to 1970, without slaughtering badgers? Since then, in spite of the test and slaughter policy for TB +ve cattle and killing badgers at tuberculosis black spots, the problem has not been eliminated. Why is TB escalating at the present time when badgers are being killed? The most obvious possibility is that there is a problem in some other species in which TB has not been detected.

Badger supporters also make the point that the tuberculin test for TB in cattle misses a significant number of positive animals and several reports suggest that the number of infected cattle testing negative could be of the order of ten per cent. These could be acting as a reservoir infecting other animals at stock markets and agricultural shows and this would invalidate all the data on badgers being the source of infection.

In 2008, the Secretary of State for the Environment announced that the government would not be issuing licences for badger culls and also stated that there would be increased investment in vaccine development.

In Britain, there was considerable public concern at the physical fitness and health of young men during the Boer War (1899-1901) when large numbers of recruits, especially those from industrial areas, failed the basic fitness tests required by the army. A major cause was tuberculosis, whose incidence was so high in the early twentieth century that the National Insurance Act of 1911 introduced specific taxes on employers and employees to raise money to pay for health and unemployment benefits. One penny from each individual's annual contribution was earmarked for the treatment of tuberculosis and research into it. This was the first example of Government money being used to fund medical research, and it led to the formation of the Medical Research Council. The targeting of tuberculosis research as the recipient of this tax illustrates the effect the disease was having on early twentieth century Britain and Europe.

The incidence rate of tuberculosis fell in Britain from the 1930s until the 1980s with the exception of the World War II years. There were numerous reasons for this fall. These include better higher protein diets, improved housing, improved working conditions, tuberculin skin testing, mass chest X-rays[145], the isolation of infected individuals into specialist hospitals and sanatoria, pasteurisation of milk, attested herds of milking cattle and the widespread use of the BCG vaccine. Wealthy patients were frequently sent to sanatoria in mountainous areas such as Switzerland and the Pyrenees, and required to sleep in the open air, even in sub-zero temperatures. The use of sanatoria started in the mid-nineteenth century, and encountered much opposition from doctors at the time, (the miasma theory again). TB also became a notifiable disease in the UK allowing it to be tracked more easily. This decline in incidence had started before any drugs were available for treatment, and to a large extent was a result of improved living conditions and better diets. There have also been suggestions that the indigenous population of Britain were becoming genetically more immune to the disease, due to natural selection between the sixteenth to the early twentieth centuries and the elimination of susceptible individuals.

A vaccine was developed against tuberculosis and first used in 1921. This is the BCG (Bacille Calmette Guérin) vaccine, so-called after the two discoverers who worked in the Pasteur Institute. It also cross-vaccinates and provides some protection against leprosy. BCG is an attenuated vaccine derived from *M. bovis*, that is, it is a vaccine of live bacteria that have been weakened by passage through laboratory culture for a large number of generations. These bacteria are no longer able to cause disease but are still able to generate an immune response from the host. The vaccine is considered low risk and is one of the most widely used vaccines worldwide, but it cannot be given to individuals compromised immunologically, for example, people who are HIV +ve, as it can cause a vaccine-related illness.

In 1924/5 in France, over thirteen hundred children

---

145   Wilhelm Röntgen discovered X-rays in 1895 and in the 1920s mass chest X-rays of the population started. This allowed lung tuberculosis to be identified before any clinical symptoms appeared.

were treated and six died. Although over forty per cent of the children were known to have tubercular relatives the deaths caused considerable mistrust in the vaccine. A further problem occurred in Lübeck in Germany in 1930. Two hundred and thirty children were immunised using a single batch of vaccine, of these seventy-five per cent developed pulmonary tuberculosis and nearly thirty per cent died. The problem has never been explained and the vaccine was not used again until after World War II when better preparations were available.

The vaccine is more effective at protecting children than adults and was first used on a large scale in the UK in the 1950s, when virtually all adolescents were vaccinated. By the early 1960s, TB had fallen to around 10,000 cases per annum. Although BCG offers considerable protection in the UK, the efficacy of the vaccine varies widely from country to country. It appears to be less effective in those countries where there is a high incidence of non-pathogenic mycobacteria, which is generally the situation in tropical countries. There has been considerable debate in the past about the reason, one common suggestion being that different strains of the vaccine were used, some of which were poor quality. However, tests in the UK, Africa and Asia involving the same strain of BCG, show that a strain of BCG protecting about 70% of children in the UK, offers virtually no protection at all to children in Malawi and Southern India. The most likely explanation is that children in the tropics build up resistance to the non-pathogenic mycobacteria in their environment, and this resistance destroys the attenuated BCG when injected, before it can initiate immunity to TB.

There is no fully effective vaccine available against the disease, and although research in this area is continuing, it is anticipated there will be no new human vaccine available for at least a decade. A major problem in developing a new vaccine for tuberculosis is the long timescale needed to prove the vaccine is effective in a disease that may take many years to develop.

THE POST WAR HISTORY OF TUBERCULOSIS

This is a difficult and emotive subject to discuss in a detached manner. The main reason is that since 1945, in most first world countries, tuberculosis has been a disease confined mainly to immigrant communities. Many attempts to discuss it in a rational and detached manner have been bedevilled by political correctness and frequently subjected to accusations of racism, in spite of the scientific facts. In the UK, so-called hot spots are found, all of which have a high ethnic minority population. It has been estimated that over fifty-five per cent of cases occurring in the UK are born outside the country, and that by 2020 tuberculosis in Britain will be more or less confined to the ethnic minority. The biggest school outbreak to occur in the UK in the last half century was in Leicester at a school with 1,200 pupils, ninety-three per cent of whom were of Asian origin. A second outbreak occurred at a school in South Wales, where over twenty per cent of the pupils were from an ethnic minority.

By the early 1970s, in countries such as the UK, much of Western Europe and the USA, TB was generally only seen in the poorest communities and amongst immigrants, and by the late 1970s it was no longer considered a problem in the West. Specialist hospitals and sanatoria were closed and there was an over-reliance on antibiotic treatment. The belief that TB was a Third World disease meant there were considerable reductions in the funding of research and very little research was carried out for about three decades from 1960.

In the USA, under the Reagan administration, it was decided that each individual was morally responsible for looking after his or her own health and public health programmes were run down. Healthy living is expensive and immigrants, the unemployed and poor frequently cannot afford expenditure at the necessary level. In the USA, as in many developed countries, there is inadequate health care for these groups. They are not insured by their employer, are too poor to purchase health care but are sufficiently solvent that they do not qualify for free government health care. By 1990, it was estimated that 37 million US citizens were without health care insurance, and by the time Obama was elected President in 2008, the figure was approximately 45 million (this figure does not include illegal immigrants). Obama's administration is attempting to deal with this problem but is meeting significant political opposition.

In the mid 1980s, TB began to increase for a number of reasons. Some of the reasons for the increase are technical and some are social. It is a major problem in immuno-suppressed people and the appearance of TB is frequently the first indication that a person has AIDS. In sub-Saharan Africa where AIDS is common, tuberculosis and AIDS are virtually inseparable and TB has risen rapidly since the early 1980s. In HIV +ve adults with latent tuberculosis, the probability of it becoming active is 5-6 times greater than for a person who is HIV -ve. At the beginning of the new millennium, some experts considered that the vast majority of people in sub-Saharan Africa were infected with TB and a further problem in the developing world is expense. People who are HIV +ve do not respond well to two of the cheapest drugs effective against TB, and the next group of effective drugs are considerably more expensive.

By the early 1990s, drug resistant TB was rampant in the US, much of this problem being due to the breakdown in health care. A further aspect was that the Reagan administration became very active against drug dealers in 1982. Large numbers of young men who were heroin or crack cocaine users were sent to prison which acts as a very efficient amplifier of TB. In the majority of cases, the TB found showed multiple drug resistance. Many of these people are serious public health risks exhaling active, drug resistant TB bacteria.

TB is now rampant in Eastern Europe and the former USSR although before the collapse of communism there was virtually no problem. The advent of AIDS and drug abuse coupled with the collapse of the medical services in these countries means that TB is out of control. It is now so widespread in the former Soviet prison system that a jail sentence virtually condemns an individual to infection, usually a drug resistant one.

In 1997, the Chairman of the British Lung Foundation blamed resistance on bacterial evolution, the lack of research for three decades and a lack of the proper use of drugs. He concluded by stating that only doctors in deprived inner city areas would recognise the disease, whereas forty years ago, the next-door neighbour could probably do so.

A recent suggestion has been made that *M. tuberculosis* is evolving to become more dangerous. There are two opposing schools of thought regarding this theory. One view is that a new strain evolved about 100 years ago in China (Beijing strain) and is now widespread. This does not appear to kill people more rapidly than other types, but does spread more easily and is more likely to develop drug resistance. It has been pointed out that when *M. tuberculosis* attacks AIDS victims it frequently kills them quickly before it can be transmitted to large numbers of new victims, hence the spread of HIV could lead to evolution of new, more infective strains of *M. tuberculosis*.

The second view suggests that *M. tuberculosis* infected humans from cattle about 20,000 years ago. It then evolved into the first true human strain that further evolved into two more modern varieties. All three varieties are still found, but the modern ones are less easily transmissible between humans. This would explain the fall in the incidence rate of tuberculosis in the UK in the nineteenth and twentieth centuries. This theory suggests that *M. tuberculosis* signed its own death warrant by developing such an impregnable cell wall that it could not exchange or scavenge DNA from other bacteria. The organism therefore cannot acquire new genetic capabilities, is aging and is doomed to a slow extinction.

Whichever view is correct, it is obvious that tuberculosis is going to remain a major infectious disease for a very long time and is going to kill millions of people in the coming decades.

CHAPTER 12

Cholera, Dr Snow and the History of Sanitation

The slogan of the UN World Environment day was *"Water: People are dying for it"*. Although many people are dying for it, many people are also dying because of it. It has been estimated that over one billion people do not have access to a supply of clean, safe drinking water, and over two and a half billion do not have access to basic sanitation and sewage disposal (UN figures 2004).

Water is probably the single most important fomite for the transmission of many diseases on a large scale, and adequate treatment of drinking water is essential to avoid the spread of epidemics such as cholera, typhoid, polio and various forms of hepatitis (this is by no means an exhaustive list). In many developed countries, the use of water is now so intensive that multiple recycling has become necessary. It has been calculated that between Oxford and the Thames estuary, a typical drop of Thames water passes through the gastro-intestinal tracts of at least six individuals. Under these conditions, it is obvious that if water is not purified extensively, then there is a very serious potential health hazard. An illustration of the huge problems faced can be highlighted by examining the history of sewage disposal in London, from medieval times until the late nineteenth century, followed by a brief review of modern methods of water treatment, before considering the history of cholera.

SEWAGE DISPOSAL IN LONDON PRIOR TO THE LATE NINETEENTH CENTURY

The description of London that follows is not unusual, it would have been very similar in most other major cities of the period, and a very full account is given by Halliday (1999). Some cities would have fared better, some would have been worse depending to a large extent on the height of the local water table. It also has to be remembered that the supply of fresh water, and the disposal of sewage or night waste, would have been regarded as two different and distinct problems, and would not have come under the umbrella of one organisation such as the modern water board authorities.

One of the best descriptions of the situation in London is given by the social reformer, Henry Mayhew, who published an article in the Morning Chronicle in 1849. *"As we passed along the reeking banks of the sewer, the sun shone upon a narrow strip of water. In the bright light it appeared the colour of strong green tea, and positively looked as solid as black marble in the shadow-indeed it was more like watery mud than muddy water; and yet we were assured this was the only water the wretched inhabitants had to drink. As we gazed in horror at it, we saw drains and sewers emptying their filthy contents into it; we saw a whole tier of doorless privies in the open road, common to both men and women built over it; we heard bucket after bucket of filth splash into it. ... We saw a little child, from one of the galleries opposite, lower a tin can with a rope to fill a large bucket that stood beside her. In each of the balconies that hung over the stream the self-same tub was to be seen in which the inhabitants put the mucky liquid to stand, so that they may, after it has rested for a day or two, skim the fluid from the solid particles of filth, pollution and disease. As the little thing dangled her tin cup as gently as possible into the stream, a bucket of night soil was poured down from the next gallery"*.

The Romans had initially piped water into a number of public buildings in London using aqueducts. Whilst much of the sewage would have been disposed of into the Thames, it would not have caused major water borne epidemics, because in common with many Roman cities, drinking water was supplied by aqueducts and was separated from sewage disposal. In Rome itself, the Cloaca Maxima or Great Sewer discharged into the River Tiber; this was begun in the sixth century BC, and was large enough to dispose of bodies. The piping of water from the mountains or countryside via aqueducts into cities is an acceptable practice, as long as the civil or military authority controls the whole area. It is obviously not a safe practice in military terms if there is any possibility of the aqueduct being cut by a besieging force, and hence many cities relied on wells for their water supplies[146]. The first aqueduct in Rome was constructed in 312 BC using lead pipes, and the city had a water commissioner who had the power to order the death penalty for polluting the water supply. By the time of Christ, there were six aqueducts, and by the second century AD there were ten, providing an estimated two hundred and fifty million gallons of water per day, to one million inhabitants, much of it going to the public baths.

The Romans were by no means the first people to move water over considerable distances. The Chinese, Egyptians, and the early civilizations of Harappa, Knossos, Iraq and Iran were building irrigation systems, utilising clay water pipes sealed with bitumen, and using water wheels and later Archimedean screws, in series, to raise water to considerable heights. Many of these would have been driven by slave power. The Inca of the New World were also capable of moving water over great distances for irrigation purposes and had an advanced public health system before Columbus reached the Americas.

In London, during medieval times, water was obtained from a number of sources including the Thames, its various tributaries and a large number of wells. Most citizens collected their own supply, although wealthy households had it delivered by water-carriers who were important enough to have their own guild. Lead pipes were being used to convey water to Cheapside from Tyburn by the middle of the thirteenth century, and in 1582 a waterwheel was constructed under one of the arches of London Bridge. This pumped water from

---

146   This was by no means a theoretical problem, in 536AD the Byzantine general, Belisarius, captured Naples by sending his troops crawling through a disused aqueduct.

the Thames and piped it into various premises in the City of London. The New River Company, directed by Sir Hugh Middleton, constructed an aqueduct between 1609 and 1613 to bring water into London from Hertfordshire, a distance of about twenty-three miles, but it was not a financial success. Seven water companies were pumping water from various parts of the Thames by the early nineteenth century and supplying much of London.

The disposal of sewage was a problem of a different order of magnitude to the supply of water. Early sewers were not designed to remove household waste, but merely to allow the runoff of surface water following rain. Most households would have had a privy in the garden, and in 1189, Henry Fitzalwyn, the first Mayor of London, ordered that cesspits should be a certain minimum distance from neighbouring buildings. Sewage and waste disposal were becoming major problems in the towns by the end of the twelfth century. The problem was that people were living in what was effectively an urban environment, but the life style was still rural, and it was common to keep farm animals in houses, even in the cities. Nearly two centuries later, Edward III gave instructions that sewage should be removed on a specified day each week, with the City of London providing the necessary carts and householders being fined for not cooperating. At the end of the fourteenth century, Richard II ordered that no-one was allowed to throw rubbish or sewage into any ditch or waterway near a city or town[147], and in 1358, there was an inquiry into the state of the ditch around the Fleet Prison. This should have been ten feet wide, and deep enough to float a boat carrying a tun of wine (252 imperial gallons) weighing just over a ton. The ditch however, was so badly choked with sewage and

---

147 The Romans had enforced street cleaning over fifteen hundred years earlier. A group of officials known as the *aediles* not only supervised cleaning of the streets, they also checked the food supply enforcing the freshness of perishable foods.

rubbish that there was no flow of water, from the Fleet Stream, around the prison.

Household waste was stored in cesspits that were dug out at intervals by labourers known as rakers or gong men, but the system broke down in 1349 during the Black Death. This was not just due to the rakers and gong men being dead, but also the logistics of removing thousands of bodies to mass grave pits. Gong men were obviously well paid, earning several times the normal labourers wages, and they were also able to sell the product of their labours to local farmers for use on their fields. Later, sewage was also sold for the extraction of saltpetre (potassium nitrate) for making gunpowder.

This removal of sewage was not always carried out at sufficiently frequent intervals. Cesspits were intended to release liquid waste and retain only solids. Not surprisingly, as early as 1328 there were complaints about them overflowing onto neighbouring properties, and in 1660, Samuel Pepys complained in his diary that, *"on going into his cellar, he put his feet into a great heap of turds which had overflowed from his neighbour's house of office"*. Civil engineering reports of the mid-nineteenth century mention cellars three feet deep in *"night soil"* from the overflow of cesspits, which had not been emptied for years. Henry VIII made the first serious attempt to control the problem. He appointed eight authorities within London to regulate the sewers in their area, enforce rules and fine offenders. The law however, did not allow houses to drain waste into the sewers, but required the building of cesspits, as sewers were still only required to deal with storm water. The formation of these eight authorities, and the powers delegated to them by various Acts and Bills over a period of time, became a serious bureaucratic impediment during the nineteenth century, when attempts were made to bring them into a unified system.

Further complaints followed during the reigns of Elizabeth I (when the Mayor was ordered to clean up London as a precaution against plague), and Charles I, who complained about the filth on the streets of London, and ordered something to be done about the problem. In 1634, the architect, Inigo Jones, was commissioned to cover the Moor Ditch to stop the smell arising from it.

By 1810, there were over two hundred thousand cesspits in London for a population of about one million, and by 1840, they were being dug sufficiently deeply to reach the sand substratum. This meant the liquid contents were able to flow away more rapidly, and leave only a small amount of solid waste. The cesspit therefore did not need to be emptied so frequently, thus saving the householder a considerable amount of money. It did mean, however, that wells and aquifers, especially shallow ones, became contaminated with sewage more quickly and efficiently.

The problems of London increased during the first half of the nineteenth century for a number of reasons. The first of these was the steady rise in population. The 1801 census recorded a population of approximately 960,000, whilst by 1861, it had risen to over 2,800,000, and London was probably the largest city in the world at that time. As London grew, so the fields became further away from the city centre, and it became necessary to transport sewage dug out of cesspits a greater distance to farms. Thus the cost increased, and poor householders, who could not afford to have them dug out, did not bother. As a result, by the 1840s, it was still common practice to empty waste into the street and hope it found its way into the sewers or rivers. This particular problem was exacerbated in 1847, by the collapse of the agricultural market for human sewage, caused by the importation of guano from South America, which was both cheaper and considerably more pleasant to handle.

During the 1850s and 1860s, John Mechi, an agricultural reformer, advocated the use of human sewage for agricultural fertilizer, and patents were taken out in 1860 for a dry earth privy, where human waste was mixed with clay to deodorise it and then used as fertilizer; soot and ashes instead of clay were also suggested. In 1876, it was concluded that although this idea was useful in rural environments, it could not deal with the quantities of sewage produced in cities.

Contemporary reports of the 1800s, write of urban dunghills as large as houses and sanitary inspectors frequently claimed they were sources of local infections. The last of them was not removed until the second half of the nineteenth century.

A change of the law, in 1815, caused a further problem as it allowed householders to connect their household drainage system to the sewers. In 1846 the volume of sewer gas (methane) generated was so great that it blew apart the covering that had been placed over the Fleet River in 1732 and destroyed several houses. A bill, in 1847, specified that all new properties should have their privies and cesspits attached to the sewage system, and by the time of the cholera epidemic of 1848-9, laws were in place compelling the owners of properties to connect them to the drains. Very little had been achieved however by the mid-1850s.

Although these factors all placed severe pressure on the sewage system, it was the development of the modern water closet (WC) that brought matters to a head. Evidence for the earliest flushing toilets have been found in the Minoan palace of Knossos on Crete, dated to around four thousand years ago. The concept then vanished for three thousand years, although a number of civilisations used running water to flush out sewage. These included the Harappan civilisation of the Indus valley around 2,500 BC. Every house had its own toilet connected to the sewers, and waste was deposited onto the fields outside the cities. The Romans used running water to clean sewage out of latrines, especially in military camps, and the medieval monks did the same in many monasteries, with the effluent in many cases passing into local rivers and streams. The ruins of

Pompeii and Herculaneum, destroyed by the volcano Mount Vesuvius in 79 AD, show both cities had complex systems of water channels for the removal of sewage.

A small number of WCs were introduced into England in the late sixteenth century by Sir John Harrington, who installed a flushing toilet for his godmother, Queen Elizabeth I, at Richmond Palace. Harrington wrote a book on the subject called *"A New Discourse on a Stale Subject: The metamorphosis of Ajax"*. It is thought that the name Ajax was a pun on the old English slang word for an outside toilet, *"a jakes"*. His idea was ridiculed and he was banished from court ostensibly for his risqué stories but more probably for his political comments. The idea was then more or less ignored for another two hundred years although Harrington became tutor to Henry, Prince of Wales, the elder son of James I.

A more widespread use of WCs started in the late eighteenth and early nineteenth centuries, although numbers were still relatively small and only found in the houses of the very wealthy and during this period, a number of improvements were patented. However, the contents were still flushed into cesspits and generally filled them up a lot faster than previously. WCs received a considerable boost when Prince Albert had them installed for public use for the first time during the Great Exhibition[148] of London in 1851[149]. In 1861, Thomas Crapper started a company making sanitary ware that eventually traded for over a hundred years, and sold so many WCs that his name became forever associated with faeces[150].

The Victorians were so proud of their WCs that the St. Frideswide's window in Christchurch Cathedral in Oxford, designed by Burne-Jones in 1858, shows the eighth century saint on her deathbed, surrounded by her acolytes and in the

---

148   They cost a penny to use, hence the euphemism of *"spend a penny"*.

149   Rome had public toilets in the first century AD.

150   The word "crap" is an old English word meaning the chaff produced when wheat is threshed, and as such it had nearly fallen out of use until Mr. Crapper appeared on the scene.

corner of her cell is one of Mr. Crapper's pieces of sanitary ware.

The widespread use of large volumes of water in WCs naturally put a very serious strain on the sewage system. An average household in London in 1850 was using up to 60 gallons of water per day, which by 1856 had risen to nearly 250 gallons per day. Furthermore, the number of households had also risen approximately 15%. The combination of the WC, the linking of household drains to the sewers, and the rise in population led to a huge increase in the volume of effluent going, via the sewers, into the River Thames. Not unexpectedly, there was a very rapid deterioration in the quality of water in the Thames, finally culminating in the *"Great Stink of London"* in 1858.

Many of the sewage outlets into the Thames were in a tidal area, and hence could only empty at low tide. Attempts to empty them at high tide resulted in the sewage backing up into houses, and when released at low water, the incoming tide washed it back up the river. *The Times* described it as *"no filth in the sewers,* [it's] *all in the river"* and Disraeli referred to London and the Thames as a *"Stygian pool reeking with ineffable and unbearable horror".* Sewage was frequently washed so far back up the river, that it reached a point above where water was being drawn out of the river for drinking purposes. The population was effectively drinking, washing and cooking in their own sewage, and by 1850, water companies were pumping water, without any treatment, into many middle-class homes. One doctor and scientist, Arthur Hassal, made the cynical comment in 1850 that, *"it is beyond dispute that a portion of the inhabitants of the metropolis are made to consume in one form or other, a portion of their own excrement, and moreover, to pay for the privilege".*

The quality of the water was extremely poor, one water company, the Southwark and Vauxhall did not filter its water, and John Snow (see later) claimed that many people who received water from the Southwark and Vauxhall tied a piece of linen or fabric over the tap, and in two hours they would collect about a tablespoon of dirt containing a variety of water insects, whilst the strained water was still cloudy.

The state of the water supply meant that a number of alternatives were used. Small beer was commonly drunk in Britain specifically to avoid the problem of poor quality water. Small does not relate to the size of the measure, it describes the relatively low alcohol content. Small beer was frequently an element of a servant's wages, the amount involved usually being about one gallon a day. Brewing beer involves heating the water to make a mash of the partially germinated barley and this would have destroyed many of the harmful bacteria. The addition of hops also has a mild antiseptic effect, although this is frequently over-rated. The beer would have contained large quantities of yeast, and this would have provided a useful vitamin supplement.

Widespread distillation of alcohol[151] started in the sixteenth century and produced drinks that were mainly used as medicinal tonics[152]. In the late seventeenth century, a tax on the malted barley used in beer making meant that the poor turned to drinking gin. This was a Dutch drink that became popular when William of Orange came to the throne in 1689, as it was considered a patriotic alternative to brandy (French). Consumption also increased greatly amongst English troops during the War of Spanish Succession (1701-1714).

Brandy and whisky were expensive, as one was distilled from wine and the other from un-hopped beer. Gin, however, could be made from anything that could be fermented and distilled, such as rotten fruit and vegetables, and hence was a lot cheaper to make. Sawdust or wood shavings were sometimes added to bulk out the fermenting liquid, however these produce

---

151   The word alcohol is derived from an Arab word meaning anything that can be distilled. Distillation was carried out widely by Avicenna who distilled volatile oils from a wide variety of plants as part of his pharmacopoeia.

152   The Company of Distillers received a charter in 1638. The name whisky is derived from a Gaelic word "usquebaugh" meaning "water of life".

methanol or wood alcohol instead of ethanol (drinking alcohol). Methanol is converted in the body to formaldehyde, the chemical used to pickle biological specimens. The first thing to get pickled is the optic nerve and the result is that the earliest symptom of drinking wood spirit is blindness, the second is madness followed by death. The provisions of the Gin Act of 1751 stopped a lot of the illegal distillation. After this date, most of the gin available was made by reputable distillers using cereal crops and the alcohol synthesised was flavoured with juniper berries. When gin is mixed with water, the alcohol has a sterilising effect on the water, and much of the over-indulgence in alcohol in the eighteenth and nineteenth centuries was due to the poor quality of drinking water. By 1721, magistrates were complaining that gin was, *"the cause of all the vice and debauchery committed among the inferior sort of people"*, and the Bishop of Sodor and Man stated in 1736, that it produced, *"a drunken ungovernable sort of people"* [153]. The prints of *"Gin Lane"* by William Hogarth depicting the lethal effects of large quantities of gin were first published in 1751, and had some influence on the publication of the Gin Act of that year.

There were a series of bad harvests in the late eighteenth century reducing the amounts of cereal crops available for fermentation, and this probably did more to reduce the level of gin consumption than any legislation, although it rose again during much of the Victorian period.

The Beer Act of 1830 attempted to reduce the quantity of gin drunk by allowing any householder to buy a cheap licence to brew and sell beer. This led to a massive increase in the number of public houses causing a large increase in beer consumption. By the mid-1870s beer consumption had reached about a gallon per person per day.

---

153   He was not the first person to complain about heavy drinking. St. Boniface wrote to Cuthbert, Archbishop of Canterbury, in the eighth century, complaining, *"in your dioceses the vice of drunkenness is too frequent. Neither the Franks, Gauls, Lombards, Romans nor Greeks commit it"*.

The result was the rise of the Temperance Movement, supported by many of the Non-Conformist churches, which initiated a number of measures to limit drinking, such as Sunday closing and forcing local authorities to control the issue of licences. The first Licensing Act was introduced in 1904, and the opening hours of public houses were reduced in World War I by Lloyd George, who claimed, *"Drinking is doing us more damage than German submarines"*. For obvious reasons, it was necessary to control drunkenness in industry, drunks packing shells and grenades with high explosive are not conducive to safety.

In the USA, the sale of alcoholic drinks was banned in 1920, the result was a huge increase in the availability of medicinal whiskey tonics containing over 20% alcohol. Regulations imposing the level of alcohol in these drinks to 0.5% were introduced in 1921. The result was the rise of the bootleg liquor industry in which alcoholic drinks were produced in illicit stills, or smuggled over the border into the USA from Canada by criminal gangs. The law was finally repealed in 1933.

The other drink that rose to prominence during the eighteenth and nineteenth centuries was tea that was drunk widely by the middle classes in Britain. The preparation of tea involved boiling water that killed harmful micro-organisms, and the tannin present in tea is also a mild antiseptic in its own right. Tea drinking started in the mid-seventeenth century but became more popular after the Portuguese princess, Catherine of Braganza, married Charles II in 1662. A chest of tea was part of her dowry. It became popular in the coffee-houses and Pepys wrote, *"I did send for a cup of tee (a China drink) which I have never drunk before"*.

By the mid-eighteenth century, huge amounts, over two thousand tons per year, were being imported (legally) in addition to that being smuggled into the country as the tax was so high. It was so expensive that it was kept in locked boxes to which the mistress of the house kept the key, and one of the perks of the servants was to dry the used tea leaves and sell them second-hand to the poor.

There were three major political consequences of the tea trade. The first was the importation of large amounts of sugar from the plantations of the West Indies to sweeten tea. The other two imports that came with sugar were rum and tobacco. The importation of these commodities led to a triangular trade, sugar, rum[154] and tobacco from the West Indies to England, trade goods from England to West Africa and slaves from West Africa to the Americas.

154   Alcohol was part of a sailor's rations in the Royal Navy, and as early as the late sixteenth century, sailors received a gallon of small beer per day. Small beer did not keep well on board due to its low alcohol content, and as ships went on longer voyages, beer was replaced by spirits that kept better, the most common one being brandy. This was replaced by rum after Jamaica was captured in 1655, and half a pint of rum per day became the official naval issue in 1731. Rum was the source of the measurement *"proof"* which is used to describe the level of alcohol in spirits. Contrary to widely held public opinion, gunpowder will only explode if it is confined inside something such as a gun-barrel. If a pinch of powder is placed on an open surface and a light is applied, the powder burns with a smoky flame. When spirits are added to the powder, whether or not it burns depends on the level of alcohol in the spirits. The transition point is 49-50% alcohol, above this figure the powder burns; below it does not. The pursers of the eighteenth and nineteenth century Royal Navy were notorious for their corrupt practices, one of which was adding water to the rum to make it go further, and selling the excess to line their own pockets. The rum ration was therefore tested using the above method. If the powder burned it was *"proof"* that the rum had not been watered. The volume of *"proof"* has now been standardised in many countries at 50% alcohol, thus spirit that is 80% *"proof"*, is 40% alcohol.

The drinking of rum in the Royal Navy has given rise to several phrases still used in Britain today. Sailors were traditionally given an extra ration of rum before battle, or after some strenuous labour such as repairing the mainbrace, hence *"splice the mainbrace"* became a euphemism for extra drinks. The Admiralty ordered that officers were not allowed alcoholic liquor until the sun had risen over the yardarm on the foremast. This did not occur until about noon in home waters, and the phrase, *"the sun is over the yardarm"*, came to mean that it was time for a drink.

The second major political consequence was the Boston Tea Party in 1773, an event that was one of the main catalysts of the American Revolution. The Stamp Act (1765) and the Townshend Act (1767) both caused serious protest in the American colonies, as both were aimed at raising taxes at a time when the colonies were not represented politically in Westminster. The British East India Company was importing tea, subject to high taxes, into the Americas and substantial amounts were also being smuggled in to avoid these taxes. A number of smugglers were charged, their ships were confiscated by customs, and some of the most influential smugglers retaliated by organising a boycott of the tea being imported by the East India Company. The British Government responded by removing the taxes that the company had to pay, thus allowing them to undercut the smugglers. The result was that the next East India Company ship, arriving in Boston in December 1773, was attacked by a group known as the Sons of Liberty, disguised as Mohawk Indians, who threw about forty-five tons of tea into the sea.

The third major consequence of tea drinking in Britain were the Opium Wars of 1839-42 and 1856-8. Britain was purchasing large amounts of tea (*Camellia sinensis*) from China, and there was also a substantial demand for silk and porcelain. This produced a serious trade imbalance as there was no demand in China for British trade goods, and the only commodity China would accept in exchange was silver. The British had no access to an easy supply of silver and had to purchase it on the open market, which was expensive. Britain and the East India Company therefore started smuggling opium, grown in India, into China, against the laws of the Qing Dynasty, to pay for their tea. The amounts involved were large, 1,400 tons per year by 1839, and when the Chinese attempted to stop the trade, the Opium Wars broke out. The result of both of these wars were defeats for China, and the annexation of ports such as Hong Kong by the British, and Macau by the Portuguese.

Speed was of the essence when importing tea to avoid it deteriorating, and this led to the development of the tea clippers, which represents the zenith of sailing ship construction. The most famous of these in Britain was the Cutty Sark, although this was by no means the fastest. In the famous race of 1872 between the Cutty Sark and the Thermopylae from Shanghai to London, the Thermopylae won by seven days.

A *"Report on an Inquiry into the Sanitary Condition of the Labouring Population of Great Britain"* was written by the social reformer, Edwin Chadwick, President of the Board of General Health in 1842. This argued that the economic costs of the problems created by smells and miasma were very high, and that society would gain by creating a healthy environment. Chadwick's influence caused the passing of the 1848 Public Health Act, and another Act (the so-called Cholera Act) for the Removal of Nuisances and Prevention of Contagious Diseases. Nuisances meant sewage, and this was the act that required existing properties to be connected to the sewage system. The result of this attempt, to reduce the problem of sewage smells and miasmas, increased the probability of diseases such as cholera and typhoid, as all the sewage went into the Thames. The Thames deteriorated very rapidly and effectively became the cesspool for London.

A Royal Commission on the state of housing and drainage was established in 1848, and a series of six commissions met over the next seven years. Typically, all were seriously under-funded, although the first initiated a survey of the existing sewers that formed the basis for much of the later work. Several different plans were submitted for intercepting effluent before it reached the river, but arguments between members of the various committees led to the scrapping of each one.

In 1849, Joseph Bazalgette was appointed Assistant Surveyor to the second commission, but discussions proved so acrimonious that it had to be dissolved, and the main protagonists were barred from serving subsequently. Further commissions followed, the third of which involved a number of engineers including Robert Stephenson of railway fame. During the fourth commission, Bazalgette was promoted, following the death of his predecessor, whilst the fifth one collapsed because of financial problems when Lord Palmerston, the Home Secretary, refused to consider the budget they had prepared. The sixth commission, appointed in 1854, had extended powers enabling it to purchase land close to the mouth of the Thames, to act as the sewage outfall. This last group was disbanded in 1855, and in 1856, the Metropolitan Water Board was formed which took over responsibility for the sewers.

It is obvious from the preceding paragraphs that one of the main obstacles to any serious work commencing was the political infighting and vested interests that had to be overcome. As the philosopher observed, *"Nothing changes"*. By this time, there had been several epidemics of cholera (1817, which did not reach Britain) and (1831, 1848-9, which both did), whilst Dr Snow (see later) had carried out his studies on the epidemiology of the disease, although typically, the importance of this was not realised until several years after his death.

An agreement had been reached in principle, by the mid-1850s, that there would be a network of sewers intercepting household waste from within the London metropolitan area, before it reached the Thames, and depositing it further downstream. Bazalgette, now Chief Engineer to the Metropolitan Sewers Commission, presented plans in 1856. These covered both sides of the river and involved building a gravity-driven, sewage disposal system that ultimately became the biggest engineering project of nineteenth century Britain, taking eighteen years to complete.

The plans were stalled for a long time by arguments over

where the sewage outfall would be situated, the cost, and who would pay. Matters were eventually brought to a head in the hot, dry summer of 1858. In June, Members of Parliament were driven out of the Committee Rooms and Library of the Palace of Westminster, by the smell arising from the river. As one paper wrote, *"Gentility of speech is at an end ...it stinks and whoever once inhales the stink can never forget it and can count himself lucky if he lives to remember it"*. A Punch cartoon of the day shows a top-hatted Michael Faraday (1791-1867), who frequently acted as scientific advisor to the government, especially over the *"Great Stink"*, holding his nose with one hand whilst presenting his visiting card to Father Thames, who is rising out of the river covered in slime and rubbish.

The Metropolitan Board of Sewers agreed to defer any further consideration of the matter until October, in an attempt to put pressure on Parliament to resolve the issue of who paid. However, at the end of June, Goldsworthy Gurney, the surgeon and scientist in charge of heating, lighting and ventilation at the Palace of Westminster, wrote to the Speaker of the House, to inform him that, *"he could no longer be responsible for the health of the House"*. It must be remembered that at this time, most doctors and MPs still thought that diseases were spread by miasmas, indeed the windows of Parliament were being screened with curtains soaked in chloride of lime to kill the miasma.

Parliament eventually passed an Act in 1858, resolving the problem of the outfall, and giving the Metropolitan Board of Sewers[155] the power to raise the necessary funding. Work was eventually started in the late 1850s, under the supervision of Joseph Bazelgette who was later knighted. The project involved a series of massive sewers running parallel to the river, which intercepted both household waste and rain water before they reached the river. The main sewers built by Bazelgette run

---

155   The Metropolitan Board of Sewers evolved into the London County Council in the late nineteenth century.

under the Victoria and Chelsea Embankments on one side of the river, and the Albert Embankment on the other side.

In addition to the sewers, it was necessary to build pumping stations to deal with sewage produced in low lying areas, and finally reservoirs to hold the effluent until it could be released at the correct state of the tide. The northern outfall was eventually located at Barking and the southern one at Crossness.

When the system was designed, the population of London was approximately 2.8 million people each using 20 gallons of water per day. Bazalgette built a system large enough to cope with a population of 3.5 million each using 30 gallons per day. By the time Bazalgette died in 1891, the population had risen to approximately 4.3 million, and the per capita use of water had more than doubled. The system was able to cope with this increased load, although considerable extensions were necessary in the twentieth century, due to the inexorable rise in the population of London. The Victorian sewers were built to such a high standard that much of the network is still operating today, nearly one and a half centuries later. However, sections are beginning to come to the end of their useful life, and a major capital investment in the sewage disposal system in the UK will need to be made in the next couple of decades.

The sewage system is now inadequate for the numbers of people involved and the Thames Water Board regularly discharges raw sewage into the River Thames to avoid it backing up into houses. Several measures to deal with the problem have been suggested but it is probable that the minimum investment that will be needed is about £2.5 billion and it will take at least eight years to construct. Whichever solution is chosen, it will require the approval of a large number of councils and local authorities that will no doubt generate more political infighting.

The first complaints about sewage being discharged into the lower reaches of the Thames were (predictably) from the Vicar of Barking in 1868. More followed about various aspects of the discharge until the mid-1880s, by which time Barking had changed from a small village to a large suburb of London. Several suggestions for dealing with these problems were made. The proposal finally adopted was one in which the solid waste in sewage was precipitated, compacted and removed by barges for disposal at sea. The remaining liquid, after various treatments, was pumped into the river. This process continued until 1998, when European Union directives forbade the discharge of sludge at sea. It is now incinerated and the heat formed is used to generate electricity.

Numerous other cities and towns followed the example of London and the result of these steps was a general improvement in public health across the country, a fall in child mortality and an increase in life expectancy.

WATER TREATMENT

Sewage treatment and water purification are now treated as integral parts of the same process. The two major objectives of water treatment are to remove poisonous chemicals and dangerous micro-organisms, such as those found in raw sewage. The removal of noxious chemicals is outside the scope of this book, although many of them will be removed, or reduced, by the treatment described for the removal of micro-organisms. An examination of water treatment is a useful exercise, as the complexity of the process enables one to realise the fragility of the infra-structure supporting many of our large cities.

Sewage and wastewater treatment require the large-scale use of micro-organisms and may be regarded as an early example of biotechnology.

Two tests widely used as a measure of water quality are the Biological Oxygen Demand (BOD) and the Chemical Oxygen Demand (COD). BOD measures the amount of oxygen required by micro-organisms to oxidise all the bio-degradable, carbon-containing chemicals in the water to carbon dioxide. The COD measures the amount of oxygen required to chemically oxidise all the carbon-containing chemicals in the water to carbon dioxide. If the BOD and COD are both low, then the water is good quality, if both are high, then it is poor quality. Occasionally there is a large discrepancy between the two values, the BOD is low but the COD is high. If this occurs, it suggests that the water is poor quality and that a large amount of the chemicals present in the water will be resistant to degradation by the bacteria in the sewage treatment system.

One problem that may occur, if the levels of chemicals in waste water are too high, is what is known as shock loading. This occurs when the sewage treatment system is not sufficiently robust to deal with high levels of chemicals delivered over a short period, and the system collapses, a problem frequently leading to pollution of local water courses.

Water effluent from industry may contain toxic chemicals that could kill the micro-organisms used in treatment, and as a result, this water is frequently subjected to specialist pre-treatment by the industry involved before it enters a municipal sewage treatment plant. One of the worst polluters however, is the agricultural industry with their use of fertilizers, pesticides and herbicides, which frequently penetrate ground water and shallow aquifers. Many pesticides and herbicides are only degraded with considerable difficulty by bacteria during the water treatment process.

Once wastewater enters the treatment plant, it is subjected to a number of procedures known as primary, secondary, and occasionally, tertiary processes. In the primary process, the effluent passes through a series of screens and sieves to remove large objects before being run into a sedimentation tank, where it is held for a period of time to allow suspended matter to settle. This process produces an insoluble sludge and a liquid containing soluble matter, both of which are then usually subjected to secondary treatment.

The insoluble sludge has a high concentration of large molecules, for example, cellulose, from industries such as food and paper processing plants. This sludge is passed to an anaerobic digester (a closed tank from which air is excluded) that contains large numbers of different types of bacteria working as a community. Some of these bacteria break down the large molecules to small molecules, whilst others convert the small molecules to methane (natural gas) and water. The methane is usually burnt to form power to run the treatment plant, and any excess power is sold to the National Grid. Chemically and biologically, the whole process is very similar to that found in the stomachs of ruminants, such as the cow. The remaining sludge is then either burnt, or may be used as fertiliser, after it has been heated to 50⁰C, to kill any dangerous bacteria that might have survived, and turned into pellets. Legislation requires that the bio-solids, as the pellets are known, can only be applied to soil, they cannot be applied to growing crops. The use of sludge pellets as fertilizer has increased significantly in recent years because of the increasing cost of nitrogen and phosphate based chemicals. One of the main problems of using this type of fertiliser is the presence of heavy metals such as cadmium, which can build up to toxic levels over a period of time.

The liquid from the primary process is subjected to aerobic secondary digestion. Two common methods are used, the trickling filter or the activated sludge system. The trickling filter consists of a bed of gravel, usually six to eight feet thick, over which the wastewater is sprayed and allowed to trickle down through the bed. Over a period of time, a bacterial community establishes itself on the gravel (this usually takes a couple of weeks initially, but is then self renewing), and it is these bacteria that break down chemicals in the wastewater as it passes through the gravel.

The second option, the activated sludge process, consists of piping the effluent into a large tank (the aerobic digester), and forcing air through it. Large masses of bacteria known as flocs form, and these degrade chemicals in the water being treated, ultimately to carbon dioxide. The process usually takes six to twelve hours depending on the temperature. At the end of this time, the effluent and floc are passed to a settling tank to allow the floc to precipitate. Some of the floc is returned to the aerobic digester to initiate the next batch and the rest is passed back to the anaerobic digester.

Many treatment plants chlorinate the effluent water at this stage before releasing it to the environment. The whole process is shown in Figure 12.1.

Figure 12.1. Water Treatment

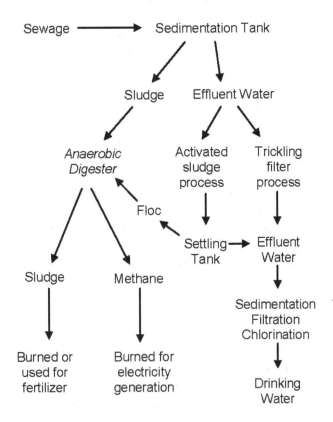

In a few cases, the effluent is subjected to tertiary treatment. This is a series of physical, chemical or biological processes, such as ultra-filtration and reverse osmosis, which removes chemicals from the water. These include phosphate and nitrate, as they can act as nutrients for algal blooms (Ch 4). Tertiary treatment is not used widely as it is energy intensive and very expensive on a large scale.

The amounts of water treated using these systems are huge; for example, it is estimated that in the USA, approximately one hundred and fifty billion litres (*ca* thirty-four billion gallons) are treated daily.

Some of the above treatments are being replaced with more environmentally friendly methods, such as the passage of polluted water through natural reedbeds and constructed wetlands, which are not only highly effective, but also considerably cheaper than conventional methods. Reedbeds in Europe consist of a bed of gravel, sand or soil in which the common reed, *Phragmites australis,* is growing, but other species may be used in different parts of the world. Polluted water is pumped into the reedbed and flows across it until reaching an outlet, the speed of flow being controlled by the particle size of the bed. The reeds slow down the water and silt and debris are deposited amongst the roots. Micro-organisms growing on the roots of the plants degrade the polluting chemicals as they pass through the system. Reeds are amongst the fastest growing plants in world, and reed beds are highly productive ecosystems; the reeds can also be harvested for use in thatching.

Constructed wetlands work on the same principle, except that they are much larger and use a range of plants, such as the common bulrush, *Typha latifolia*. Such systems are now in use in a number of countries to treat wastewater from a range of industries such as farming, fish farming and mining, and properly managed, they produce results that are as good as, or better than, those produced by conventional technology.

In both methods, the type of soil or substrate is important. The smaller the particle, the higher the surface area of the particles and the greater the number of micro-organisms adhering to them. The higher the number of micro-organisms, the more efficient the process becomes. The size of the particle also influences the rate of flow, the larger the particle the faster the flow. The size of particles chosen is ultimately a pay-off between the speed of flow balanced against the efficiency of the degradation process.

Variations on these themes use lagoons in which floating plants such as the water hyacinth, *Eicchornea crassipes,* is grown. These take up pollutants, and the micro-organisms associated with their root systems degrade numerous chemicals. One advantage of using floating plants is that they can be harvested at intervals to remove non-degradable pollutants, such as heavy metals.

Water treated by the above processes can be released to the environment, but is not suitable for drinking, and before it can be distributed to consumers, it is necessary for it to have further treatment. This consists of holding the water in a sedimentation tank, to allow sand and grit to settle out, before aluminium sulphate and metal-binding polymers are added[156]. The addition of these compounds causes flocculation that removes finely suspended material. The water is then filtered through sand beds and followed by treatment with chlorine, which kills most micro-organisms within about half an hour. The initial level of chlorine added is such that the residual levels, in the water, should remain sufficiently high to stop the growth of bacteria throughout the distribution network.

Occasionally people claim to be able to taste the *"chlorine"*

---

156   In 1998, a large overdose of aluminium sulphate was added to water in the Camelford area of Cornwall and contaminated the drinking water for about twenty thousand homes. There were widespread allegations of brain damage, memory loss, premature Alzheimer's disease and a number of deaths.

in the water. Levels of chlorine may be increased under certain conditions, such as a long period of drought followed by a heavy storm. When this happens, large amounts of detritus may be washed into the reservoirs leading to an overload of the system and to high levels of organic chemicals in the water that is being treated. These chemicals can neutralise the effect of the chlorine, and chlorine levels are raised to counter this problem. The excess chlorine reacts with some of the chemicals in the water to form a group of compounds known as chloro-phenols. Humans are able to taste certain chloro-phenols at levels as low as one part per billion (1 in 10^9), and it is these compounds we are complaining about when we taste the *"chlorine"* in drinking water.

Although the principles of water purification are well understood in under-developed countries, clean running water is an expensive commodity[157], and water treatment plants are frequently poorly maintained. Chlorination may be carried out irregularly, with no monitoring of the system to ensure it is being done in an efficient manner, something that requires human resources with the appropriate level of technical skill.

Some micro-organisms, such as *Cryptosporidium* (see later), are resistant to chlorine treatment and have caused serious outbreaks of disease. Also a number of viruses are not killed by levels of chlorine that kill most bacteria, and in some countries, especially in the tropics, there have been numerous outbreaks of viral diseases, such as polio or hepatitis, linked to poor quality water, that have not been accompanied by outbreaks of the water borne bacterial diseases, cholera and typhoid.

It is obviously essential that this complicated process continues to operate efficiently, and in all developed countries, potable water is tested at frequent intervals (daily, or even

---

157   Many consumers in the developed world have difficulty in understanding this concept. They assume that running water, which is safe to drink, is part of the infrastructure, one just turns on the tap, and out it comes, at little or no cost.

more frequently, if the water is being distributed to a large community), for the presence of bacteria that might indicate contamination of the water by sewage. In the UK, this testing is mandatory and subject to strict government regulations.

An example of how the system can go wrong in even the most advanced countries was seen in the USA in Milwaukee in 1993. There was an outbreak of the disease Cryptosporidiosis, which caused the largest epidemic of a water borne disease ever seen in the USA, with an estimate of over 400,000 people infected and some fifty dead. The disease organism was the protozoan, *Cryptosporidium parvum,* which causes a severe, prolonged diarrhoea that may be fatal in people compromised immunologically. The symptoms are generally very similar to those of cholera. The disease has been known for many years in the farming industry, where the organism responsible and its relatives have caused major epidemics of a disease known as coccidiosis in poultry. It is also found in small animals, such as mice and rabbits, and a number of farm animals such as cattle. Although it had been described in humans before the Milwaukee outbreak, nothing on this scale had ever occurred previously.

The outbreak came after heavy spring rain around Lake Michigan, and it is possible that the epidemic was caused by runoff from farms in the area. The problem was difficult to solve, as the protozoan forms cysts that are highly resistant to the levels of chlorine normally used to purify water, and it was necessary to advise the public to boil drinking water. One contributing factor to the size of the epidemic was the long interval between family doctors treating infected people, and the public health authorities being informed of the problem. Further smaller outbreaks have occurred since then, and the conclusion has been reached that the standard water treatment methods do not eliminate *Cryptosporidium*. It would probably be possible to eliminate it using advanced filtration techniques, but these are expensive and would not be viable for large-scale use.

A similar problem with *Cryptosporidium* occurred in the UK in 2005, although on a much smaller scale, when the Llyn Cwellyn reservoir in North Wales became contaminated and 70,000 customers were forced to boil their drinking water for six weeks. A further problem with the same organism occurred in Northamptonshire in 2008.

One of the major factors in dealing with this problem is that the resistant cysts are only present at very low levels. They do not grow in the laboratory, therefore the cultural techniques applied to detect bacteria are useless, and it is frequently necessary to examine as much as a thousand litres (*ca* two hundred gallons) of water, using advanced filtration and microscopic techniques to obtain a positive result. These methods are time consuming, very expensive and require highly trained technical staff.

Cryptosporidium is not the only problem in drinking water in the USA. In 2004 there were complaints, from the orthodox Jewish communities in New York, that water coming out of the taps was not kosher. The problem was caused by small crustaceans known as copepods that are less than one millimetre long. Jews are forbidden to eat crustaceans (animals with skeletons outside their bodies) under Talmudic law. To date, the city authorities have refused to deal with the problem on the grounds that it would be too difficult and expensive. They have also pointed out that copepods are part of the cleansing process, as they graze on a number of more harmful species.

CHOLERA

Cholera initiated one of the first serious studies of epidemiology in Western Europe[158], and contributed heavily

---

158   Semmelweis had already carried out a less rigorous epidemiological survey on puerperal fever in Vienna (Ch 3). Semmelweis's views were ridiculed by the medical opinion of the day, but were vindicated after his death by the experiments of people such as Pasteur, Lister and Koch.

to the development of modern ideas of public health, sanitation and our concepts of contagion and the transmission of diseases.

As mentioned earlier, there are a number of diseases spread by polluted water, and of these, cholera is almost invariably the first to appear when there is a major breakdown in public health systems involving the production of clean drinking water and the disposal of sewage. It is one of the most dangerous bacterial diseases recorded in history, and when it does appear, it usually does so on a grand scale.

Cholera first appeared as a pandemic in the Ganges region of India in 1817. There are differences of opinion about whether it was a new disease, or an old one that had previously been highly localised within certain areas of the Indian sub-continent. Modern day usage limits the word *"cholera"* to the diarrhoeal disease caused by the bacterium *Vibrio cholerae,* which was previously known as *Vibrio comma.* In the past, the disease went under several names, Asian cholera, Indian cholera, Black cholera and Cholera morbus.

The name is derived from a Greek word meaning bile and some authors think that Hippocrates was describing cholera, when he mentions diarrhoea causing death through dehydration. Celcus mentions severe outbreaks of diarrhoea in Rome, and Thomas Sydenham described an epidemic very similar to cholera in London in 1669. Literary sources in India have described epidemic diarrhoea for about two thousand years and several Portuguese physicians described epidemics in India before 1817. Most experts accept that these are descriptions of genuine cholera. In 1503, it is reported to have killed 20,000 soldiers in the Calicut army, many of whom died within eight hours, and in 1543, it killed so many in Goa that it was impossible to bury them. The Portuguese doctor, Garcia D'Orta, described the symptoms of cholera in Goa in 1620, and in 1629, a Dutch doctor, Jacob Bontius, described something very similar in Indonesia. Several other epidemics in the seventeenth and eighteenth centuries occurred whose descriptions match cholera closely, including one in 1783 that killed 20,000 pilgrims near Calcutta within a few days.

It would therefore seem that cholera was a fact of life in India before the nineteenth century, and a number of British army doctors mention it occurring in the delta region of Bengal in the late eighteenth century. In 1817 however, the pattern of behaviour started to change in that the disease moved out of India, a fact that led some authors to consider that a new disease had appeared. The reason for its change in behaviour is not known, but in 1816, the volcano Tambura exploded in Indonesia, causing a summer with very little sun in many parts of the world. In India, it produced a very hot, dry summer followed by exceptionally heavy rains, which possibly displaced rodents and similar pests. By this time, Calcutta at the mouth of the Ganges was the biggest city in British India, the centre of a world-wide trading network, and in a key position to export cholera over a large area.

There is some evidence that cholera was a disease of cattle and buffalo and may have reached humans from drinking water polluted by animals. Transmission then took place from human to human, by the diarrhoeal cycle of infection, which includes drinking polluted water, personal contact with a diseased person and fly-borne contamination of food.

Cholera is an extremely dangerous bacterial disease for a number of reasons. In India, the water table of the Ganges delta is high, meaning that wells become contaminated very easily. The carrier state is also common in individuals recovering from the disease, and may persist for some weeks, making them highly infectious for a relatively long period. In common with many other diseases, it is considerably more dangerous during periods of mass famine. Unlike many bacterial diseases, infection does not produce a long-term immunity, and re-infection is commonly found. Finally, the vaccine against cholera, which is a vaccine of killed bacterial cells, is not very effective, and immunisation only provides limited cover for a few months. The vaccine is of little use at preventing or controlling an epidemic.

The ability of the cholera organism to cause disease is controlled genetically. Virulent organisms produce pili (flagella on their surface) allowing the bacterium to attach to the wall of the small intestine of the host. Non-virulent *Vibrio* lack these pili. When the virulent organism attaches to the intestine, a toxin is secreted which changes the permeability of the intestinal wall and causes vomiting and diarrhoea[159]. The diarrhoea is frequently a greyish coloured liquid known as *"rice water stools"*, with very little smell, and a large number of small white flecks in them. These white particles are bits of tissue shed from the lining of the intestine. There is a massive excretion of water into the gut that flushes away bacteria that cannot attach to the intestinal wall and this creates a virtual mono-culture of *V. cholera*. This loss of fluid and salts via the gut is so great that the person becomes comatose and the body goes into shock. People who survive the early stages develop a prolonged fever and during this stage they are highly infectious.

The volume of liquid lost is large, frequently amounting to as much as 15 to 20 litres (3 to 4 gallons) in 24 hours, with the victim losing as much as thirty per cent of their body weight within a few hours. Basically death is by dehydration. The blood more or less coagulates causing the heart rate to rise, vital organs such as the kidneys shut down in attempt to conserve water, the body darkens (hence the name occasionally used "Black cholera") and death ensues. The victim remains mentally alert until very near death, a situation that *The Times* described as, *"a spirit looking out in terror from a corpse"*. The death rate is frequently 20-50% of those infected in the absence of antibiotics and rehydration therapy.

---

159   The word diarrhoea is derived from a Greek word meaning "to flow through". A more apt description is hard to imagine in the case of cholera.

Cholera kills very rapidly, frequently within a few hours. There are many well-documented cases in India (where it is traditional to cremate, or bury the dead on the day that they die), of people who were apparently healthy at dawn, being dead and buried by dusk. The massive dehydration and loss of salts from the body can cause violent convulsions both before, and after, death. There are numerous accounts of corpses kicking off their shrouds or knocking on the inside of their coffins. These are the source of many of the apocryphal stories relating to this disease suggesting that people were buried before life was extinct.

Cholera is a disease of population growth, and by 1820, the world population had grown to almost one billion. London, for example, had grown from an estimated population of half a million in 1700, to approximately two and a half million by 1850. In 1817, the first epidemic of cholera killed 5,000 British troops in Calcutta in a few weeks. At this time, the treatment was emetics such as castor oil and rhubarb, and purging and bleeding of the victims. One of the purgatives used was calomel, a particularly nasty concoction of mercury chloride. It is difficult to think of a more unsuitable treatment, or one more guaranteed to kill the infected individual. Attempts to treat patients by bleeding them would have been more or less impossible as the blood had effectively coagulated. The only other treatment occasionally used in the nineteenth century was opium. This works by suppressing the contractions of the gut, thereby reducing diarrhoea and effectively reduces the water and salt loss. One doctor, Thomas Latta, tried curing patients in 1832 by injecting them with saline. This is basically rehydration therapy and is the treatment used today, but he did not use enough. Modern rehydration therapy uses litres of glucose/saline drip to treat severe cases.

From the port of Calcutta, cholera spread to the rest of India, Nepal, Afghanistan, China, Japan, South-East Asia and Africa. On reaching Mecca it was then carried throughout the

Arab world by pilgrims. The first pandemic lasted for six years, but stopped in 1823 before reaching Europe.

A second, more widespread pandemic started in 1826, reached Europe in 1830, and lasted until 1837. It killed an estimated four thousand people in London, over twenty thousand in England and Wales, seven thousand in Paris in less than two weeks, and large numbers in Stockholm and Moscow. It then travelled to Ireland from England and from there to the USA via Irish immigrants. This pandemic caused widespread panic in Western Europe[160], as there had been no lethal epidemic in England since The Great Plague of 1665, and France had only experienced typhus during the French Revolution and Napoleonic wars. Traditional British phlegm and black humour gave rise to a popular music hall song of the 1830s.

> *The cholera's coming-*
> *oh dear, oh dear,*
> *The cholera's coming, oh dear*
> *To prevent hunger's call*
> *A kind pest from Bengal*
> *Has come to kill all*
> *With the cholera, dear*
>
> *The people are starving-*
> *oh dear, oh dear,*
> *The people are starving, oh dear*
> *If they don't quickly hop*
> *To the parish soup shop*
> *They'll go off with a pop*
> *From the cholera dear.*
>
> *The cholera's a humbug-*
> *oh dear, oh dear,*
> *The cholera's a humbug oh dear*
> *If you can but get fed*

---

160   Crowds gathered in 1830 in the churchyard in Salzburg where Paracelsus is buried, to pray for a cure, when an epidemic of cholera struck the region. Given his personality, Paracelsus would no doubt have relished the situation.

> *Get a blanket and bed*
> *You may lay down your head*
> *Without any fear.*

Cholera mainly attacked the poor and initially was not thought to be contagious. When it was realised that it was, the public in many countries demanded quarantine regulations to control the disease, but these stopped travel and trade, resulting in a rise of staple food prices. Riots began when it was rumoured that cholera was being spread deliberately by the rich to eliminate the poor. This type of reaction frequently happens during epidemics; for example, in the Middle Ages, the Jews were frequently blamed for plague and massacred, and in the present day, black Americans have claimed HIV is an instrument of racial germ warfare.

One comment on quarantine is by Charles Darwin, whose diary, *"The Voyage of the Beagle"*, states they were not allowed to land in Tenerife on 6th January 1832, *"by fear of our bringing the cholera"*.

Cordons sanitaire were introduced in Russia to control the epidemic. These provoked widespread riots resulting in doctors and magistrates being massacred for trying to enforce the quarantine laws. One hundred thousand died in Hungary in 1831, and the peasants rioted, sacking castles and killing members of the aristocracy and middle classes. The same problems occurred in Prussia. In India, the English were accused of deliberately starting and spreading cholera to kill troublesome peasants, whilst in various European countries doctors were accused of spreading it to provide corpses for dissection.

It should be remembered that at this stage, the driving force for a sewage system disposal system in London was solely the smell and the state of the River Thames. Any suggestions that disease could be transmitted through water were ignored. In 1848, the miasma theory was still widely believed and was being blamed for the transmission of cholera[161]. Politicians

---

161   It also led to the spontaneous generation theory gaining strength,

such as Edward Chadwick were urging that cesspits should be connected to the sewers transporting waste to the Thames, in an attempt to reduce the smell in residential areas. Not surprisingly, the result was the *"Great Stink"* of 1858, and Disraeli, who was Chancellor of the Exchequer, introduced a bill to deal with the problem. The result was the sewage system described earlier in this chapter.

The second cholera pandemic disappeared from Europe in 1837, but was followed by a third pandemic lasting from 1848 to 1862. These pandemics reached Britain through trade with the Baltic, the city of Hamburg being a major focus of the problem. The third pandemic was much worse: in London, whereas approximately four thousand had died in 1832, over eleven thousand died in 1848 during the cholera months (basically the summer). An estimated fifty thousand died in England in 1848-9[162], whilst in France, the death toll rose to one hundred and forty thousand, and when the epidemic peaked in Brazil in 1855/6, it killed an estimated two hundred thousand.

One memorial to this epidemic is found in Lichfield Cathedral to the officers and men of the 80th Regiment of Foot who were on active service in Burmah (*sic*). It states that three hundred and sixty-nine officers and men died between March 1852 and November 1853, of these ten were killed in action; *"The remainder were carried off by cholera, dysentery and other diseases of the country".*

Cholera is interesting as it was the first disease on which

as all attempts to enforce quarantine laws were ineffective.

162   In the city of Kingston upon Hull, one record (1864) states that during the cholera epidemic of 1849, 1,860 citizens died; *"1,738 belonged to the labouring classes and 122 to the gentry, traders and well-to-do classes".* An obelisk in one of the cemeteries where over seven hundred victims were buried in a grave pit commemorates *"this dreadful visitation"* and puts the figure higher stating that, *"during the months of July, August and September, upwards of 2,000 of the inhabitants fell victims to that fearful disease".* One pharmacist claimed that he had spoken to a lady in the street who was *"as well as he was"* but within twelve hours he found that she had not only died from cholera, but she had already been interred.

a thorough epidemiological study was carried out. This was done in 1854 by John Snow (1812-1858), a London physician specialising in anaesthesia, but with a keen amateur interest in epidemiology.

Snow started his career as an apprentice to a surgeon in Newcastle, but moved to London at the age of twenty-three, where he enrolled in medical school. He qualified as a doctor at the age of twenty-five and practised successfully, obtaining an MD in 1844. At this time, the only two anaesthetics available were alcohol and opium and all surgery was carried out as quickly as possible to minimise shock. Ether was introduced in 1846, and Snow started to specialise in anaesthetics, carrying out a lot of early work (including self-administration) to standardise dosage and efficacy. In 1847, chloroform was introduced which was considerably more reliable than ether, and in 1853, he anaesthetised Queen Victoria for the birth of one of her children, which did a considerable amount to making anaesthesia more socially acceptable[163].

In 1848/9, there was a major outbreak of cholera in London, and Snow started to investigate the victims and their lodgings. By the middle of 1849, he was suggesting that cholera was transmitted by the oral faecal route, with drinking water as the fomite or intermediate. His first epidemiological survey was small-scale, but he then moved to a larger scale, finding that the number of cholera deaths south of the River Thames was eight times higher than the number north of the Thames. People living south of the river got their water from the river as it passed through central London. Those living on the north bank got their water from several cleaner sources, some of them piped in from rural areas. Snow published a monograph on cholera in 1849 that was sent to medical journals, but received very little attention, and medical and public opinion generally remained sceptical.

---

163   The church disapproved of the use of anaesthetics in childbirth as it claimed the pain of childbirth was ordained in the Bible, *"in sorrow thou shalt bring forth children"*, Genesis 3, 16.

At this time there were many theories about the source of cholera. Most people, including many doctors still believed in the miasma theory, and powerful supporters included the Sanitation Commission of London, Edwin Chadwick, a major figure in the struggle for social reforms, and William Farr, the Registrar General. Another supporter of the miasma theory was Florence Nightingale, one of the nurses in the local Middlesex Hospital. A few months after the Broad Street outbreak, she went to Scutari to nurse the wounded and sick from the Crimean War[164].

Snow realised that he had the ideal experimental situation by comparing the victims of cholera against their water supply during the 1848 and 1854 outbreaks. He compared water supplies from two different companies, the Lambeth, and the Southwark and Vauxhall, and found that in 1848-9, the death rate from cholera was very similar for both companies. A major problem was sorting out who supplied whom with water as Snow found that the two companies frequently supplied houses in the same street, and householders did not know who their supplier was, they just paid landlords or their agents[165]. However, Snow realised that water from the Lambeth company was taken from upstream and was low in salt (sodium chloride), whilst water from the Southark and Vauxhall company was high in sodium chloride, as it came from the tidal basin. He could therefore distinguish between the two suppliers by adding a solution of silver nitrate to a water sample; this is the standard chemical test for chloride ions.

By the summer of 1854 when cholera reappeared, the Lambeth Company had cleaned their water supply by filtering it, the Southwark and Vauxhall had not. Throughout the

164   Nightingale believed that by eliminating dirt from hospitals, she would also eliminate miasmas and that would reduce the appalling death rate of wounded soldiers. Her attitude to cleanliness did improve the survival rate, but for the wrong reason.

165   The big advantage of this experiment, was that it would compare like with like. If the miasma theory was correct, then the death rate would be same for every house in the street. If the miasma theory was not correct, and the cause of the disease was some other factor, then different rates would be seen.

epidemic, the death rate from water supplied by the Southwark and Vauxhall ranged between eight and fourteen times higher than that of the Lambeth Company. One interesting point is that Snow had identified the epidemiology and risk of cholera without identifying the agent responsible. He was just about to publish his results when the Broad Street outbreak occurred.

There were numerous pumps in the Soho area of London, but the water from the Broad Street pump, in the Golden Square area, was considered to be high quality. The well went down twenty-five feet, through a layer of gravel, to a layer of sand containing the ground water. The water from this well appeared much clearer than water from other local pumps.

The month of August 1854 was very hot and dry, and the smell in Soho was so bad that one doctor complained the air was hardly breathable. The first case was a baby taken ill on 28th August 1854, who died on 2nd September. On the 31st August, over two hundred people became ill within a few hours, and within ten days of the outbreak starting, over five hundred were dead, and the count was rising[166]. This appeared to be centered on the Broad Street pump. The final death toll was nearly seven hundred individuals within a fortnight[167], the vast majority of them living within 250 yards of the pump. Snow started investigating the outbreak, visiting all the houses in which cases had occurred and making enquiries about their water supply.

On Thursday 7th Sept 1854, Snow addressed the governors of St James Parish, who were responsible for the public health of the parish, and informed them of his findings. On Friday morning the handle of the pump was removed. The irony is that by this time the number of cases had started to subside

---

166   Undertakers struggled to keep up with the number of dead, and some corpses were buried so quickly it gave rise to the usual rumours of people being buried before life was extinct.

167   This is almost certainly an underestimate, many people fled and died elsewhere, as did a number of people working in Soho but living outside the area.

anyway. The epidemic ended as quickly as it began, by the end of September it was over.

St James Church set up a committee to examine the outbreak in the parish. Snow was a member, as was Henry Whitehead, a local priest with an intimate knowledge of the area. The committee found that the first case or index case was a baby girl born to Sarah Lewis, the wife of a policeman living at 40, Broad Street. The six month old baby had an attack of diarrhoea in August and died five days later, but it is not known how the baby contracted the disease. Her nappies were soaked in buckets of water, which were then thrown into the cesspit, in the cellar of the house, which was connected to the sewer. The church committee arranged for a surveyor to examine the cesspit and he was able to show that the bricks lining it were rotten, the well was less than three feet away from the rotten brickwork[168] and the water level in the well was eight feet below that in the cesspit.

The Church committee produced a reasoned report stating that the cholera outbreak, *"was in some manner attributable to the use of impure water from the well in Broad Street"*, and suggested that water from shallow wells was not safe to drink. This report was criticised strongly by a Board of Health report published some weeks later stating, *"We see no reason to adopt this belief"*, and it went on to express the opinion that the epidemic was due to a localised miasma. The Board of Health report was very much a case of forcing the facts to fit a pre-determined theory, rather than using the facts as established by Snow and the church committee to construct a theory.

Snow prepared a map of the epidemic in the autumn of 1854 using dot mapping. This was a new method that consisted of taking a map and placing a dot or bar at the site of each case. It enables the relationship between the location of cases and the

---

168   A cartoon of the time published in the "Illustrated London News", shows a cloaked skeleton wearing a crown, operating the pump handle whilst small children queue up to fill containers with water. It is labeled, *"Death's Dispensary, open to the poor, gratis, by permission of the Parish"*.

location of key elements, such as pumps, to become obvious. Unlike some of the earlier maps that had been produced, Snow eliminated all the extraneous material from his maps, except for the pumps in the Soho area and the bars showing each case. It immediately became obvious that the vast majority of cases were centred on the Broad Street pump. On the basis of his experience of the behaviour of gases in anaesthesia, Snow argued that if the epidemic had been caused by a miasma emanating from the pump, then these cases should fall into a perfect circle in the absence of wind, or a plume downwind if there was a breeze.

The cases did not form a perfect circle around the pump, but Snow then produced a second version of his map, which he modified, to show the length of time it took to walk from each of the houses where a case had occurred, to the pump. When this was done the map showed that in the vast majority of cases the nearest pump was Broad Street.

Snow realized that there were individuals or groups of people who appeared to be anomalies, some had died unexpectedly, and others lived whom he would have expected to die. Two obvious examples were the inhabitants of the St James Parish Workhouse that had over 500 inhabitants. A few died, but nothing like the numbers expected on a pro-rata basis as the workhouse had a reliable private water supply and did not use water from the Broad St pump. The other example was the Lion Brewery, with seventy workers, which had its own well and the workers also received a daily ration of beer. Not a single brewery worker died!

On the other hand, Eleys, a factory making percussion caps for ammunition[169], had many employees dying of cholera, due

---

169   The modern equivalent would be an explosives factory on a housing estate. Eleys is mentioned by Conan Doyle, in one of the Sherlock Holmes short stories, *"The Speckled Band"*. Holmes asks Watson to slip his revolver into his pocket stating, *"An Eley's No. 2 is an excellent argument with gentlemen who can twist steel pokers into knots"*. Conan Doyle got it wrong, Eleys did not make revolvers, only ammunition and percussion caps.

to the fact that they kept barrels of water from the pump on the premises for their workers to drink when thirsty. The brothers who owned the factory also used to send containers of the water to their mother who lived in Hampstead, a considerable distance away. She died of cholera, as did a visiting relative.

Snow published his work on cholera in January 1855. This was the second edition of his 1849 monograph, "*On the Mode of Communication of Cholera*", but it is a great deal longer than the first edition, with a large amount of extra data. He claimed that cholera is contagious, that it is an intestinal disease spread through the oral/faecal route by contaminated water. He also recognised that the vomiting and diarrhoea caused dehydration, leading to the coagulation of the blood and death. The work contains his map of the Broad Street area, and also his comparison of the houses supplied by the Southwark and Vauxhall, and Lambeth companies in 1854, and compares this with the 1848-9 outbreak. He then makes the point that cholera can be avoided by taking a few simple precautions such as improved hygiene and clean drinking water. Snow claimed that the poverty of victims was an important factor in the spread of the disease and stated that, "*amongst the poor...there is very often little cleanliness...when typhoid or cholera enters such a dwelling it is very apt to go through the house...in cleanly families where the nursing, cooking, sleeping and eating go on in separate compartments, it is hardly ever found to spread*"[170].

The work of John Snow was the first scientifically based survey in epidemiology, a science that involves analysing unusual statistical patterns during the course of an epidemic.

---

170   One outbreak occurred in Barnard Castle in County Durham in 1849. The town is built on a steep slope, the gentry and professional classes lived at the top, well-to-do traders lived halfway down, and the labouring classes who lived at the bottom, against the river, obtained their water from five public pumps. The church and cemetery were halfway down the hill. A total of 275 died, two members of the gentry out of a population of ninety-five (2.1%) nineteen members of the traders families out of one thousand, two hundred (1.6%), and two hundred and fifty-four out of approximately three thousand labourers (8.3%).

"The Lancet", the premier medical journal of the day, took nearly a year to review it!

Snow died on 16ᵗʰ June 1858, at the age of forty-five, from a stroke which may have been a result of his early self-experimentation with ether and chloroform, by great irony in the week that the Great Stink of London was starting. Snow would no doubt have appreciated the fact that although the smell was worse than anything that had gone before, the number of deaths during the Great Stink was lower than average, a mortal blow to the miasma theory.

A number of personal obituaries were highly complimentary, but the one in *"The Lancet"*, read as follows, *"This well known physician died at his house in Sackville Street from an attack of apoplexy. His researches on chloroform and other anaesthetics were appreciated by the profession"[171]*.

Many of Snow's contemporaries considered his views on cholera wrong and ignored his findings for a considerable period of time. His theories were eventually accepted by most people[172] (although not until after his death), and made a significant contribution towards major improvements in both sewage disposal and water provision in London.

Snow was given the final accolade when a pub in Soho was named after him; he is one of the few non-aristocrats in Britain to have ever received this honour. It was perhaps the final irony, Snow was a lifelong teetotaller!

In August 1854, Edwin Chadwick was replaced at the Board of Health. He was an extremely unpopular, highly opinionated lawyer with little or no knowledge of medicine, and had upset most people with whom he had come into contact. He was also a champion of the miasma theory. In spite

---

171   Although some of Snow's contemporaries may have regarded him as a crank, the importance that is now attached to his work on anaesthetics, can be seen by the fact that he is one of the two supporters of the heraldic shield of the Royal College of Anaesthetists.

172   A number of supporters of the miasma theory, such as Chadwick and Nightingale, died still believing in it, Chadwick in 1890 and Nightingale as late as 1910.

of having no medical qualifications, he had refused to listen to any alternative suggestions and had thoroughly alienated the medical establishment.

He was replaced by Sir Benjamin Hall, after whom Big Ben is named. Hall found that government at a local level was in absolute chaos and mired in bureaucracy. One of his first moves was to appeal to Lord Palmerston, the Home Secretary, for the power to deal with the local authorities and send medical officers into every parish where there was cholera, over the heads of the local politicians and doctors, if necessary. Unlike Chadwick, Hall realised he could not afford to alienate the medical profession, and appealed to senior doctors at the Royal College of Physicians and the Royal College of Surgeons, for help in establishing a medical committee to study the problem. A committee was set up and a number of eminent doctors were appointed, but not Snow, even although several committee members were aware of his work. One had even published a report claiming that Snow's theories were untenable. One committee member was William Farr, a doctor who later became a statistician, at the Register Generals Office, using Snow's methods of dot mapping to identify and track epidemics. When the Broad Street epidemic started, Hall sent a team of inspectors to visit every property and record everything, the number of occupants, the number of sick, the number of dead, information on their living conditions and surroundings, and the state of the drains, privies and local sewers.

The Hall Committee of Scientific Inquiry into Cholera reported in 1855. The report was huge, over 300 pages long, with 350 pages of tables, charts and appendices. Their conclusion; cholera is caused by a miasma, the effects of which can be exacerbated by hot weather!

One member of Hall's committee, microbiologist Arthur Hassall, who examined water samples for various parts of London, found that the Southwark and Vauxhall supply was full of micro-organisms and commented that the water was probably unfit for drinking. Hassall also examined rice-water stools from cholera patients microscopically. He found vast numbers of what he called *"vibriones"*, elongated motile micro-organisms. He stated however that they were, *"possibly of importance"*, and assumed that they were the result of cholera rather than its cause.

Cholera was the driving force behind the start of various Public Health campaigns and the establishment of Health Boards, and when the fourth pandemic broke out in 1863, and cholera returned to England in 1868, there were fewer fatalities. This outbreak subsided in 1874, having been spread world-wide by Muslim pilgrims attending the Hajj[173]. Marc Ruffer, a pupil of Pasteur, who became Professor of Bacteriology at Cairo School of Medicine, later played a major role in ridding Egypt of cholera by the rigorous enforcement of quarantine at relay stations on pilgrim routes.

In spite of all the evidence, the International Sanitary Conference held in Istanbul in 1866, announced that the spread of cholera was due to a miasma in the air and had nothing to do with water.

Many European and US cities followed the example of London, and when the fifth pandemic broke out from 1881-1896, these cities were almost untouched by cholera, although a major outbreak in Hamburg reinforced Snow's findings. The German city of Hamburg drew its water from the River Elbe, upstream from the city, and did not treat it. The nearby area of Alton also drew water from the Elbe, below Hamburg, but filtered it. Similarly, Wandsbeck, an area of Hamburg took water from a lake and also filtered it. In 1892, cholera

---

173   "Life Magazine" in 1883 depicts cholera as a skeletal Arab immigrant dressed in rags, complete with fez, carrying a scythe over one shoulder, wearing a sash round its body labelled cholera and riding the bowsprit of a immigrant sailing ship. The level of political incorrectness in many of these early cartoons is such, that if repeated today, the cartoonist and editor would probably find themselves charged under the Race Relations Act.

broke out in the area, and approximately eighteen thousand cases occurred in Hamburg, with eight thousand fatalities. The number of cases in Alton and Wandsbeck were both very low. Although the water intake of Hamburg was above the city, the water was presumably contaminated by cases of cholera occurring on the barges passing up and down the Elbe.

By 1892, during the fifth pandemic, the city of New York was using laboratory based tests, in one of the first examples of public health screening, to identify cholera cases on newly arrived immigrant vessels, and taking appropriate precautions by quarantining victims when positive results were obtained.

The sixth pandemic of 1899-1923 did not reach Western Europe, but ravaged Russia during World War I and during the revolution which followed, reaching a peak in 1921/2. One of the major logistical problems of World War I was supplying troops on the Western Front with clean drinking water.

In the 1840s, William Budd had shown that typhoid[174] was spread by contaminated food and water, and had also demonstrated the presence of bacteria in the stools of cholera victims. In 1854, a scientist Filippo Pacini, from the University of Florence, described the cholera bacterium clearly in the autopsy of cholera victims. Snow was not aware of these results and the information was lost for thirty years.

Pasteur sent Emile Roux and Louis Thuillier to Alexandria in 1883 to investigate a major outbreak of cholera. The attempt was unsuccessful as they concentrated on the victims only and Thuillier died of the disease. Koch also sent a team to investigate, but it did not arrive until the epidemic was over, so they continued to Dar es-Salaam in German East Africa, then onto Calcutta in India. They concentrated not only on

---

174   Typhoid is alleged to have been the disease that killed Henry, Prince of Wales, the elder son of King James I. Henry was widely regarded as brilliant by his contemporaries, and his death meant that James was succeeded by his younger, weak and vacillating son, Charles, who became Charles I. His inept policies, stupidity and stubbornness were major factors leading to the English Civil War, his execution and a Commonwealth from 1649-1660.

examining the corpses of cholera victims, but also on the corpses of people who had died from other enteric diseases. They were able to isolate the bacterium *Vibrio cholerae* from about thirty live patients suffering from cholera, and from the autopsies of about sixty dead ones, but were unable to isolate the bacterium from the autopsies of thirty people dying from intestinal diseases other than cholera. They also examined the water supplies, basically replicating the work carried out by Snow, and were able to show that if *Vibrio* was present so was cholera, no *Vibrio*, no cholera. The reason for Koch's success was superior technology to that of Pasteur's team. They had perfected the use of solid media for growing bacteria (Ch 3) whilst Pasteur's research group was still using liquid media.

As a result of his work on both cholera and anthrax, Koch enunciated a set of rules in 1891, now known as Koch's postulates, although he did not state them as categorically as they are usually quoted in modern textbooks. These postulates are as follows:

- The disease organism must be found in all cases of the disease, and its distribution through the body of the victim should be in accordance with the lesions found. The converse of this statement is not necessarily correct. It is frequently assumed that if the person does not have the disease, then the micro-organism is not present; however, the micro-organism may be present, but the host is in the carrier state (Ch 1).
- The disease organism should be cultivated outside the body in pure culture for several generations.
- Pure cultures of the isolated organism should be able to reproduce the disease if it is introduced back into the body of a susceptible host.

Certain technical problems made it difficult to demonstrate these postulates in all cases, but it must be remembered that Koch was working before the discovery of viruses.

A number of other bacteriologists challenged Koch's findings, and tried to prove that they were not true by drinking cultures of *Vibrio cholerae*. Some, but not all, were infected, which led to considerable disagreement over the validity of Koch's work. It is now known that the dose of *V. cholerae* needed to initiate an infection varies considerably, depending on the acidity of the stomach, whether or not the bacteria were ingested with food and a number of other factors. Under most normal circumstances, it would appear that approximately one million bacteria are needed to initiate an infection[175], but if the stomach acid is neutralised with bicarbonate[176], then a dose as low as one thousand bacteria may suffice to cause a clinical case of the disease.

The treatments of drinking water, described earlier in this chapter, have now more or less eliminated cholera, typhoid and various other water-borne diseases in Western Europe and North America, and most cases which do arise in these countries can usually be attributed to individuals arriving from areas where they are still endemic. Water-borne diseases are still found widely in many developing countries, and also in the Muslim world, where diseases of this type are frequently regarded as the Will of God. Even although the relationship of contaminated water to intestinal diseases has been recognised for well over a century, a substantial percentage of the world's population still have no, or at best inadequate, sewage disposal facilities and safe drinking water. Gastro-intestinal diseases are a major cause of death in children under the age of five in the developing world, probably causing at least five million deaths

---

175   Whilst this might seem to be a large number, there are no signs of bacteria in water until they reach a level of about 10 million per ml, when the water starts to become visibly cloudy. Therefore a half-pint glass of water, which is equivalent to 284ml, could contain up to 2.84 billion (2.84 x 10^9) bacteria before they become visible to the naked eye.

176   Our ancestors would have frequently fed on carrion and rotten meat, and evolved numerous defensive mechanisms to deal with the problems such a diet entails. One such mechanism is the acid of the stomach, but this can be bypassed by drinking too much water or eating alkaline food.

per year. Diseases of this type, especially cholera, are almost always the first to break out when disruption of a water supply occurs, either through war, or some natural disaster.

The great cholera pandemics of the nineteenth and early twentieth centuries were caused by a variety of *Vibrio cholerae* known as the Asiatic, or classical, strain. In 1961, a variety of the cholera bacterium known as the El Tor vibrio appeared in Indonesia, and reached twenty-nine countries in Africa, killing approximately ten per cent of its victims. An outbreak of the El Tor strain in Rwanda, in the early 1990s, as a result of the inter-tribal wars in that region, caused an estimated fifty thousand deaths in refugee camps within a few weeks. The El Tor vibrio causes a milder form of cholera than the classical strain, which can kill up to fifty per cent of untreated victims. Whereas the classical strain is very virulent, the El Tor variety is less virulent but much hardier, survives longer in water supplies and is extremely difficult to eliminate once it has entered the environment.

In 1991, the El Tor strain reached Peru where population movement to urban areas has been exacerbated by a long and bitter civil war. The population of Lima has risen from one to seven million in 20-30 years, in a city whose sewage system was built in the 1920s, and designed for a population of around a quarter of a million. The provision of clean water, and the sewage disposal systems are now totally inadequate for a city of this size. There has been no modernisation of the water supply or sewage disposal systems, and in 1991, chlorination of the water supply was stopped on cost grounds. The excuse used was that the US Environmental Protection Agency had linked the chlorination of the water supply to a remote risk of colon or rectal cancer.

This of course totally ignores the fact that water that has not been chlorinated is a much greater risk than water that has been chlorinated. Not surprisingly, the result in Lima was an epidemic of cholera, with one hundred and fifty thousand cases between January and April of that year, with a death rate of approximately two per cent. It was estimated that only two per cent of actual cases were reported. This latter figure is in line with other gastro-intestinal diseases, for example, it is known in the UK that only between one and ten per cent of all food poisoning cases are reported to the medical authorities. The death rate in Peru was kept so low by the use of rehydration therapy. However, the use of these rehydration packages containing salt and glucose was opposed by the Catholic Church, as they had been named, *"packages of salvation"*. The Church considered (naturally) that they had a monopoly on salvation. This opposition was used as an excuse by the local civil bureaucracy to do very little in attempting to deal with the epidemic. Cholera reached much of the rest of South America in 1992, causing an estimated four hundred thousand cases, which a year later had risen to two million, with the epidemic rapidly approaching the US/Mexican border.

The Peruvian epidemic probably arose from bilge water when a Chinese freighter emptied its ballast tanks whilst still in harbour. This coincided with the ceviche season; ceviche is a dish of mixed raw fish and shellfish in lime-juice, and is thus an ideal transmission system for any disease which involves the oral/faecal mode of transmission. The combination of this with the use of unchlorinated drinking water in Lima was devastating and the epidemic was then spread along the coast by the prevailing currents.

A new strain of cholera known as the Bengal strain has recently appeared in India. In 1993, this was responsible for an epidemic in Madras that resulted in a quarter of a million cases, and caused about two thousand deaths. It appears to be an El Tor strain possessing the virulence genes of the classical strain, and is significantly more virulent than the normal El Tor variety. It also lacks antigens that humans recognise and therefore even adults who have survived earlier attacks of cholera are susceptible to it.

It had been thought for many years that pathogenic bacteria would evolve over time to produce strains that were less lethal to the host. In an environment where the rate of transmission to a new host is low, the best strategy for the bacteria is a mild attack that keeps the host alive longer, thus maximizing the time over which another host can be infected. However, in a densely populated urban environment where transmission is easy, and there are plenty of susceptible victims, the bacteria can afford to become deadly very quickly as the chances of finding another host are excellent. Thus in a low transmission environment, lethal strains are at a disadvantage and the milder types become dominant, whilst in a high transmission environment, severe strains that can kill the host will evolve rapidly. When the water supply is improved, transmission is no longer easy, and bacterial strains are selected that are non-lethal, or at least do not kill the host so rapidly. The bacteria therefore survive in the individual host who is living longer, which improves their opportunities for passing to a new host.

The latest major outbreak of cholera is in Zimbabwe following the collapse of its economy and infrastructure over the last couple of decades. Many areas of Harare have not had running water since the end of 2007, sewage disposal has broken down and many local people are forced to get water from shallow wells and drains. By the spring of 2009, there had been nearly one hundred thousand cases of cholera and over four thousand deaths. These numbers are almost certainly an underestimate, and estimations by the WHO and Western health organisations consider that the true figure was probably double this number. In early February 2009, one Zimbabwean official announced, *"Cholera is under control"*.

It has now been shown that the cholera bacterium and many viruses can exist for long periods inside algae, many of which are single celled plants found in the phytoplankton. Further research has demonstrated that the toxin responsible for making cholera lethal is due to a bacterial virus, or phage, which has infected the bacterium. Phytoplankton occur widely in the sea, and may cover many square miles under ideal conditions of temperature, light and nitrogen availability. The suggestion has been made that plankton "blooms" are essentially giant, floating, gene pools containing viruses and bacteria, in which ultra-violet light speeds up mutation rates[177]. Indeed, plankton blooms in the tropics have now been shown to herald cholera outbreaks on a number of occasions. A further problem is that during periods of environmental stress, many of the algae in these blooms can encyst and become dormant, allowing the micro-organisms inside them to survive adverse conditions. Global warming will also raise the temperature of surface water causing an increase in plankton, and increased levels of *V. cholera*.

It is obvious that cholera is still evolving, and, that like many other diseases it will cause serious problems again in the future if we drop our guard. The problem is not confined to cholera. Analysis of water quality in the Chesapeake Bay in North America shows that virus numbers vary from one thousand per ml in winter to one billion per ml in summer. Much of the increase is due to both raw and treated sewage effluents being released into the environment. The result is a stew of viruses, bacteria and various genetic elements such as plasmids (Ch 4). The probability of genetic exchange between micro-organisms under these conditions is high. Micro-organisms are known to scavenge DNA coding for antibiotic resistance, and the possibility arises that these micro-organisms will be taken up by shellfish to enter the human food chain and thus cause food poisoning resistant to many drugs.

---

177   L. Margulis has stated that, *"all the world's bacteria essentially have access to a single genetic pool and hence to the adaptive mechanisms of the entire bacterial kingdom".* This allows very rapid genetic recombination between bacteria, horizontally across species, in addition to vertically down the generations within a species.

CHAPTER 13

Typhus

"So, naturalists observe, a flea
Has smaller fleas that on him prey;
And these have smaller still to bite 'em,
And so proceed *Ad infinitum*".
Jonathon Swift (1667-1745)

The more usually quoted version of this is:

"Big bugs have little bugs
Upon their backs to bite 'em,
And little bugs have smaller bugs,
and so *Ad infinitum*".

This may occasionally be followed by a second verse:

"And the big bugs themselves in turn,
have bigger bugs to go on;
and these again have bigger still
and bigger still and so on".

Enterprising biology students have been known to present these verses as an answer to an examination question on food chains. Their fate has not been recorded for posterity.

The name typhus comes from a Greek word meaning stupor or coma. It frequently occurs associated with other diseases such as typhoid with which it was often confused in early accounts. Both are found in similar circumstances of poor hygiene but they are caused by different organisms with different behavioural patterns.

Typhus is caused by a member of the bacterial group known as the Rickettsia, specifically *Rickettsia prowazekii.* In some older medical textbooks, these micro-organisms are considered to be a transitional form between bacteria and viruses. They are now regarded as bacteria that have lost the ability to carry out certain functions, such as the production of energy, and as a result have become obligate parasites. All members of the group are transmitted by vectors such as fleas, lice and bedbugs. Typhus symptoms include a headache, fever, rash and the face darkens and swells. These early symptoms are followed by a coma and sores that turn gangrenous followed by death. It is easily treated and victims are unlikely to die if the disease is diagnosed at an early stage and appropriate antibiotics given.

Several different forms of typhus and related diseases occur but epidemic typhus carried by lice is the most dangerous form of the disease. The others include endemic or murine typhus carried by rats and their fleas, and scrub typhus (also known as tsutsugamushi disease) carried by mites. There is also a form of rickettsial disease known as Rocky Mountain Spotted Fever carried by ticks. All these diseases are characterized by a severe headache, chills and fever with a characteristic rash appearing about the third to fifth day after infection. If the victim recovers, the disease terminates after about twenty days but leaves the patient extremely tired and depressed. In fatal cases the patient becomes progressively worse, ultimately becoming delirious and comatose with this being followed by cardiac arrest. In some cases of epidemic typhus, the bacteria may survive in the body for years and reappear in a mild form, known as Brill-Zinsser disease, if the immune system of the victim weakens or is stressed.

By contrast, typhoid (which is frequently known as enteric fever in older texts) is caused by the bacterium *Salmonella typhi.* This is an atypical member of the genus *Salmonella*, all the other bacteria in the group cause food poisoning. Typhoid is usually spread by contaminated food and water. It establishes itself in the intestines and may cause intestinal perforation leading to peritonitis. Typhoid has a death rate of about ten per cent in the absence of treatment. Typhus was frequently mistaken for typhoid in the nineteenth century and the difference was not fully understood until the end of the first decade of the twentieth century.

Clothes are a relatively new environment in terms of evolution, and allow humans to survive in extreme weather conditions such as the Arctic. However, they also enhance the survival of a number of ectoparasites (parasites living on the outside of the body), such as lice, fleas, and bedbugs, many of which carry various diseases. Ectoparasites have developed specialised modifications allowing them to hold onto body hair and feed on blood, thus enabling them to parasitise the host animal. Modifications of this type take a long time to develop, and probably originated in the rubbish in caves used as living quarters by both animals and early humans.

Human fleas rarely transmit diseases although rat fleas can carry bubonic plague. The main disease associated with bedbugs (also known as the assassin bug), is Chagas disease (American sleeping sickness), a protozoal infection of the tropical Americas. Lice are probably a long-standing parasite inherited from primate ancestors. One type has developed to grip hair on the head, whilst a second type developed to grip hair in the pubic region. Body lice (*Pediculus humanus corporis*) diverged from head lice *(Pediculus humanus capitis)* to live in clothes. Their existence was helped by overcrowding, thick clothing and the host not bathing frequently. Etiquette lessons for European royalty, as late as the seventeenth century, taught them how to crush and dispose of lice politely.

Typhus is spread by the body louse, the disease is transmitted when the louse bites an infected human to obtain blood and ingests bacteria that then multiply in the cells lining the louse's gut. These bacteria are not injected when the louse bites a second person, instead the louse defecates at the site of the bite after feeding. This releases bacteria onto the skin, and the person scratches the louse faeces containing *Rickettsia* into skin abrasions during attempts to stop the bite itching. The bacteria may remain viable in dried louse faeces for a number of days.

Many insects that are ectoparasites carry endoparasites (internal parasites), especially members of the *Rickettsia*. Several different types are found, for example, *Rickettsia typhi* that lives in rat fleas. Normally, this organism does not harm the rat, but when the infected rat flea bites a human it causes endemic typhus that is fatal in less than five per cent of cases. It is thought that as urban crowding increased, *R. typhi* evolved into *Rickettsia prowazekii* that causes epidemic typhus. The organism was named after Howard Ricketts and Stanislaus von Prowazek, both of whom died of typhus whilst researching the disease during the early twentieth century.

R. prowazekii is able to live in ticks without causing disease but rats and rat fleas become ill when infected with this organism and then recover. When the micro-organism attacks human lice and humans, the louse always dies after about fifteen days and the human frequently does. This pattern of behaviour suggests successive transfers from a stable existence in the tick, to a less stable one in rats and their fleas, to an unstable relationship in humans and lice. It is therefore presumably a recent transmission (in evolutionary terms) from ticks to lice and humans.

The French doctor, Charles Nicolle, demonstrated that typhus is transmitted from person to person by the body louse in the first decade of the twentieth century, a discovery for which he received the Nobel Prize for medicine in 1928. Following this discovery, the *"nit nurse"* was a regular visitor to British schools to examine pupils for lice until well after World War II.

Typhus is also known by a variety of other names, prison fever, ship fever, camp fever, spotted fever and occasionally famine fever. In the nineteenth century, the German epidemiologist, August Hirsch, pointed out its association with famine, overcrowding, war and revolution, especially during cold weather. The louse requires human clothing for shelter and therefore soldiers and sailors wearing heavy clothing, and crowded together in cold weather in ships or barracks, with little opportunity to wash and change, create ideal conditions for the transmission of the disease.

Typhus probably evolved around a thousand years ago as a result of warfare and larger armies. Developments in defensive warfare such as fortifications made sieges and campaigns longer, and both defending and attacking soldiers were forced to spend longer periods in crowded quarters, with poor hygiene and inadequate food. Although the Romans had significantly larger armies than many medieval ones, they also had much better organisation over hygiene and the provision of supplies.

Zinsser suggested that typhus may have caused an epidemic in Salerno Monastery in 1083 and a few authors have suggested it caused the Plague of Athens. The first undisputed outbreak occurred in 1492 at the siege of Granada, the last Moorish stronghold in Spain. The Spanish used mercenaries from Cyprus who had fought in the East against the Turks, and it is thought that they imported the disease into Spain. During the siege the Spanish lost 20,000 men, 3,000 in battle, and 17,000 to typhus. The physician, Girolamo Fracastoro, who wrote *"On Contagion"* (1546), which is one of the founding classics of infectious diseases and their spread, believed that typhus came from the East. When it first appeared, it behaved in the typical manner of a disease attacking a new host in that it killed a very large percentage of those infected.

It killed approximately fifty per cent, about 30,000 troops

(14,000 in one month alone) of the French Army besieging Naples in 1528. The result was that Spanish and Imperial troops under Charles I (who was also the Holy Roman Emperor, Charles V) were able to hold Italy and retain control of the Papacy. This enabled the Spanish to coerce the Pope into refusing to divorce the English king Henry VIII from his wife, the Spanish princess, Catherine of Aragon, who was the aunt of Charles I. Henry responded by declaring himself Head of the English Church, triggering off the English Reformation, and leading to a massive boost for the Protestant faith throughout Northern Europe. Some years later in 1552, the position was reversed, when typhus caused Charles and the Spanish to abandon the siege of Metz, after losing 10,000 men.

In addition to entering Europe through Spain in the 1490s, typhus also appeared in the Balkans in the early sixteenth century. In 1542, it killed 30,000 Christian troops fighting the Turks in Hungary, and in 1546, it destroyed the Turkish army besieging Belgrade. Epidemics do not stop at borders or ask your religious or ethnic affiliation before they kill you! The disease forced the Holy Roman Emperor, Maximilian II, to make peace with the Turks in Hungary in 1566 and when his troops scattered after the campaign, they spread typhus across Europe. As a result of this, typhus also became known as *morbus Hungaricus* (the Hungarian disease).

Typhus played a major role when it attacked the combined Christian fleets of Venice, Spain, the Knights of Malta and the Papal States, the so-called Holy League, put together by Pope Pius V in an attempt to stop the Ottomans capturing the island of Cyprus from Venice. The combination of procrastination followed by typhus, which killed about twenty thousand men, allowed the Ottomans to land unopposed and capture the city of Nicosia in September 1570. The Pope managed to hold the Holy League together for the year of 1571 and gave command to Don Juan of Austria, the illegitimate half-brother of Philip II of Spain. The fortress city of Famagusta was captured by the Ottomans in August 1571, but in October, the Christian fleet managed to trap the Ottoman fleet at Lepanto, near the entrance to the Gulf of Corinth.

The Christian fleet numbered just over two hundred galleys whilst the Ottomans had about three hundred, although these tended to be smaller, lighter and faster. Galleys of this period had a small number of cannon pointing forward, and galley fighting tended to consist of one volley fired at close range, followed by a technique best described as ram and board. The Christian fleet however was reinforced by four large Venetian galleasses that were basically floating gun platforms. These were placed in the vanguard of the Christian line of battle, and their firepower shattered many of the Ottoman ships before they could come to close quarters. Over half the Ottoman galleys were captured, many more were sunk and twenty-five thousand Turks were killed, including their admiral, Ali Pasha. The Spanish lost about fifteen thousand men[178]. The defeat of the Ottomans at Lepanto, coupled with their failure to capture Malta from the Knights of Malta in 1565, effectively stopped Ottoman expansion into the Western Mediterranean. After Lepanto, Spanish naval interest shifted from the Mediterranean to the Atlantic seaboard.

Typhus then caused major epidemics in Europe during the Thirty Years War (1618-1648), which was fought initially between German Protestants and Catholics but then escalated to eventually cover much of Europe, except Britain.

It was also widespread in England. During the "Black Assizes" in Cambridge in 1522 it infected judge, jury, witnesses, and spectators in addition to the prisoners. In another outbreak at Oxford Assizes in 1577, one condemned prisoner is reputed to have cursed the judge, jury and lawyers to the effect that

---

178   Luckily one of the Spanish survivors of the battle, although he was badly wounded, was Miguel de Cervantes, who later wrote the classic, *Don Quixote*. The Spanish leader, Don Juan, died of typhoid in Flanders in 1578, attempting to suppress a revolt by the Dutch.

they would be in hell before he was. The disease was the origin of the traditional nosegays of sweet smelling flowers given to judges, at the start of the Assizes in England, to ward off the stench of jail fever. The problem was so bad in certain jails in England during the eighteenth century that it was claimed that four condemned prisoners died of jail fever for every one executed.

It occurred widely in England during the Civil War (1642-1649), fought between the King and Parliament, when it caused significant losses on both sides. There was also a major outbreak at the *"Bloody Assizes"* of Judge Jeffreys in 1685, following the *"Monmouth Rebellion"*, the unsuccessful attempt by James, Duke of Monmouth (the illegitimate son of Charles II), to dethrone his uncle James II.

In the eighteenth century, typhus played a major role in both the Austrian War of Succession (1740-1748) fought between Austria and Prussia, and the Seven Years War (1756-1763) fought between Britain and France (this is known as the French and Indian Wars in North America).

In England, by the 1750s, military hygiene had improved significantly, new recruits were deloused and washed, given new uniforms, and their old clothes were burned. The latrines were located away from the kitchens and diets became regulated to control deficiency diseases such as scurvy. Many armies started training military doctors and developing medical policies to keep their soldiers in good health, as European nations realised that diseases could destroy an army more effectively than battles and war. It was however approximately another hundred years before the civilian authorities started to copy many of these ideas.

Typhus took a major toll during the French Revolution (1789-1793), and the Napoleonic Wars that followed. In 1798, Napoleon invaded Egypt, which he intended using as the launch pad for an attempt to reach India and cut the British off from the wealth generated by trade with the Indian sub-continent. That venture came to an end when Nelson defeated the French navy at the Battle of the Nile (1798), and Napoleon abandoned his army and made his way back to Paris.

In 1808, the Spanish rebelled against French rule when Napoleon tried to foist one of his brothers onto them as king and Britain landed an expeditionary force in Portugal, in what became known as the Peninsular War. One of the major features of the Peninsular War was that Britain was able to supply her army by sea, the French however faced the problem encapsulated by the comment that, *"in Spain, small armies are defeated, large armies starve"*.

In retrospect, it seems obvious to us that Napoleon should have dealt with the threat in the Iberian Peninsular before attempting any further military adventures in the east. In 1812 however, he launched an attack on Russia, stripping thousands of his most experienced troops from Spain to join the Grand Army (also known as the Army of the Twenty Nations), whose numbers were estimated at over six hundred thousand men. Napoleon started the Russian campaign in June 1812, claiming that he would defeat the Russians in a matter of weeks. It was a very hot summer, the food supply broke down (the French Army of this period was notorious for *"living off the land"*, [a polite euphemism for theft and looting]), and much of the water supply was polluted. Enteric diseases and typhus became widespread and nearly a third of his men died of disease and starvation before the first battle. Once they entered Russia, their problems were exacerbated by the lack of food, as the retreating Russian armies carried out a scorched earth policy to deny the French supplies. A number of major battles were fought and although the French won them all, there was serious attrition of their numbers and each time the Russian armies were able to disengage and avoid being encircled and destroyed.

By the time the French fought the Battle of Borodino, just

outside the gates of Moscow, they were down to about 130,000 men, and lost another 30,000 at Borodino. Again, although losing the battle, the Russians under Prince Kutusov were able to withdraw with their army intact, and on 14th September 1812, Napoleon's army entered Moscow unopposed. The city had been evacuated, all the stores and munitions had been removed, and three quarters of Moscow had been torched. The autumn was very warm and, although warned repeatedly by French diplomats who had first hand experience of the severity of a Russian winter, Napoleon refused to believe them claiming that it would be no worse than a winter in Fontainebleau. The French spent five weeks in Moscow trying to pin down the Russian armies and bring them to battle, but failed, and on October 19th with the Russians threatening to encircle them, the French retreat started. By 5th November, several indecisive battles had been fought resulting in heavy French losses, the weather had turned bitterly cold and it had started to snow heavily. The winter of 1812-3 was one of the coldest on record, and the French were constantly harried by Cossack cavalry and guerrillas. Napoleon reached his base at Smolensk on 8th November only to find that most of the food and supplies had been used, and the hospitals were full of typhus cases. The city was evacuated five days later leaving twenty thousand men dying in the hospitals. The next base on their line of retreat, at Minsk, had already been captured by the Russians and the French were forced to march to Vilna which they reached on 8th December, only to find there was no food left there either and again, thousands were dying of typhus. On December 5th, Napoleon deserted his army to return to Paris to foil an attempted *coup d'etat*. By the time the remnants of the Grand Army crossed the River Niemen on their way back into Poland on 14th December, only about 20-30,000 men were left, and many of them were sick and dying. It was claimed that only one thousand of them were ever fit for service again. Marshal Ney wrote, *"General Famine and General Winter have defeated the Grand Army".* He left out the most potent enemy of all, disease especially typhus, which should have been given most of the credit. Even the Russians lost an estimated 300,000 men from disease, mainly typhus, and they were the winners! The same thing happened with another large army Napoleon raised in 1813, typhus again killed approximately half of them during the winter of 1813/4[179].

Typhus began to wane in the mid-nineteenth century, probably due to increased hygiene, and it killed relatively few combatants in the American Civil War of 1861-5, and the Franco/Prussian War of 1870-1.

It did however play a major role in the Eastern European revolutions of 1848, and the Crimean War (1854) fought between Russia on one side and Britain, France and Turkey on the other. The losses of the British army from diseases such as typhus at Scutari, where wounded troops were evacuated, were appalling. These losses from disease, in both the British and other armies, were probably the origin of much of the *"spit and polish"* seen in many modern armies. It was realised widely by the end of the

---

179   I have never understood why Napoleon was considered such a great general. Although he won a number of important battles against considerable odds, he also made a number of basic mistakes. In 1798, he launched a sea-borne assault on Egypt without first securing supremacy at sea and consequently had his fleet smashed at the Battle of the Nile. He attempted to fight a war on two fronts at opposite ends of Europe simultaneously. He under-estimated both the Russians and the Duke of Wellington, claiming that the Russians could be beaten in a matter of weeks and that Wellington was merely a sepoy general who could only fight defensive battles. He ignored the advice of informed diplomats regarding the severity of the Russian winter and he was extremely careless with the lives of his men. It has been claimed that the cost of keeping Napoleon on the throne of France was 10,000 men per month. Given the death toll of the Grand Army, this would seem to be a considerable underestimate, the events of the second half of 1812 alone was about five years worth. He also abandoned two armies, one in Egypt and one in Russia; to paraphrase Oscar Wilde, *"to lose one army is a misfortune, to lose two armies looks remarkably like carelessness".*

nineteenth century that when large armies congregate, hygiene and cleanliness are essential to reduce the risk of epidemic diseases.

Typhus (also known as ship fever) occurred widely in navies when large numbers of men were crowded together, especially in old style warships, which needed large crews to handle the sails and guns. The British naval surgeon, James Lind (1716-94), is best known for his work on scurvy and the use of lime-juice to control it. He also studied typhus, and found that in the fleet it could be controlled to a large extent by stripping new recruits, giving them baths, haircuts and new clothes. The resulting reduction in the death rate, from both typhus and other diseases, may have given the British a considerable edge during the Napoleonic wars; even so, the death rate from disease in the British navy during these wars was estimated to be several times higher than the death rate from battles and accidents. The effect of short hair and clean clothes had been well known for some time. Pepys commented that he found he had lice in 1669, and solved the problem with the above measures.

Numerous epidemics of typhus and other diseases were carried to the Americas by ship. In addition to the problems it caused in the Old World, typhus also killed large number of Amerindians in Mexico; the number of deaths was estimated at over two million by the end of the sixteenth century. The Plymouth colonists were attacked by typhus in both 1629 and 1634, and as a result of a serious outbreak in Philadelphia in 1754 caused by German immigrants, screening of immigrants and newly arrived ships was introduced. Numerous ship-borne epidemics also occurred in the nineteenth century.

From 1892 to 1954, immigrants into the USA were processed through Ellis Island. Over twelve million immigrants passed through its doors during this period, most of them only staying a few hours. More than three thousand died in the hospital however from some infectious disease.

In the mid-nineteenth century, a German doctor named

Virchow published a report on typhus stating it was a disease of the poor and uneducated and found in filthy unhygienic conditions. This report called for democracy, education and public health as the best treatment for the disease. It was suppressed for political reasons.

During the First World War both sides carried out major delousing exercises. Typhus did not appear on the Western front, where a mild rickettsial disease called trench fever (caused by *Rickettsia quintana*[180]) infected one million men, and probably gave some resistance to typhus through cross immunity. Typhus did appear as a major disease on the Eastern front, when army discipline broke down, and it killed 150,000 troops in Serbia alone in 1915. There were major epidemics in 1916 during the Russian retreat, and in 1917 during the Russian revolution and the civil war that followed. In places it killed up to 70% of the people it infected. After the collapse of the Russian Empire, it spread widely through Eastern Europe; the estimated numbers of dead vary widely, from three to twenty million. The state of Russia at the time makes a more accurate estimate impossible, but Lenin commented, *"Either socialism will defeat the louse, or the louse will defeat socialism"*. Socialism won but most experts think it was only by a small margin.

By World War II, an effective typhus vaccine was available. Allied troops were immunised and there were only about one hundred cases of typhus in the US army during the whole war. DDT, which is a long lasting insecticide (Ch 16), was used widely, and the massive use of this chemical stopped an outbreak in Naples in 1943/4 as the Allied armies advanced through Italy. This was the first time a major epidemic of typhus had been stopped in its tracks.

A few outbreaks of scrub typhus killed a number of troops in the Pacific but there were outbreaks of typhus in Japan, Korea and on the Russian front. Severe epidemics also occurred amongst civilians in the Balkans, in most of the concentration

---

180   In the 1960s, this was removed from the genus *Rickettsia* and placed in the genus *Rochelina*.

camps in Germany and also in Italy. It was generally however, the first time in 400 years that a major war had been fought without the intervention of typhus. Between 1490-1920, it is estimated to have killed far more soldiers than any military action.

Zinsser who wrote *"Rats, Lice and Disease"* described typhus as, *"the inevitable and expected companion of war and revolution"* and in 1934 he wrote, *"Soldiers rarely win wars. They mop up after epidemics; typhus, plague, cholera, smallpox, typhoid and dysentery have decided more campaigns than all the generals of history. Epidemics are blamed for defeats and generals are credited with victories. It should be vice versa"*. He also commented, *"Swords and lances, arrows, machine guns and even high explosives have had less power over the fates of nations than the typhus louse, the plague flea and the yellow fever mosquito"*.

Typhus frequently co-existed with other epidemics, not necessarily human ones. The Potato Famine in Ireland in the 1840s was a classic example, and is seen as a major turning point in Irish history. A major problem appears that Ireland was notorious for lice. Giraldus Cambrensis (Gerald of Wales 1146-1220) a cleric who visited Ireland with Strongbow, the Earl of Pembroke, wrote that, *"the whole of Ireland is infested with lice"*, whilst some centuries later a Dr Moffat (1590) stated that, *"All Ireland is noted for this that it swarms with lice"*.

There were numerous epidemics in Ireland before the 1840s. An outbreak of plague occurred between 1649-52, and there were major epidemics exacerbated by famine and war throughout the 1650s, during the aftermath of the English Civil War.

The first evidence of the use of the potato *Solanum tuberosum* is dated to about 10,500 BC from the site at Monte Verde (Ch 2) and it was introduced into Europe from South America in the mid-sixteenth century. The first report of its cultivation in the Old World appears to be in the Canary Islands in 1567. Eight different species with varying numbers of chromosomes are cultivated in South America, some are diploid, some triploid whilst *S. tuberosum* is tetraploid. There are approximately five thousand cultivated varieties and a number of wild species with many of these producing considerable quantities of toxic alkaloids rendering them uneatable.

The varieties of potato grown in Europe are descendants of *S. tuberosum* subspecies *tuberosum,* a variety adapted to producing high yields in the long daylight hours of a Northern European summer. Although a large number of cultivated varieties are found, they are derived from a very small genetic base, which means they are all highly susceptible to the same diseases. By the late seventeenth century, potatoes were replacing oats as the staple crop in Ireland and changing agricultural practices. During the winter of 1739/40, there was a very severe frost lasting seven weeks, most of the potato crop froze in the ground and was destroyed. This was followed by a cold spring with no rain, a cool summer and then the coldest autumn for two hundred years with heavy snow the following winter. The normal rainfall pattern only reappeared after two years. Seed corn was eaten to prevent starvation, and the acreage of cereals and potatoes planted in the 1740s was low. Food could not be imported as the problem was occurring throughout the whole of Europe, in addition, Britain and Spain were at war in 1740 and this disrupted trade. It is estimated that out of an Irish population of approximately 2.4 million in 1739, some four hundred thousand may have died from a series of epidemics of typhus, dysentery and other diseases compounded by starvation. If these figures are correct, then about fifteen per cent of the population died, which proportionately is considerably greater than in the Potato Famine of the 1840s.

Between 1810 and 1845, there was a decline in the potato varieties grown in favour of a small number of high yield varieties that required very little manure and were able to tolerate poor soils. This created large areas of monocultures of a small number of varieties, rendering them even more susceptible to disease.

Other problems followed, there was economic depression following the Napoleonic wars, the winter of 1815-16 was very bad, and the summer of 1816 was poor following the explosion of Tambura in the East Indies. This reduced the sunlight significantly and became known as *"the year without a summer"*[181]. By the winter of 1816-17 famine and disease were common throughout Europe. Attempts to alleviate the problems, by providing soup kitchens, only exacerbated them by attracting large numbers of starving and diseased vagrants into the towns. Between 1817-19, it is estimated that 25% of the population were suffering from one epidemic disease or another.

The problems continued into the 1820s. The price of agricultural produce halved, the herring catch collapsed when the shoals disappeared from the west coast and the weaving of linen, which was the main cottage industry, was under-priced by factory production.

The Potato Famine however, started as a crop failure. When a single crop dominates the ecosystem, serious problems occur if that crop fails, and in the 1840s, Irish agriculture was dominated by the potato. By this time, oats had become a cash crop. Peasant farmers relying solely on potatoes were eating up to 15 lbs (7 kg) per day. Potato blight caused by the fungus, *Phytophthora infestans*, which comes from South and Central America destroyed the crop. The fungus grows well in warm damp climates, and Ireland was very wet from the middle of the 1840s to the end of the decade.

By the 1840s, the population of Ireland had reached nine million, approximately 50% higher than it is today. Land

---

181   Many of the paintings of Turner showing beautiful sunsets are attributed to the spectacular effects produced by the amount of volcanic dust in the upper atmosphere.

reforms were badly needed, as the Celtic rules of inheritance that were applied produced very small holdings, incapable of supporting a large family, even in a good year. These inheritance rules divided the land owned by a man equally between all his sons, including illegitimate ones, as long as they had been acknowledged by their father. Over a relatively small number of generations, subdivision of land holdings in this manner creates an impoverished class of peasant farmers with tiny holdings. The situation amongst the land holding classes in England was very different, the eldest son took virtually everything and subsequent sons went into the army, navy or church. The result was that estates were not divided.

The potato blight of 1845 caused mass starvation not just in Ireland but also across much of Europe. The summer of 1846 was very wet and the winter of 1846/7 was the worst for nearly a century. The result was famine fever, which is a mixture of typhus, dysentery and scurvy followed by pneumonia. Thousands died whilst emigrating, so many, that the vessels carrying them were known as *"coffin ships"* and the disease was carried to England, the United States and Canada. The years 1847 and 1848 were just as bad, and in January 1849 an epidemic of cholera broke out killing tens of thousands. In addition, an extremely virulent form of smallpox appeared. In the second half of the decade, an estimated one million Irish died, and two million emigrated (the so-called Irish diaspora). Once again, overpopulation was solved by nature's cure, disease.

Famine is usually considered a natural disaster, but most twentieth century famines reflect war, poverty, poor food distribution, poor government planning, incompetence and corruption. There was some food in Ireland in the 1840s, for example oats and wheat, but very few people could afford them. Social welfare was regarded as the prerogative and responsibility of the Church and parish, and governments did not do much even to help their own poor and starving, let alone those of other countries. The potato blight was a combination of many problems, too high a population, single crop farming, old-fashioned land tenancy systems, several years of bad weather and political incompetence. It is a classic example of how a biological problem can mix with man-made problems to either cause epidemics or make them significantly worse.

S. tuberosum is now facing an even bigger problem than it faced in the 1840s when it was first attacked by the fungus, Phytophthera infestans[182]. Some potato varieties showed a certain amount of resistance to the 1840s blight, and breeders used these in the second half of the nineteenth century in an attempt to develop resistant commercial varieties. Wild species of potato native to Mexico showed high levels of resistance, and when crossed with domestic varieties yielded potatoes immune to the disease. Further studies showed P. infestans existed as a spectrum of races, and the wild potato species from Mexico were resistant to the race of P. infestans causing the Irish potato famine. However, within a few years, a race of fungus appeared which could attack the new varieties of potato, and when these immune varieties were used on a commercial scale, the fungus rapidly overcame resistance. It developed into a biological arms race between fungus and potato growers that the fungus won. Commercial growers eventually gave up attempting to develop resistant potatoes, and after 1880 the disease was controlled with Bordeaux mixture (which is based on copper salts) and later by the use of fungicides.

The problem took a serious new twist in 1976. In Mexico, where Phytophthera evolved, the fungus is found as two mating types A_1 and A_2, both of which are required for it to reproduce sexually. The sexual stage is the oospore that is very resistant and can survive in soil for many years, so initiating a new infection every year. Prior to 1976, only the A_1 mating type had been found in the rest of the world and the fungus had no sexually reproductive stage outside Mexico. It was therefore

---

182   Although Phytophthera is generally regarded as a fungus, it is closely related to certain types of algae.

effectively a clone that caused infections by over-wintering on seed potatoes, but could not survive over winter in soil.

In 1976, Europe experienced one of the hottest, driest summers of the twentieth century, the potato crop was very poor and large quantities of potatoes were imported. These included many from Mexico that were carrying the A_2 form of the fungus, thus enabling the fungus to reproduce sexually for the first time in Europe. Since then, the fungus has caused earlier and more severe attacks of potato blight. The sexual stage now over-winters in soil, causing soil to be infective for many years and this is causing serious problems about crop rotation involving potatoes. This problem has now spread world wide, leading to much greater diversity of the fungus and the development of new fungal races with an altered and increased potential for infecting potatoes. As potatoes are one of the twenty or so crops that provide a major portion of the calories that the human species requires, the problem is obviously a very serious one. Research is proceeding in attempts to develop new types of blight resistant potatoes and related plants, such as the tomato and aubergine, which are also attacked by relatives of *Phytophthera*.

CHAPTER 14

Syphilis (The Great Pox)

INTRODUCTION

Syphilis was one of two apparently new diseases that appeared in Europe in the 1490s, both of which became very serious problems; the other one was typhus (Ch 13). Syphilis is a venereal disease, named after Venus, the Roman Goddess of Love (a singularly inappropriate term), the more modern terminology is STD (sexually transmitted disease) or STI (sexually transmitted infection). As such, it is transmitted by coitus (so-called horizontal transmission [no pun intended]), but can also be transmitted congenitally, that is from mother to offspring (vertical transmission) either *in utero,* or during birth. Numerous cases of this occurring are known in history. Some doctors thought that it could also be caught by infants being breast fed by an infected mother, and in the nineteenth century, it was considered that it could be transmitted by *"arm-to-arm"* vaccination against smallpox using a child with congenital syphilis as the donor (Ch 10).

Syphilis is caused by bacteria of a type known as spirochaetes. These are thinner and longer than most other bacteria and have a corkscrew structure. The one causing syphilis is called *Treponema pallidum.* It enters the body through the mucous membranes of the genitals, mouth or anus and infection can take place either by homosexual or heterosexual transmission. This bacterium is not particular in its habits. *Treponema* remains in the body of the victim for their lifetime unless killed by antibiotic treatment. It requires moisture to survive and dries out and dies very quickly once it leaves the body, so the hoary old excuse that, *"I must have caught it from the toilet seat",* causes most doctors considerable exasperation.

There are three distinct phases during an infection of syphilis, although at the present time only a relatively small percentage of victims proceed to the tertiary stage. Initially, the bacterium causes a small ulcer or chancre (lesion) at the point of entry (the primary stage), about two to six weeks after infection and this heals about a month later. There is then a latent period of several weeks to a few months before the secondary phase of symptoms appears. These are very variable, they include fever, severe pains in the joints, headache, a rash, pustules and lesions that may be found anywhere on the skin. This secondary phase is highly infectious, but the symptoms slowly disappear and are followed by a second latent period that may last for years or even the lifetime of the victim. Cases are known of the second latent period lasting as long as twenty-five years before any symptoms reappear. Finally, there is a tertiary phase developing over a period of years, in which lesions known as gummata may appear anywhere on the body, including the internal organs and skeleton. These may destroy bone tissue, which attempts to heal itself by producing new bone on the side opposite the lesion, so that the bone becomes progressively more deformed. If this occurs in the legs it produces a noticeable waddle and in many cases, the damage to the bone is sufficiently characteristic to allow skeletons in archaeological sites to be identified as having contracted syphilis.

Frequently, the tertiary phase attacks the central nervous system causing paralysis of the face and lower limbs, and the victim may become blind. It may also attack the heart causing an aortic aneurysm that can rupture causing instant death. This complication is rarely seen these days because of treatment with antibiotics. In the final stages, lesions may appear in the brain leading to dementia and death.

In a significant percentage of congenital cases the foetus is stillborn but in those that survive, the disease develops through childhood and the tertiary form appears at an early stage. Children suffering from congenital syphilis frequently have what is known as Hutchinson's triad, first described by Johnathon Hutchinson in 1861. This consists of blindness, deafness and deformed teeth that are one of the most characteristic features of the congenital form of the disease and which can be used diagnostically in skeletal remains.

The organism responsible for syphilis was discovered in 1905 by Fritz Schaudinn and Eric Hoffman who identified *T. pallidum*. It is a long, very thin bacterium twisted into a spiral, the name *Treponema pallidum* meaning a pale twisted thread. It grows very slowly and is extremely difficult to culture in the laboratory. In 1906, August von Wasserman developed the Wasserman reaction, an immunological test that allowed victims to be identified before the symptoms became obvious, although it was not a cure. A number of variations of this are known, but a problem commonly occurring with these tests is the interference of malaria with the interpretation of the results. This can cause serious problems in the diagnosis of syphilis and the determination of its frequency in areas where malaria is endemic. A number of more advanced tests are now used in the developed world. Venereal syphilis also has the distinction of being the first bacterial disease to be treated by a synthetic drug, the arsenic containing compound salvarsan, developed by Erhlich (Ch 3).

WHERE DID IT COME FROM?

What is recognised as the modern clinical form of syphilis first appeared in Western Europe in the early 1490s, more or less coincidentally with the voyages of Columbus to the New World. Columbus returned from his first voyage in March 1493, and some authors consider that it was brought to the Old World by Amerindian slaves that Columbus and his men transported from the West Indies. A number of these authors have specifically suggested it came from Hispaniola, the island that is now divided between Haiti and the Dominican Republic. In 1526, Gonzalo Fernandez de Oviedo (1478-1577) stated categorically that it came from the New World, whilst Astrac (1684-1766) considered one of the ways of contracting it was by eating the meat of the American iguana.

If it did originate in the Americas, it was the only disease that came east to the Old World, all the rest went westwards to the New World. Given that guaiac wood (see later) was being touted as a cure in the first decade of the sixteenth century, it is obvious that the idea of a New World origin was circulating at an early stage. This theory does follow the xenophobic pattern mentioned later, that syphilis was the fault of everyone except the ethnic group to which the victim belonged.

One major factor against the theory that it came from the Americas is that the Amerindians were extremely susceptible to syphilis. If it had originated in the Americas, one would have expected the local inhabitants to have been highly resistant to it, especially as the disease altered its behaviour so rapidly after appearing in Europe. Several authors have claimed that pre-Columbian Amerindian skeletons from archaeological sites show lesions typical of syphilis, but they could have been yaws or pinta (see below).

There have been suggestions that it was in Europe in a mild form before 1492 (i.e. pre-Columbus), and there was then a mutation leading to a more dangerous form. Again the skeletal evidence is not convincing. Some experts claim to have recognised syphilitic lesions in Old World skeletons dated to before the fifteenth century, but these are almost certainly the remains of individuals who were suffering from leprosy, which was common in the twelfth and thirteenth centuries. No contemporary sources before the last decade of the fifteenth century contain descriptions of any disease with the sequence of genital sores, joint pains, skin eruptions, the various secondary and tertiary lesions and dementia, which were described widely by physicians of the early sixteenth century. Syphilis may have existed in Europe before 1492, but obviously in a much less virulent form that we cannot recognise today. There have been suggestions that there are references to syphilis in the Talmud, but these are not precise, and are probably descriptions of chancroid sores, possibly caused by bacteria of the genus *Haemophilus*.

Gruner (1744-1815) wrote a general history of pox in 1789, in which he claimed that it had been spread by the Marrani, a term used to describe the Jews and Moors who had fled from Spain in 1492, to escape the religious persecutions and inquisitions started by Ferdinand and Isabella. He considered that the Marrani had had the disease in Spain, but because they were culturally separated from the Spanish, it had not spread to the general community. He argued that syphilis had appeared in Italy at the time the expelled Marrani had arrived there in 1492-3, and claimed that the dislocation of the Marrani caused inter-ethnic sex leading to syphilis appearing in French soldiers and hence to all of Europe.

The Portuguese doctor, Antonio Sanches, claimed it had started in Italy before June 1495, whilst the Papal Secretary also stated it was transmitted by the Jews driven out of Spain by King Ferdinand. Parallels were drawn between the arrival of the pox in Italy, and leprosy being carried around Europe by the Jews, when they were expelled from the Holy Land by the Romans in the first century AD. Senarega, from Genoa, claimed, "*Many say it came from Ethiopia*", and numerous later authors also suggested Africa as the source. It was a common European view in the eighteenth century that Africa was the origin of all skin diseases. This theory was an extension of the Roman proverb, "*Always something new out of Africa*".

There were of course the usual astrological reasons given for the appearance of syphilis. One doctor claimed pox was due to a conjunction of Saturn and Jupiter in 1484, followed by a solar eclipse the following year, giving rise to pestilence, wars, famine and finally pox. A frequently published wood-cutting by Albrecht Dürer, dated 1496, shows a mercenary covered by pock marks. Above him is a globe with zodiac signs and the date 1484, alluding to the claim that syphilis was caused by the planetary conjunction that occurred in that year.

Some Italian doctors stated that it was caused by warm humid weather in the spring of 1496, and they also connected the humidity to a high number of earthquakes that year. However, given that a major epidemic had started in 1494 at the siege of Naples, the dates do not fit. The miasma theory was also invoked with the suggestion that it was caused by bad air from receding floodwater. Girolamo Savonarola, a radical cleric who established a republic in Florence, had warned in 1495 that God was about to punish the great and good of Italian society with, *"a great scourge"*. However, this was again a case of being wise after the event.

In Germany at the Diet of Worms[183] in 1496, it was described as God's punishment for blasphemy, whilst in 1497, The Holy Roman Emperor, Maximilian I, declared it was God's punishment on wicked men. Because the disease was considered as divine punishment or generated by the conjunction of the planets, it was thought that the scope for any doctor to cure it was limited.

Many doctors also believed it was a form of leprosy that had interacted with the Black Death to generate syphilis, and in the early years of the epidemic there appears to have been considerable confusion between syphilis and leprosy by many Arab and European doctors. It is interesting that doctors of the period considered lepers to be extremely lecherous, and were of the opinion that leprosy was spread by sexual contact. The obvious conclusion therefore was that syphilis was a venereal form of leprosy.

Two modern hypotheses have been proposed for the spread of syphilis, the first suggests that there is only one treponematosis. This is caused by one pathogen, *Treponema pallidum,* which

---

183   A meeting of the provinces of The Holy Roman Empire.

takes up varying clinical forms under different sociological, cultural and epidemiological conditions, with syphilis being one extreme of a spectrum of the disease symptoms. Four forms are found, known as syphilis, yaws, pinta and bejel (an Arab word for non-venereal syphilis). Infection by one of them seems to provide considerable protection against being infected by any of the others, and it is also impossible to distinguish between the four diseases immunologically. These two facts suggest that they are extremely closely related, if not identical. There must be some difference as the yaws and bejel forms of treponematosis do not invade the spine and brain, whilst syphilis does, but what this difference is, is uncertain.

The second hypothesis considers that the different forms of the disease mentioned above are mutations from an ancestral form of *Treponema* that has disappeared. It suggests that there was a mutation leading to a dangerous form of syphilis at the end of the fifteenth century, this mutation being favoured by the social and environmental conditions of the time. It suggests that *Treponema* had infected the genitals and, coincidently, was beginning to develop a sexual mode of transmission when Columbus discovered America. It is possible that there was some precursor venereal disease in classical times, which mutated to a more destructive form, ultimately producing the epidemics of the late fifteenth and sixteenth centuries. A variation of this theory suggests that possibly it was infections of yaws coming into contact with a new community. It became less destructive over three to four decades for reasons discussed later.

The generally accepted version suggests that *Treponema* infected humans about twenty thousand years ago, and spread throughout the Old World as pinta, crossing from Siberia to the Americas with the migrations across Beringia (Ch 5). Pinta is a mild skin infection that is now found mainly in Central America. Several thousand years ago, pinta in sub-Saharan Africa evolved into yaws. This is a more serious disease attacking the skin and skeletal tissues, especially in young children, and persists in Africa and Latin America to the present day. Both pinta and yaws are transmitted by skin-to-skin contact through minor abrasions.

The organism then spread to Neolithic communities in colder climates, where people were fully clothed and therefore protected from many minor skin abrasions. It infected the mouth and started spreading by kissing to give bejel or non-venereal syphilis. This form of the disease can damage both the heart and bones, but virtually never progresses to paralysis or insanity, and lesions on the genitals are uncommon. It also infects children as well as adults. Bejel was once widespread, but has now faded to a large extent in the Old World, except in desert areas of Asia and Africa.

Bejel (or possibly yaws) probably adapted to urban life in the Middle East about six thousand years ago as cities started to grow. Transmission from one victim to another was poor and the organism therefore needed to survive in the body for long periods thus causing damage to the heart and nervous system. It had thus evolved over a long period of time from a relatively mild rural disease, usually of children, to a serious urban disease of adults. This is an unusual evolutionary pathway for a pathogen and there must have been some advantage for the bacterium in taking this route, probably one that related to the rate or method of infection of a new susceptible individual.

Syphilis is spread by sexual contact and it requires a situation in which a considerable percentage of the population must have sex with more than one partner. This is more likely to happen in cities, where there is a considerable degree of anonymity, rather than villages where everyone knows everyone else's business. It may possibly be linked to the appearance of the Black Death in the fourteenth century that caused several generations of general movement and unrest. Many families were disrupted, and a huge influx of people into the cities occurred. When syphilis first appeared, it was also rumoured that people suffering from it did not catch plague, that is, one poison drove out the other, a common misconception at this time. Such an attitude would have greatly encouraged promiscuity, and in these conditions multiple partner sex may have reached a critical level, allowing *Treponema* to develop into a more lethal form.

One problem that is difficult to explain is why yaws or bejel from Africa, did not make the jump to syphilis in Europe before the fifteenth century, as there was plenty of contact between the two continents before this date. However, yaws and leprosy both produce skin disfigurations that contemporary doctors may have had difficulty distinguishing, so the misdiagnosis of yaws as leprosy was a distinct possibility.

Yaws, pinta and bejel appear to be more or less mutually exclusive within a given region, and each gives some immunity against the others. There have also been reports of them changing into each other depending on the climate. It is claimed that if a person moves from tropical lowland to a cooler mountain area, yaws can change to bejel, whilst it has also been suggested that bejel and syphilis can change into each other.

History

Syphilis has been called the great masquerader as the wide range of symptoms it produces, especially in skeletal tissues, mimic several other diseases. Skeletons from before 1490 showing traces that might be interpreted as syphilis are very few, in both the Old and New Worlds. Descriptions of venereal diseases before 1495 tend to be very vague, and contemporary accounts suggest it may have been confused frequently with leprosy, however skeletal remains from lazar house cemeteries show no signs of syphilis, although the signs of leprosy are very obvious.

The most severe symptoms are so obvious that people such as Galen, Hippocrates and Avicenna would have mentioned them if they had been present. The fact that these physicians of antiquity had not recognised syphilis, caused the doctors of the fifteenth and sixteenth centuries considerable problems. Niccolò Leoniceno (1428-1524), Professor of Medicine at Ferrara wrote, *"I cannot believe that this illness is born suddenly now and has infected only our own epoch and none of the preceding ones"*. If a disease had been described by the ancients, this provided more kudos and gravitas for the physician of the sixteenth century who could treat it. Many physicians did not believe that there could be a new disease that had not been described by Hippocrates or Galen, as they considered that the achievements of the ancients represented the pinnacle of human medicine. As all cures were based on the descriptions of the ancients, if Hippocrates and Galen had not recognised the disease, then logically it did not exist and therefore it was not possible to treat it.

Numerous explanations were proposed to explain why descriptions of syphilis did not appear in ancient literature. Common ones were that Hippocrates had described it without naming it, secondly it was an ancient disease but only in the New World, thirdly it had been a trifling disease in classical times but the degradation of modern man made it serious and finally, it was a new combination of old diseases. However, a number of contemporary Italian writers describe the epidemic of pox as one of the main events occurring in the last decade of the fifteenth century, many of them recognising that it was new and unknown to any doctor of the period.

When syphilis first appeared, it was known to the medical fraternity as *Morbus Gallicus* (the French disease, although occasionally translated as the French pox or the French distemper). It was widespread throughout Europe by 1500, and regarded as an occupational disease of soldiers, seamen and students (by 1585, one London doctor estimated that fifty per cent of students suffered from it).

By 1520, it had reached Japan, China, India and the

Portuguese colonies of Africa. The French called it the Neapolitan disease or less frequently the Spanish pox, whilst Italy, Germany and England called it the French disease. It was known as the Spanish disease in Holland, the Castilian disease in Portugal, Polish disease in Russia, German in Poland, Christian or European in Turkey, Turkish in Persia, and Portuguese or Chinese disease in Japan, whilst in the Indian sub-continent it was known as the Frankish disease. It has been described as the most unwanted and xenophobic disease in history.

When it first appeared, the descriptions of it were variable, causing one cynic to remark that the only constant factor about the disease, was the wish of every ethnic group that acquired it, to blame it on somebody else.

In England, the French disease was known in the vernacular as the pox or the Great Pox, to distinguish it from smallpox. In Elizabethan times, the curse, *"a pox on you"*, expressed the wish that the recipient of the curse contracted syphilis and the resulting disfiguring sores. In England, it was also cynically known as the *"Bishop of Winchester's bumps"*, as the Bishop had a controlling interest in all the brothels in Southwark, and prostitutes were known as *"Winchester geese"*. British troops in the Peninsular War called it the *"Black Lion"* and it has also been referred to as *"Cupids measles"* (the Flashman novels).

Two contemporary Florentine writers called it the *"bolle francaise"* (French boils) and *"rogna franciosa"* (French itch). It also became known as *"Mal Napolitano"* due to another contemporary belief that it had been brought to Naples by the Spanish. At this time there were close political and commercial connections between the kingdoms of Naples and Spain. There are claims that Spanish sailors from the fleet of Columbus were sent to Naples to help defend it against the French and they took it with them. The French naturally encouraged this last name as it removed some of the stigma for spreading the disease from them.

The name syphilis first appears in a poem written by Fracastorius describing the disease, *"Syphilis sive morbus Gallicus"* (Syphilis or the French Disease) published in 1530, although it was probably written several years earlier. In this poem, a shepherd boy, Syphilis, supposedly complained to Apollo, the Sun God, about the heat, and in protest started a cult of a mortal king. Appollo punished him by a pestilence that produced ulcerations of the body that could only be removed by washing with quicksilver (mercury). The name is possibly derived from an Alexandrian Greek word, *syphlos,* which means maimed with especially reference to blindness (one of the symptoms of tertiary syphilis). Fracastorius also suggested that a nymph called Ammerice had indicated that people should look for the cure in Haiti, a suggestion related to the idea that it had originally come from Hispaniola. Unusually for the time, Fracastoro recognised that pox could be caught by a perfectly healthy person and was not as a result of an imbalance of the humours of the body.

The term syphilis did not come into widespread use until the late eighteenth century, from the late sixteenth to the early eighteenth centuries, the disease was more generally known to the medical fraternity as lues venerea (venereal buboes or venereal disease).

The first known description appeared in 1495 by a Spanish doctor in Barcelona, one Nicholas Squillacio, who wrote a report on the disease for Ludovico Sforza, Duke of Milan, and commented that it was widespread. Squillacio implies that it had been known for at least one year, and suggested that the local people thought it came from France. The Spanish physician, Gaspar Torrella (*ca* 1452-1520), published an account in 1497, suggesting it appeared in 1493 in France, and then spread to Spain and Italy, whilst in 1498, another Spaniard, de Villalobos, wrote a poem on the *"French pockes"* and suggested that it was a new disease. The Spanish doctor, Roderigo de Isla, claimed to have treated members of Columbus's crew after their return from the Americas, but this claim was not made until 1539, some forty-six years after the event. However, Gonzalo de Oviedo y Valdes claimed to have seen the Indians, who returned with Columbus, at the Spanish court, and makes no mention of any skin rash.

Torrella also considered that the *Morbus Gallicus* was a single disease. This was a somewhat unusual view in the early sixteenth century as gonorrhoea was frequently confused with the early stages of syphilis when it first appeared. This confusion became worse when the behaviour of syphilis moderated in the mid-sixteenth century. Gonorrhoea had been known for a long time, and was mentioned by numerous writers and cultures including the Assyrians, Egyptians, Chinese and Hippocrates. As late as 1736 however, Astrac published an account, *"De Morbis Venereis"*, suggesting that venereal diseases such as gonorrhoea and genital warts were the preliminary stages of lues venerea.

Many doctors had realised, even before 1500, that syphilis was transmitted by sexual contact and was exacerbated by prostitution, and a number of states, especially in Italy, had recognised the venereal origin of the disease and begun to expel prostitutes or control prostitution. As early as 1497, Torrella, who became Papal physician, was urging men to avoid sex with infected women, and by 1500, he was advising the city states of Italy to deal with infected prostitutes by isolating them in sanatoria and treat them at public expense. Many Italian states and cities legalised brothels and taxed them and they were only required to close during Mass on Sundays. Apprentices were not allowed to marry until they qualified as journeymen or masters and prostitution was tolerated as an acceptable safety valve for young men.

Once it had been realised it was a sexual disease, women were blamed for transmitting it, although it was considered that women did not suffer from syphilis. It was thought that a woman became a carrier if she had sores in her womb and had sex with a man suffering from leprosy[184]. The front piece of one contemporary German book on the pox, shows the Christ-child throwing thunderbolts at infected women, and the great Protestant reformer, Martin Luther, suggested that, *"syphilitic whores should be broken on the wheel"* (not much Christian charity there).

Fracastorius later mentioned in his book *"On Contagion"* published in 1546, over fifty years after the appearance of syphilis, the suggestion that it came from the Americas. Later writers were sceptical about the American origin, and it became a hotly debated issue. As stated earlier, it is probable that it was present in Europe prior to 1492 in a mild form we cannot recognise today, and then altered or mutated in some way. It was also argued that it may have spread as leprosy faded.

When Fracastorius wrote *"On Contagion"*, he commented that syphilis had become less dangerous than when it first appeared, it caused fewer deaths and the symptoms were also milder. When diseases first attack a species, they frequently damage many organs and cause numerous unpleasant symptoms. As the host and pathogen adapt to each other over generations, the disease becomes less severe with milder symptoms. Syphilis is a classic example of this type of behaviour. When it first appeared in the late fifteenth century, it caused pustules all over the body and attacked many internal organs, especially the nervous system, frequently causing death within months or a few years. Within a relatively short space of time however, the effects were limited to the face, genitals and central nervous system and the victims frequently survived for a number of years.

As early as 1519, Ulrich von Hutter in Germany stated that the pox was not as severe as it had been and also suggested that it had a venereal origin. In 1529, Sir Thomas More wrote a tract arguing against the suppression of the monastic hospitals. In

---

184   There does seem to be some sort of basis for this, modern studies suggest that men are three times more likely than women to contract syphilis from an infected partner.

this, he stated that there was only one patient being treated for syphilis for every five treated in 1499. Contemporary sixteenth century medical documents from numerous sources, including Asian ones, agreed with these opinions. It suggests a new disease whose severity abated rapidly as the host and parasite become more tolerant of each other.

Some physicians declared it was a disease of the Indies that thrived in the sun, but declined in European weather. Fracastoro thought syphilis was a disease in its old age by 1546, and would disappear within a short period of time. Other sixteenth century doctors thought it was changing into another disease, whilst Astrac writing two centuries later thought it was declining to the point where it would become extinct.

There may have been considerable evolutionary pressure on the bacterium to mutate to cause a less disfiguring form of syphilis. When a bacterium, spread by sexual contact, produces repulsive sores on an infected individual, then that individual is likely to be rejected as a desirable sexual partner. The bacterium is thus reducing its own chances of spreading through the human community. In such a situation, it obviously makes evolutionary sense from the point of view of the micro-organism to become less dangerous and produce less obvious symptoms in the target species.

The first major epidemic of syphilis appeared at the siege of Naples by Charles VIII of France in 1494. The various city-states of Italy were at war with each other, and the French invaded and besieged Naples with 50,000 troops, many of them mercenaries, and a large number of camp followers (frequently a euphemism for prostitutes). The Kingdom of Naples was controlled by the Spanish, who were alleged to have chased infected prostitutes into the French camp. This technique had first been suggested by Kautila (Ch 2) in the fourth century BC, when he advocated the use of, *"poison maidens"*, to destroy an enemy army.

The French position eventually became untenable and they were forced to retreat. The mercenaries pillaged and plundered the countryside and then dispersed, spreading the disease all over Europe. The winter of 1495/6 was very severe with heavy snow and flooding, exacerbated by severe earthquakes in Italy. There were serious food shortages followed by numerous epidemics, and a number of contemporary sources started to describe this new disease, which everybody agreed had been introduced by the French. To compound the misery, plague also reappeared in 1496.

When syphilis first appeared it was deadly although the symptoms described by early writers vary considerably. Many physicians considered that this variation in the symptoms was caused by different humours in different people. The priest, Ser Tommaso di Silvestro, who wrote from personal experience, commented as follows *"some had sores with pains, some had sores without pains, and some had pains without sores"*. Symptoms mentioned frequently by most writers include fevers accompanied by severe pain in the joints. There were also sores known as bolle or buboni over the whole body and at this point the bacteria began to destroy the body, attacking both flesh and skeletal tissue, hence the perceived similarity to leprosy. The afflicted person began to smell, which many people considered to be one of the prerequisites for an epidemic to begin (the miasma theory again). Ser Tommaso gives a very graphic description of his symptoms stressing the boils and pains, but emphasises that these were not continuous, there were periods of remission, a point frequently made by other contemporary writers.

Perhaps one of the most graphic descriptions of syphilis is given by Joseph Grunpeck in 1496, *"In recent times I have seen scourges, horrible sicknesses and many infirmities afflict mankind from all corners of the earth. Amongst them has crept in, from the western shores of Gaul, a disease which is so cruel, so distressing, so appalling that until now nothing so horrifying, nothing more terrible or disgusting, has ever been known on this earth".*

Ulrich von Hutter also described the symptoms from personal experience in 1510, stating, *"Boils the size of acorns......* *so great a stench". "If anything may cause a man to long for death, truly it is the torment of this illness".*

A later description is given by Voltaire in his political satire, "Candide" or "The Optimist" probably written about 1758. This is a considerable time after the worst effects of syphilis have disappeared. Candide meets his old tutor, Pangloss, who has contracted syphilis. *"Candide was out walking, he met a beggar covered with scabs, his eyes sunk in his head, the end of his nose eaten off, his mouth drawn to one side, his teeth as black as a cloak, snuffling and coughing most violently, and every time he attempted to spit, out dropped a tooth".*

Some of the early treatments were bizarre by the standards of today. Mercury ointment was used (the first recorded use of mercury was in 1496), as were arsenic and vitriol (acid). These treatments were frequently accompanied by heat to induce profuse sweating, causing one contemporary writer to comment that the cures killed more people than the disease. However, the prevailing opinion in the mid-sixteenth century regarded infection with syphilis as a sign of sin, and painful treatments such as mercury, were the necessary price to be paid for being cured. Mercury treatment was certainly painful, it included loss of hair and teeth, ulcers in the mouth, excess saliva and severe stomach pains. The amount of saliva produced was such that the treatment was sometimes referred as *"salivation"*. The use of mercury led to the cynical contemporary comment that, *"A night with Venus meant a lifetime with Mercury".* It was not just European doctors who used mercury, Arab doctors treated syphilis by making patients breath fumes of heated cinnabar (mercuric sulphide), which releases pure mercury vapour, and also used mercury in frankincense, wax and oils as an ointment to be applied to the joints several times a day. One contemporary comment by Jean Fernel (1506-58), a Professor of Medicine in Paris mentions mercury, which our predecessors, *"took from the school of the Arabs"* and mercury containing ointment was known as, *"Unguentum Saracenicum"* (ointment of the Saracens).

By the early sixteenth century, guaiac wood or guaiacum (also known as "Holy wood" [Legno Sante] or lignum vitae [wood of life]) was being imported from the West Indies (Hispaniola) in large amounts, specifically as a cure for syphilis, as bark infusions were claimed to be effective against it. This related to the contemporary idea that illnesses from a specific location could only be treated with a remedy from that location, and it was thought at that time that syphilis originated from the Americas (specifically Hispaniola). Frascatorius writing in 1546 suggested both mercury and guaiac wood as remedies.

Guaiacum was in use in Spain and Portugal as early as 1508, but did not appear in much of the rest of Europe for about another decade. The wood was used by converting it to shavings and sawdust and boiling it in water. The foam was removed and dried to a powder to treat sores, and the mixture was drunk. In addition, the patient was starved and purged, and placed in a sweat room, the treatment continuing for up to thirty days.

A merchant banker family, the Fuggers, controlled the guaiacum trade and had a virtual monopoly throughout Europe and it was alleged that they were in conspiracy with the medical establishment to promote it. The Fuggers obtained the monopoly to import the wood from The Holy Roman Emperor, Charles V, (who was also infected) in return for a substantial loan to the Imperial treasury. It certainly made a major contribution to their wealth to the extent that they established a hospital in Augsberg, known as the Woodhouse. In spite of the large amounts imported into Europe, it proved to be completely ineffective; the treatment with guaiac wood was however considerably more humane than some treatments, a number of them appear to be more akin to torture.

Torrella claimed to have cured a number of patients including the infamous Cesare Borgia, Cardinal of Valencia, son of Pope Alexander VI (Rodrigo Borgia). He used a programme of blood letting, sweating and the removal of skin lesions using chemicals such as mercury, sulphur, ammonia, vitriol (acid) and aqua fortis (sulphuric and nitric acids, a mixture so powerful it will dissolve metallic gold) in preparations of myrrh, incense and turpentine.

The sweat boxes were barrels big enough for the patient to sit in except for the head, and were heated by throwing water onto hot stones. The patient (victim) was then sweated for 20-30 days to purge the body of corrupt material.

A number of doctors, including Torrella, were aware of the dangers of mercury, but thought these could be alleviated by combining it with other chemicals. If the skin lesions were resistant to treatment with caustic chemicals, it was suggested they could be removed by cautery. One suggested cure was cautery applied to the top of the head, the rationale being that it would stop the production of excess phlegm, which is one of the side effects of mercury treatment.

One suggested treatment was immersion of the victim in olive oil containing various herbs and spices, and in 1498, the Health Board of Venice was forced to prohibit the resale of olive oil used for this purpose! Folklore amongst the peasants suggested that the cure was to apply a freshly killed, decapitated pigeon or chicken to the sores on the penis when it would act as a poultice, and suck the poison out! This was also a suggested cure for the plague, in this case, application to the buboes. The alternative variation was to pluck the feathers from around the vent of a live chicken, and to apply the chicken's vent to the sore or bubo, and the chicken would suck out the poison and die. This had to be repeated until the chickens stopped dying when a cure would have been affected.

Perhaps one of the most unusual cures was developed during the early twentieth century, when it was realised that the bacterium, *Treponema,* was very heat sensitive and that patients could be cured by inducing a high fever (Ruy Diaz de Isla had commented on this as early as 1539). Julius von Wagner-Jauregg in Vienna, noted patients with the paralytic and neurological symptoms of syphilis frequently showed considerable improvement when they had malarial relapses. He deliberately infected patients with malaria to send them into a high fever, thus raising their temperatures and curing them of syphilis, and then dosed them with large amounts of quinine to cure the malaria. He received the Nobel Prize for medicine in 1927 for developing this technique which was still in use as late as the 1940s.

Although some physicians thought that syphilis was incurable, others thought that the death rate was relatively low. It probably depended on which social class the sick person came from, the wealthy would have obviously received better treatment. However, even those doctors who thought it was fatal agreed that the victim might survive for a considerable time. The result was that the numbers of sick and poor became very visible, with many of these living by begging in the cities. The doctors of the sixteenth century generally dealt with patients sufficiently wealthy to pay their fees, and not the proletariat suffering from epidemics such as syphilis.

The civic authorities in the Italian city states especially, but also in other parts of Europe, asked advice from physicians on the control of epidemic diseases. As a result it was in these urban centres that public health measures first evolved, as a response to diseases such as leprosy, syphilis and plague. Numerous Italian cities established hospitals in the sixteenth century to treat the poor who were the biggest social group affected by syphilis and who could not afford doctors. These were known as Incurabili hospitals, and specialised in patients with *Morbus Gallicus.* The first of these was in Genoa, and was followed by a hospital in Bologna, dedicated to St Job, the patron saint of pox sufferers (he is also the patron saint of lepers). The hospitals were seen as having an important religious role, and had the blessing of Pope Leo X, who offered a papal indulgence to all who supported them financially above a certain figure, and granted those hospitals in the Papal States freedom from taxes.

The hospitals for the incurables admitted all people of either sex suffering from *Morbus Gallicus* and other incurable diseases, but not those suffering from epidemic diseases such as plague and leprosy. There were already pest houses and lazar houses catering for these in most Italian cities. In many cities, the authorities had the power to search the city and forcibly hospitalise the incurables if necessary. There are numerous contemporary comments on the smell of the incurables (the miasma theory), and the aggressive begging tactics they employed, and forcing them into hospitals would have been perceived as improving the health and social comfort of the tax-paying public. In Venice, those incurables who refused to enter hospital were seen as a threat to the health of the community, and the authorities had the power to expel them from Venetian territory at public expense. The records show that in Rome in the mid-sixteenth century, twenty per cent of the men admitted to incurables hospitals were soldiers and over two-thirds of these had syphilis.

Mercury is effective against syphilis, but it is a question of finding the correct dosage as Paracelsus (who has also been called the Luther Medicorum) suggested. It is a poison in excess, but medicinal if taken in moderation in the correct formulation. A number of chemists, such as Paracelsus, were starting to appear who recognised that metallic mercury was dangerous, and advocated the use of various combinations of mercury with other chemicals. They argued that it was useless to use the methods of Galen to treat a disease that Galen had not known, and stronger medicine (e.g. chemical distillates) were needed to deal with them.

Paracelsus himself thought that syphilis was a new disease transformed from an older one and therefore needed a fresh remedy. He published the first chapter of an *"Essay on the French Disease"* in 1529, the other two chapters were censored by town authorities at the instigation of the local doctor's guild. He found a publisher who was prepared to circumvent this censorship and then had to flee from Nuremberg, following complaints from the doctor's guild that thought his views too radical. He also published a pamphlet opposed to the use of guaiac wood, which also involved him in political controversy, this time with commercial overtones.

Syphilis rapidly spread outside the confines of Europe. There was a major epidemic in Japan in 1512, which was reported as infecting possibly half of the population of Tokyo, and by 1520, it was widespread in China, India and the Portuguese colonies of Africa. The Portuguese explorer, Vasco da Gama (1469?-1524), was the first known European to round the Cape of Good Hope and reach India by sea in the last few years of the fifteenth century. The Portuguese took syphilis with them on their voyages of exploration. da Gama returned in 1502 and established a Portuguese trading empire defended by forts along the coasts of Africa and India, but his administration was extremely harsh and soon caused problems with the local inhabitants. At one stage, the ruler of Calicut was unable to lead his army against the Portuguese, as he had the French disease, and had it in the throat!

By the early sixteenth century, it was so widespread throughout Europe that the Dutch scholar Erasmus (1466?-1536), cynically commented that, *"a nobleman without syphilis was either not very noble or not much of a gentleman"*.

It was also widespread amongst the ruling families of Europe, both Charles VIII and Francis I of France were victims as was Lorenzo de Medici (Lorenzo the Magnificent), ruler of Florence. Henry VIII probably had it and may have passed it to his wife, Jane Seymour, who transmitted it to their son, Edward VI, during pregnancy or childbirth. If this is correct, it certainly had a significant effect on England, as Edward VI died young, and the throne passed to his half-sisters, initially Mary Tudor (Bloody Mary) and then Elizabeth I. It also occurred in the Russian royal families, including Ivan the Terrible, Peter the Great and Catherine the Great. When the body of Ivan was exhumed, the skeleton showed definite signs of syphilis, and given his behaviour in the final stages of his life, he was probably suffering from the tertiary stages including dementia. He personally murdered one son, and the son, Fedor, who succeeded him, was a congenital idiot due to syphilis; on the death of Fedor, the Romanovs became rulers of Russia. Numerous Ottoman sultans also suffered from it, and individuals rumoured to be victims included Durer, Cellini, Cardinal Richelieu, Goya, Keats, Schubert, Lord Randolph Churchill, Gauguin, and Oscar Wilde. It was not just the great and good of Europe who suffered, Al Capone was also a victim.

The disease had become a major problem in London by the eighteenth century and Cruikshank considers that one in every five women in London was a prostitute. The centre of the sex trade was Covent Garden, and Harris published a *"List of Covent Garden Ladies"* that listed the attributes and prices charged by the various prostitutes. William Hogarth engraved a series of six morality prints known as *"The Harlot's Progress"* in 1732. The first shows a country girl arriving in London and being propositioned by the madam of a brothel. In the second, she is portrayed as the mistress of an elderly man with a younger lover on the side, whilst in the third she has become a common prostitute and a magistrate is shown arriving to arrest her. In the fourth she is doing hard labour in the Bridewell Prison and in the fifth she is dying of syphilis. The last print shows her funeral at the age of twenty-three with her friends holding a wake and using her coffin lid as the bar.

Gonorrhoea, also known as clap (from an old French word, *clapoir,* meaning venereal buboes), was frequently thought to be one of the stages of syphilis, the confusion being worst when the severity of syphilis began to wane. It was not until the mid-eighteenth century that doctors started to distinguish between the various venereal diseases. The process was not helped by the Scottish doctor John Hunter (1728-93) who infected an unnamed patient (possibly himself), with pus taken from a patient suffering from gonorrhoea. The symptoms of both gonorrhoea and syphilis appeared, leading Hunter to consider that they were the same disease. In retrospect it is probable that the donor was suffering from both diseases. The problem was finally solved in 1879, when the German doctor, Albert Neisser (after whom the organism is now named), identified the gonococcus bacterium, *Neisseria gonococcus,* finally establishing that gonorrhoea and syphilis were two different diseases.

The first major breakthrough in the fight against syphilis was made by the German doctor, Paul Ehrlich (1854-1915) in 1910, with the development of the arsenic containing drug, salvarsan. Ehrlich had researched a large number of drugs for their anti-microbial action and salvarsan was occasionally known by its number 606[185]. Although salvarsan was effective in the treatment of syphilis, it did produce some unpleasant side-effects and it was later modified to a derivative, neosalvarsan, which was used until the advent of penicillin. Ehrlich shared the Nobel Prize with Elie Metchnikoff for their work on immunity in 1908, but Ehrlich is remembered today for his work on chemotherapy. Salvarsan is interesting in that it does not kill the spirochaete causing syphilis, it only stops it growing which gives the immune system time to counter it.

The moral lobby campaigned against this type of drug saying that by curing syphilis, Ehrlich was removing fear of

---

185   The Germans had a long history of research into synthetic drugs and dyes that started in the mid-nineteenth century.

fornication and this would result in the gross moral turpitude of society. However, society already had a serious problem; by 1910 it was thought that as many as sixty thousand adults per year were dying in the UK from syphilis.

During World War I, it is estimated that 25% of all troops in Europe were incapacitated by venereal diseases of one type or another. Different armies dealt with it using different methods, the British made contracting a venereal disease a military offence leading to a charge, with propaganda statements claiming, *"A German bullet is cleaner than a whore"*. The Americans closed the brothels and invoked the spirit of Panama (Ch 17), *"to drain a red-light district and destroy thereby a breeding place for syphilis and gonorrhoea is as logical as it is to drain a swamp and thereby a breeding place of malaria and yellow fever"*. The French took the pragmatic attitude, *"boys will be boys"*, licensed the brothels, issued condoms to the troops and carried out regular medical examination of all prostitutes.

The Oxford Dictionary claims that the etymology of the word condom is unknown, however two suggestions are that a Dr Condom prepared them for King Charles II of England in the seventeenth century, making them out of sheep gut tied at one end with a ribbon. The second suggestion is that condom is derived from the Latin word *condere* that means to hide. The first rubber ones became available in the mid-nineteenth century. In England they became known as *"French letters"* as the English gentry obtained them by post from France, whilst the French returned the compliment by calling them *"capotes Anglaises"* (English overcoats).

In 1916-7, laws were passed in the UK enabling local authorities to deal with problems such as syphilis. The main emphasis was on sexual continence, and the National Council for combating Venereal Diseases was formed to, *"fight the terrible threat to our imperial role"*. The Royal Commission reporting on the problem recommended the formation of specialist clinics attached to hospitals, and strongly emphasised that anonymity was essential in dealing with the patients, who otherwise would be frightened away.

In 1917, the USA cancelled German patents on numerous items under the "Trading with the Enemy Act", and US manufacturers began to synthesise salvarsan and its analogues. The second major breakthrough in controlling syphilis was in the 1940s when it was found that *Treponema pallidum* was susceptible to the new antibiotic penicillin, which proved to be a very effective method of treating non-advanced cases.

Treponema pallidum has a very small chromosome, only about one third of the size of the chromosome of *Escherichia coli,* and does not have the genetic resources to make the enzyme, β-lactamase, that destroys penicillin. It is unable to exchange genetic information with other bacteria and thereby acquire the necessary genes. The result is that penicillin is still as effective today as when it was first used, and mutant strains of *Treponema* resistant to penicillin have never arisen.

One of the most notorious incidents involving syphilis was the Tuskegee study carried out from 1932 to 1972 by the US Public Health Service. This study involved the progress of untreated syphilis in Afro-American men from Alabama. A group of about four hundred infected black patients were compared with an uninfected control group, the infected ones not being told that they had syphilis or that it could be transmitted by sex. The initial study was on treatment of the disease and involved chemicals such as mercury and arsenic, and also studied the progress of tertiary symptoms such as neurological and cardiac damage. The initial study failed to produce any useful information and it was therefore decided to withhold any further treatment and just follow the course of the disease in infected individuals. Even when penicillin became available in the 1940s, patients were not treated in spite of the fact that US government legislation had made the treatment of venereal disease mandatory. Over one hundred of those suffering from syphilis are thought to have died from the tertiary symptoms. The experiment was finally halted in 1972 when the press exposed the affair. A major lawsuit followed which was settled out of court and the US Congress introduced legislation requiring all experiments involving human subjects to be reviewed and approved.

The incidence rate of syphilis fell sharply after World War II due to a programme of education and treatment much of which was based on the introduction of penicillin. However it reappeared in the 1960s in homosexual men and then became widespread amongst drug addicts trading sex for drugs. The sexual permissiveness of the 1960s was also an important factor in the increased incidence. Figures from the Center for Disease Control in the USA show that the incidence increased by over eleven per cent between 2005-6, and US health workers reported over 36,000 cases in 2006. It is also increasing significantly in the UK. Many of the new cases are appearing in older age groups, people who have divorced in middle age and are re-entering the dating game. Much of this rise is due to the fact that they are not taking precautions against pregnancy as the woman is no longer fertile.

One of the main problems of contracting syphilis, at the present time, is that the lesions produced greatly increase the probability of a person exposed to HIV contracting this also (Ch 18).

CHAPTER 15

Influenza (Flu)

The word influenza comes from an Italian word meaning influence and is probably related to astrology, horoscopes and the movement of the planets and stars. Italian doctors realised that the appearance of flu was seasonal, and considered it was due to solar movements, hence the name that appears to have first been used in the sixteenth century. It was almost certainly an Old World disease originally as the indigenous populations of the Americas and Pacific had very high death rates when they first came into contact with it, compared with the inhabitants of the Old World.

Flu is one of the world's worst epidemic diseases, it kills large numbers of people and is the infectious disease highest in the league table of the causes of death in the developed world. Outbreaks are divided into seasonal and epidemic flu. Seasonal flu is a relatively low number of annual cases that rises in the winter months and follows a predictable pattern.

In England and Wales, flu is considered to have reached epidemic levels when there are over 400 cases per week per 100,000 people. The death rate of most forms of epidemic flu is less than one per cent of the victims. This is low for an infectious disease, and death frequently occurs amongst the elderly from a secondary infection of pneumonia, or problems such as heart attacks or strokes. The number of dead is so high because so many people become infected. Some estimates suggest there are as many as five million serious cases of seasonal flu per year causing quarter to half a million deaths worldwide. The mortality rate for flu can be controversial as it is measured by excess deaths, that is, the number of deaths above those who would normally be expected to die at that time of the year. The base line is derived using data from the same weeks in years when there were no influenza epidemics. The system is obviously not foolproof, but most medical workers accept that this treatment gives a good indication of excess deaths. The number of deaths from seasonal flu in the UK varies from about four to eight thousand per year, most of them being the old and frail.

In humans, flu is a viral infection of the respiratory tract spread by inhalation of infected droplets resulting from an infected person coughing and sneezing. The virus attacks the host cells lining the respiratory tract, bronchial tubes and trachea. The symptoms range from trivial with a slight fever, to a high fever with headaches and severe pains in muscles and joints that usually last four or five days. This is followed by fatigue and depression during convalescence which lasts several weeks. The highest risk is related to people with respiratory diseases, heart problems, diabetes, those compromised immunologically, very young children and the elderly. Vaccination of these high-risk groups reduces the death rate. Another group who experience a higher death rate are pregnant women as pregnancy suppresses the immune system. Whilst antibiotics are frequently prescribed for flu victims, antibiotics are useless against flu because it is a viral infection. They are given as prophylactics to prevent secondary infections such as pneumonia and bronchitis caused by opportunistic bacteria attacking a weakened host.

Flu is easily transmitted by droplet infection and contact with fomites, and the incubation period is short, taking only two days. The disease therefore spreads very rapidly and it would be expected that the entire world population would catch it within a few years. The susceptible members of society would be killed, leaving an immune population and flu would rapidly become a childhood illness. Flu is however, a microbial chameleon with the ability to evade the human defence systems periodically. The ultimate source is farm animals and epidemics often coincide with, or follow rapidly after, outbreaks in species such as pigs and poultry (both domestic and wild). The disease in humans probably dates back to the domestication of these types of livestock around 8,000 BC.

Many people think that the virus is clever or ingenious in the manner in which it circumvents our immune systems, an opinion frequently fostered by inaccurate press reports. The virus is neither clever nor ingenious, it makes a lot of mistakes when copying itself and produces a large number of mutations and it is this inaccuracy that gives it an evolutionary advantage. Evolution is a game of numbers. The larger a population is and the greater the number of generations there are, the more mutations appear and the higher the probability of natural selection favouring a beneficial mutation and eliminating a deleterious one. As pointed out earlier, what is advantageous and what is deleterious depends on the perspective from which the mutation is viewed.

Flu is caused by an RNA virus with a very high rate of mutation and genetic re-assortment, which accounts for repeated epidemics, and the fact that immunity to this disease is not lifelong. The replication of RNA is a lot more error prone than the replication of DNA, as there is no proof-reading mechanism of the type that occurs in DNA synthesis. This means that during the synthesis of DNA and DNA viruses it is possible to check whether mistakes have been made, and if so, they can be corrected. This does not occur during the synthesis of RNA viruses, such as flu and HIV. These both mutate at a very high rate, and if a mistake (mutation) is made, the mutants produced either survive or are eliminated by evolutionary pressure. If the mutation survives, it generates a new strain, the key question being whether the new strain can evade the antibody response produced by the host? The range of new viral combinations produced is so great that although the vast majority of them are destroyed, there is an excellent chance that sooner or later one of these new combinations will evade the host immune system.

The disease is caused by viruses from the orthomyxovirus group. Three major types of flu virus are found, types A, B and C. These produce similar symptoms, varying in their severity, but they are completely unrelated antigenically so that infection with one type gives no immunity against the others. Type A is highly variable antigenically, causes most epidemics and pandemics and is found in birds, especially aquatic ones, cats, pigs, horses and some aquatic mammals as well as humans. Not all strains of the virus infect all the species mentioned.

Type B occasionally has antigenic changes, but usually causes milder, small local epidemics and the immune system of anyone who has previously experienced it will recognise it easily. Type C is antigenically stable, is found in humans and pigs and causes only mild illnesses, which are frequently mistaken for the common cold. It has been described in the past as, *"a virus looking for a disease".*

Type A and type B viruses each contain eight separate segments of a single stranded RNA molecule, each strand coding for one or two viral proteins, the total being ten. Type C only contains seven strands. Two important proteins, haemaglutinin (H) and neuraminidase (N) are found on the surface of the virus. These determine the antigenic variation of the virus and when the human immune system reacts to a flu infection, antibodies to these two flu antigens are formed. Haemagglutinin holds the red blood cells of the host together to form clumps of cells. Neuraminidase pinches off pieces of host cell membrane and wraps them around the virus to form a coat that protects the virus and allows it to attack a new host cell. The virus cannot infect a host cell without these two proteins, yet these are what are recognised by a successful defence system.

Fifteen different sub-types of haemagglutinin have been isolated to date, labelled H_1, H_2, H_3 etc. Similarly nine sub-types of neuraminidase have also been isolated, N_1, N_2, N_3 etc. The two antigens H and N are able to vary independently of each other, thus producing a large number of variants of the virus. The H_1, H_2 and H_3 sub-types are those that normally infect humans.

Two types of antigenic change can be recognised in influenza, the first of which is known as antigenic drift. After a pandemic, the virus undergoes a series of minor genetic mutations, at frequent intervals, for a few years as it responds to changes in the immune pattern of the human population. This produces small changes in the viral proteins. These changes are recognised by most people who experienced the pandemic and developed immunity to it. A number of mutations are needed before the appearance of a new epidemiologically significant strain, and an accumulation of appropriate mutations may take some years to evolve. Once a sufficiently large drift has taken place, most people who survived the pandemic would produce antibodies that only partially recognise the modified H and N antigens and as a result they get a mild dose of flu. Those who had not experienced that strain before, usually small children born after the previous pandemic, will get a more serious infection. Only the old and those with underlying health problems will die.

The second type of change is known as antigenic shift. In this case there is a re-assortment of RNA segments in host cells with a double infection of virus. When the cell is infected with two different strains of flu virus, the parental gene segments of RNA may become mixed to produce novel combinations that effectively become a new sub-type. This process is termed genetic re-assortment and it causes large, unpredictable and sudden changes in the antigenic pattern of the virus. The most probable scenario is a re-assortment of genetic material from human and non-human viruses in a single host. This host may not be human, pigs for example are infected by both human and avian forms of the flu virus. The mixing of human and non-human strains of virus may cause a major recombination, frequently showing no cross-immunity to previous epidemics and producing a virus to which very few people are immune. This can lead to deadly new pandemics such as that of 1918-1920. Only type A viruses show antigenic shift, it is not found in either type B or C viruses.

The flu strains causing the 1957 (Asian flu) and 1968 (Hong Kong flu) pandemics were both results of an antigenic shift. The 1957 virus H_2N_2 contained five human and three avian strands of RNA, whilst in 1968, the virus H_3N_2 had six human and two avian strands. Although both of these pandemics infected large numbers of people, the infections were generally mild and death rates were relatively low, only approximately two million died world-wide in 1957 and one million in 1968 and deaths were generally confined to the very old and those already sick.

The behaviour of two different strains of the virus in one host explains why most of the major flu epidemics originate in rural areas, for example, rural China, where humans live in close proximity to pigs and birds such as ducks. It also explains the epidemiological features of influenza and creates serious problems for companies involved in vaccine development, as any vaccine can only be developed on a reactive basis rather than a pro-active one.

HISTORY

Hirsch claimed that the first identifiable flu epidemic occurred in 1173 in Italy, Germany and England, although some authors have suggested that flu slowed the conquests of Charlemagne in the eighth and ninth centuries. There may have been epidemics in Italy in the fourteenth century, and France and Italy in the fifteenth century, but contemporary accounts are vague. It is difficult to be certain whether they were flu as there are problems in distinguishing it from other diseases and chest infections that have similar symptoms.

In 1920, the British Ministry of Health published a compendium of flu epidemics going back over centuries. Some experts think the first recognisable large-scale epidemics were probably 1510 and 1557, but in 1580, Peter Forrest, a professor of medicine in Leyden, published a work on epidemic catarrh. The description he gives is a classic description of flu and this outbreak is considered by many experts to be the first recognisable pandemic. It is thought to have depopulated many Spanish cities and this, and the epidemics that followed, are considered to have been major factors in the start of the decline of Spain as a world power.

There were a number of outbreaks of epidemic catarrh in the seventeenth and eighteenth centuries whose descriptions also match that of modern day flu. There was a recognisable epidemic in 1647 that killed a large number of European settlers in the New World, and in 1658 the English doctor, Thomas Willis, gave a description of an epidemic that would be recognised as flu by most people today. *"It was sent by some blast from the stars, which laid hold of very many together, that in some towns in the space of a week above a thousand people fell sick together. The particular symptom of this disease, which invaded the sick as a troublesome cough, with great spitting, also a catarrh falling down on the palate, throat and nostrils: also it was accompanied with a feverish distemper, joined with heat and thirst, want of appetite, a spontaneous weariness and a grievous pain in the back and limbs. Such as were endowed with an infirm body, or men of a more declining age, that were taken with this disease, not a few died of it; but the more strong, and almost all of a healthful constitution recovered".*

Further epidemics occurred in 1729, 1732 (described as the most universal disease upon record), and contemporary reports suggest that the 1781-2 pandemic infected seventy-five per cent of the population of Britain. In the nineteenth century there were pandemics in 1830, 1833, and 1847. The pandemic of 1833 was a very dangerous one killing tens of thousands in Europe. These were followed by a major pandemic in 1889-90 (Russian flu) that is thought to have infected about ninety per cent of the world population, which is extremely high, even for flu. This epidemic probably killed several million world-wide and at least a quarter of a million people in Europe. On the basis of serological analysis of blood samples of old people taken early in the second half of the twentieth century, it has been suggested that this was an H_2 strain. The Ministry of Health report also stated that there had been a surge in flu cases in 1895, 1900, 1908 and 1915. These were followed by the massive and deadly pandemic of 1918, which prompted the Ministry of Health report of 1920.

Richard Pfeiffer isolated the bacterium, *Haemophilus influenzae,* which became known as Pfeiffer's bacillus in the 1890s, and claimed to have discovered the cause of flu as the bacteria were found in many cases. However, it was shown in the early 1900s to be a secondary invader, which is not present in all cases, but which is frequently associated with the bacterial pneumonia that may follow flu. It was claimed that this bacterium, "*inveigled a lot of scientists into wasting a lot of time discovering its insignificance*".

By 1918, there was a strong suspicion that flu was caused by a virus, although the technology to prove it was not available at that time. The human flu virus was finally discovered in 1933 at the Mill Hill laboratories in the UK. Scientific research work on flu was difficult as it did not infect any of the common laboratory animals and experiments on human volunteers frequently proved inconclusive. Finally, ferrets were found to be susceptible to the virus, and were used as laboratory animals, not an ideal situation as anyone who has handled ferrets for hunting rabbits would realise.

THE 1918 INFLUENZA PANDEMIC

"I had a little bird,
Its name was Enza
I opened a window,
And in-flu-enza".

Children's skipping song of the 1920s.

Widespread epidemics are a feature of flu, and in 1918 the so-called Spanish flu caused the worst flu pandemic in known history and the worst pandemic in living memory. Unusually, it killed a very high percentage of young men and women especially pregnant women; it also killed extremely quickly, frequently within a few hours. There was a very high death rate, 9,000 in one week in New York alone, whilst the total number of deaths in the USA is thought to have been 500-650,000. It is impossible to obtain a more accurate figure as there was no network for co-ordinating data[186]. In India it is estimated to have killed fifteen to twenty million, somewhere in the region of five per cent of the population. The problem was exacerbated by famine as the monsoon failed, and crop production fell 20%, causing rising prices and widespread starvation. In Western Samoa, it killed nearly 8,000, some twenty per cent of the population within two months. Very high death rates were also seen in Inuit and Icelandic villages.

An estimated 250,000 died in the UK compared with 4-8,000 dying of flu in a normal year. It is however difficult to be certain as it was not a notifiable disease in Britain, and in addition, wartime censorship was being used to suppress bad news.

The estimates for the global mortality vary widely. Low figures of twenty million and high figures of eighty to a hundred million have been quoted. Most experts consider a figure of forty to fifty million dead over a period of about six months to be realistic, but the truth is that nobody knows. These figures have to be put in the context of a world population of about one quarter of what it is today, that is about 1.5 billion. The death rate therefore represents approximately three per cent of the world's population at that time. In comparison, World War

---

186   To give an indication of the scale of the problem, in Philadelphia, which was one of the most badly affected cities in the USA, over 700 died in one day; the local morgue had a capacity of only 36 bodies.

I killed an estimated fifteen million over four years. However, because of the social upheaval at the end of World War I, many of the details of the pandemic are obscure and it is a part of early twentieth century history that does not survive in the community memory. Unusually for such a massive event, there were very few novels about it, one of the few is *"Pale Horse, Pale Rider"* (an obvious reference to the Four Horsemen of the Apocalypse), written by Katherine Porter, who caught the disease, but survived.

It spread world wide, occurring as three waves of infection, the second and third being much deadlier than the first. Those who survived the first wave, in the spring of 1918, were generally not attacked in the second wave.

The epidemic was known as the "Spanish flu" or "Spanish lady", but it is almost certain that it did not originate in Spain. It has been suggested that it acquired this name because Spain was not at war, there was no censorship and the press was able to report the progress of the epidemic in full. Many experts think that it started at Etaples in Western France, which was the biggest British military camp in France. It was a large training area with a constantly shifting population of about 100,000 men from every part of the British Empire. Many of these had been there a long time, were living in overcrowded conditions and were also keeping livestock such as pigs, geese and chickens. These were ideal conditions for generating a pandemic of influenza. There were also a large number of horses present that were widely used for transport in the armies of the time, and in 1917, numerous horses fell ill with an unusual form of pneumonia. In the light of our current knowledge of flu and the inter-species transmission of this disease in particular, this type of infection would now be regarded as a very ominous portent. There were also large numbers of Chinese labourers who came to Europe to work in World War I, and it has been suggested that they may have brought the virus with them.

The 1918 pandemic appeared virtually simultaneously in a number of countries as far apart as Australia, various parts of Africa, Europe, India, New Zealand and the USA including Alaska. The question arises how did it spread so quickly over such a large area in the absence of long-distance flights and fast transport? The pattern of spread suggests that it started long before the 1918 epidemic appeared, in a form that was only recognised as flu in retrospect.

The army medical journals of hospitals in the Etaples area mention a new disease, purulent bronchitis, in the winter of 1916/7, the symptoms of which were very similar to the form of flu that appeared later. It was very infectious with a high fatality rate, many of those who died had a high temperature, were coughing up blood and showed signs of cyanosis. A number of experts consider these were the first cases of the 1918 flu. It spread through the camp, and would have been taken to the UK by soldiers on leave, and hence to the rest of the world by ship.

The first wave of the recognisable form of the pandemic started in the early spring of 1918. This was relatively mild, and initially only killed a few people, although these were mainly young adults. The second wave was much worse and began in August 1918, when it appeared in several widespread places more or less simultaneously including the USA, Sierra Leone and France. At one army camp, Camp Devens in Massachusetts, the first case was diagnosed on September 12th, six days later there were over six thousand cases and by the 23rd there were nearly thirteen thousand. Nineteen hundred of these developed pneumonia and died within 48 hrs and eyewitnesses described, *"bodies stacked like cordwood"* in the morgue. By October 1918, over twenty per cent of the US army were medically unfit and 24,000 soldiers died, only a few thousand less than American battle casualties in World War I. Most of the fatalities occurred in the autumn of 1918, but a third wave of the disease, which was milder than the second wave, reappeared in the spring of 1919. Large numbers died on the troop ships coming to Europe and were buried at sea, the conditions being so chaotic that many were dropped over the side unidentified.

It was not just the Allies who had problems, in 1918, the German commander, General Erich von Ludendorff, blamed the failure of his summer offensive on both political enemies, and the poor physical condition of his troops due to flu.

In the civilian world, schools, churches, dance halls, theatres, cinemas and public gatherings were closed in attempts to stop the spread of the disease. Whilst these measures might have slowed down the speed at which the epidemic spread, it is debatable whether they had much effect of the final total numbers of those infected

There were a number of unusual aspects to this pandemic. It was significantly more deadly than any previous pandemic of flu and the profile of those who died was different, at least half of them were in the age group 20-40 years. It has been suggested that this was because the disease evolved in an army camp containing young men in that age group. The victims displayed all the normal symptoms of flu and many recovered at this stage, but in others it progressed to pneumonia. Cyanosis was seen for the first time in flu, followed in many cases by internal haemorrhaging, coughing and vomiting blood. Once it had reached this stage the prognosis for recovery was very poor. Autopsies showed that the dead had bloody lung tissue, which was described as being like a purple jelly, and the liver and kidneys were oozing blood. Initially there was speculation amongst some doctors that the Black Death had returned. There have also been suggestions that the deadly form of flu that appeared was due to mutations caused in the virus by the use of mustard gas as a weapon. It is now known that mustard gas and related chemicals are mutagenic agents.

It killed incredibly quickly. There are numerous reliable descriptions of patients dying before the doctor arrived at the house (this was in the days when doctors did house visits), fit soldiers dropping dead on the parade ground, and young adults being taken off the train dead only a couple of hours after they had got on it in an apparently healthy condition. Numerous people died just walking along the road and there were widespread accounts of bodies lying on the streets for hours before collection. As the authorities could not cope, many bodies were stacked up in mortuaries for weeks. Individual graves could not be dug fast enough so mass graves were used.

Further outbreaks of Spanish influenza occurred in the 1920s, but the virulence of the pandemic declined sharply after the third wave in 1919.

A major outbreak of *encephalitis lethargica* (known colloquially as sleepy sickness) followed the 1918 flu epidemic, with a lag of about one year. This is also known as von Economo's disease, after the Professor of Neurology in Vienna, who recognised it at the end of World War I. Approximately one third of those suffering from this late complication of flu died, and many of those who survived developed symptoms similar to Parkinson's disease. One very unusual feature of the disease was that it was possible in a few cases to re-awaken people, who had been in a coma for decades, by giving them the drug, dihydroxy-phenylalanine (DOPA). The effects were generally short-lived and the patient relapsed into a coma over time. *Encephalitis lethargica* caused degenerative changes in the brain and spinal cord tissues that were only found at autopsy. Occasional cases had been mentioned as a late sequel of previous flu epidemics, but the epidemic following the 1918 flu outbreak produced exceptionally large numbers of the disease. Modern research has not been able to link *encephalitis lethargica* to influenza, and it has been suggested recently that it was caused by an over-reaction of the immune system to a staphylococcal or streptococcal infection of the throat.

One of the most important questions is why did the 1918

flu epidemic kill young people instead of the old, and how did it kill them so quickly? Why did the survivors survive, and why did the susceptible die? The reason for death occurring so rapidly was that the lungs filled with fluid and the victim effectively drowned. Why did this happen? Many scientists and doctors consider that it was probably an over-reaction of the immune system creating a cytokine storm that initiated an anaphylactic shock type of syndrome. The immune system of young adults in the age group 15-40 is more active than in individuals above and below those ages, and if the virus did precipitate a serious over-reaction of the immune system, the effect would have been most deadly in the age group mentioned. As it probably evolved in army camps, this might explain why it was so dangerous for young adults.

THE HUNT FOR THE 1918 VIRUS

Attempts to obtain the answers to the questions above have involved a search for the virus that caused the 1918 pandemic and the determination of its structure. The obvious goal is to discover how it differed from other strains of the flu virus and what made it so deadly. It has not been possible to obtain an intact virus, and attempts to identify it have involved piecing together fragments. The 1918 virus has been reconstructed and it has been shown to be an H_1N_1 strain. Confirmation of this has been obtained by studying blood samples from elderly people who were children at the time of the pandemic.

Various methods were used to reconstruct it, these have included studying corpses of people who the records show died of flu. It is essential in these cases to select victims who are known to have died very quickly after contracting the disease as the virus is eliminated from the body within about a week of catching the infection. It is therefore useless to examine a victim who succumbed to pneumonia two or three weeks after contracting flu. It is also necessary to study victims who have been subjected to a minimum of post-mortem change, which means the bodies of people who died in northern latitudes and were buried in permafrost. There have also been attempts to exhume the bodies of victims who were buried in lead coffins, which exclude air, in the hope that these conditions will have preserved the virus.

The first of these attempts was made in 1951, when Johan Hultin opened graves at one village in Alaska and obtained tissue. Using the technology of the time it was possible to retrieve bacteria known to cause pneumonia, but not any virus samples.

Attempts were also made to recover the virus from graves in Longyearbyen, on the island of Spitsbergen, in 1998. It was known that a number of young men had arrived from Norway in 1918 to work in the coal mines and had died of flu within a few days of their arrival. When the graves were opened, the coffins had been subjected to frost heave and the bodies were above the permafrost layer. Although some samples were obtained, the quality was not adequate for the purpose.

Jeffrey Taubenberger working at the Armed Forces Institute of Pathology in the USA approached the problem from a different direction. He was able to obtain pathology samples taken from a small number of soldiers who had died of flu and these had been kept in an archive storage facility. The main problem with examining these samples is that they are only thin slices of lung tissue, containing minute amounts of viral RNA. His team therefore developed techniques for isolating small amounts of viral RNA from highly degraded samples, and then increased the quantities using Polymerase Chain Reaction (PCR) technology. This is a technique for copying minute quantities of nucleic acid material accurately and is widely used for DNA identification in forensic cases. The material they were working with was seriously degraded with small pieces of viral RNA, 100 bases long at most (the complete flu genome is about 13,000 bases split between the various RNA strands). The virus was then reconstructed by arranging the segments obtained in a linear manner and looking for overlapping sequences. Using these methods, Taubenberger's team were able to obtain samples from the archives of two individuals and reconstruct the virus.

The next step was to obtain all the known RNA sequences of H_1 type viruses, line these up and look for the areas that were conserved, that is, those areas where the RNA sequence is identical, or very similar, from one type to another. This was then compared with the material recovered from the H_1 virus that had caused the 1918 epidemic. A structural protein known as the matrix protein was studied first. This is normally highly conserved from one flu virus to another, but the protein sequence for the 1918 virus differed in several important features. The importance of this finding was that it confirmed that they were dealing with original material and not a modern day contaminant.

The pandemic of 1918 was deadly amongst the native peoples of Alaska; the mortality rate for native Americans was on average over ten per cent. In many communities, it was much worse and at one village, Teller Mission, seventy-two individuals died in five days out of a population of 150[187]. These were buried in a mass grave in the permafrost and permission was obtained from the village elders to open the grave. One of the dead was a very obese woman, aged about thirty, whose body was in a good state of preservation; the lung tissue, protected by fat, contained a large number of virus fragments.

Taubenberger's team sequenced these fragments and reconstructed the H gene, showing that it was virtually identical to that obtained from the two dead soldiers. Comparison of the H_1N_1 strain of 1918 with non-pandemic strains of flu, suggest that it had gone through a sequence of about ten mutations. One of these mutations appeared to be the ability to switch off production of the human cytokine (Ch 7), interferon. This

---

187   This was by no means the worst death toll, in the Inuit village of Okak in Labrador, only 59 survived out of a population of 266, and many other villages in this region were attacked nearly as severely.

would have immediately compromised the ability of the host immune system to respond to the infection. H_5N_1 (bird flu) has already acquired several of the mutations found in the 1918 strain.

Obtaining the genetic sequences does not tell us how the 1918 virus killed, nor why it was so lethal. They do however, provide a considerable amount of information that will be useful in the design of a vaccine, and indicate whether the anti-viral drugs being used currently are effective.

THE 1976 FIASCO

In 1976, there was an outbreak of flu in January in a number of American military camps. Several hundred cases occurred, one of which was fatal. The majority of samples taken from these cases were typed as H_3N_2, but a small number, including the fatal one, were an H_1N_1 type that was similar to the strain causing the 1918 pandemic.

By 1976, there was a widespread assumption that the increasing human population would allow flu to mutate and evolve more rapidly, and widespread air travel would enable it to spread throughout the world faster. As a result, it was thought that the time between epidemics would decrease. There had been a pandemic caused by an H_2 type in 1957, and another one caused by H_3 in 1968. By 1976, it was assumed that the next pandemic was due.

It was known in 1957 that an H_2N_2 variety of flu was circulating, but medicine in the USA is a private matter for individuals, and the US government would not pay for mass public vaccination. Because there were no financial guarantees forthcoming, pharmaceutical companies would not make any vaccine until they were certain there was going to be a pandemic. There is a lead time of about six months for the synthesis of large quantities of vaccine, and as a result of the vacillation of both the US government and the companies involved, vaccine synthesis in 1957 did not commence until far too late. The epidemic killed tens of thousands of Americans when it arrived, and the companies lost substantial amounts of money with millions of doses of vaccine that could not be sold once the epidemic was over. In the case of the UK, mathematical modelling suggests that a flu pandemic would peak within about fifty days, compared with the six months required to synthesise sufficient vaccine. In the USA, a pandemic would peak within about three months.

Similar problems occurred over vaccine production during the 1968 pandemic, only about half as many Americans died as in 1957, but again the drug companies lost large amounts of money.

It was assumed in 1976 that flu would begin in earnest during autumn, and the pharmaceutical companies therefore had about seven or eight months from the cases in January to prepare sufficient vaccine. In addition to preparing the vaccine, it obviously takes time to administer millions of doses, and a further ten to twelve days for the effect of vaccination to become optimal in an individual.

The original scientific report suggested that there was a small possibility of a serious flu epidemic in late 1976. This report then entered the political system, and by the time it reached President Ford, less than a fortnight later, it had escalated into a prediction that the strain of flu causing the 1918 pandemic was about to re-appear and would kill at least one million Americans. It was an election year, and the President could not risk the accusation that his administration was doing nothing. He therefore agreed in April 1976 that the entire US population, over 200 million people, should be offered vaccination.

By June, it was obvious that the various vaccine manufacturers would struggle to produce even half the number of vaccine doses required in time. In the meantime, tests carried out in the UK suggested that the flu that had appeared in January was not a serious pandemic threat, and the Americans were being alarmist.

The next problem was that the insurance companies, underwriting the vaccine manufacturers, became worried about the size of the potential financial risk if anything went wrong and threatened to cancel insurance liability. They had to be placated with the promise that the government would underwrite any problems, but the pharmaceutical companies stopped production until the insurance question was solved.

In the middle of this there was an outbreak of a new unknown disease that became known as Legionnaires disease as it first occurred amongst members of the American Legion, at a conference hotel in Philadelphia. There were over 200 cases in August 1976, of whom 34 died from pneumonia-like symptoms. The disease is caused by a bacterium (*Legionnella pneumophila*) that has no relationship whatsoever to flu, and had not previously been recognised. As it did not grow in normal laboratory media, new methods had to be developed and it took some time for it to be identified. The US Congress however, assumed it was the beginning of the new flu pandemic, and tried to rush the insurance legislation through various committees. The Center for Disease Control then announced it was not flu, but President Ford held a press conference to accuse Congress of leaving the American public unprotected against a flu pandemic.

The vaccination programme started in early October and several elderly people who were amongst the first to be vaccinated died suddenly over the next few days. Typically the press over-reacted and the vaccination programme was stopped. It was eventually shown that the deaths were not vaccine related, and vaccination re-started. At the end of November, the first cases of Guillain-Barré syndrome appeared. This is an autoimmune disease that attacks the nervous system and appears in a small number of cases after flu vaccination[188]. Statistics indicate that there is about one case for every one hundred thousand people vaccinated. It causes paralysis, about 85% of cases recover completely, about 10% are permanently paralysed to a greater or lesser extent and approximately 5% of cases are fatal.

By mid-December, about one fifth of the US population had been vaccinated, approximately one hundred cases of Guillain-Barré syndrome had appeared, and vaccination was stopped. By March 1977, over four hundred cases had been linked to flu vaccination, of which about twenty to thirty were fatal. Eventually, several thousand claims were made against the vaccine manufacturers coming to over three billion dollars, and millions of doses of vaccine were left unused.

It was probably the biggest public health fiasco in history. Ford lost the election and one of the first things the new Carter administration did was to sack a number of the people involved. The scientists and doctors who give the advice in this type of situation are in a catch-22 position. They either advise vaccination because there is a possibility of a pandemic and companies lose millions of pounds or dollars if they get it wrong, or alternatively, they do not advise vaccination and tens of thousands of people die if an epidemic breaks out.

One aspect of the epidemic was that the USA reneged on commercial agreements to sell supplies of the vaccine to Canada. The sale was blocked politically when the US realised that they would not be able to produce sufficient vaccine for their own citizens. Given the events that followed, the only comment is "lucky Canadians".

One of the results of the above fiasco was that a number

---

188   It was suggested in 2004 that there may be a link between the syndrome and a food poisoning bacterium called *Campylobacter*. This is endemic in chickens and fertile eggs are used for vaccine production. It is possible that a few eggs were contaminated and some *Campylobacter* proteins appeared in the vaccine. To confuse the issue further, it has also been shown that flu itself may cause Guillain-Barré syndrome.

of companies making vaccines decided that the profit margin was not worth the risk and dropped out of the market, leaving only a handful of companies actively involved in vaccine manufacture. The result is that if one company has production problems, the output of vaccine can be seriously compromised. This happened in 2004 when the entire output of one company became contaminated and was destroyed.

VACCINES

The main problem in preparing a vaccine against flu is that, as seen in the previous sections, it is impossible to be pro-active. One can only be reactive once it is known which particular strain of flu has appeared. There is no cross-immunity between various types of virus, and both personal immunity and the vaccine become obsolete as the virus mutates.

The vaccine to seasonal flu usually contains two or more of the type A strains known to be circulating, and frequently type B also. The vaccine for 2008/9 for example, contained H_1N_1, H_3N_2 and influenza B. The protection provided by one vaccination seldom lasts more than a year due to the rapid mutation of the virus, and is usually repeated annually for susceptible individuals. There have been several occasions when the flu vaccine manufactured has been wrong and has proved useless against the strain that eventually appeared. The vaccine mentioned above is a case in point. The H_3N_2 strain, known as Brisbane flu, was prevalent in Australia in 2007 and it was assumed that it would be the predominant strain in the Northern Hemisphere the following winter. In the event, very few cases of H_3N_2 appeared in the Northern Hemisphere in 2008 and the inclusion of this strain in the vaccine was superfluous to requirements.

One serious problem occurring in recent years has been that Indonesia has refused to send samples of the bird flu (H_5N_1) known to be circulating within its borders to the WHO. Indonesia claims that the country is too poor to buy vaccine and demands that free vaccine is supplied in return for providing the samples.

Once a new strain has been identified, it can take up to six months to get the appropriate vaccine made, tested and distributed, compared with a period that could be as short as a few weeks for the virus to initiate a pandemic. Synthesis of the vaccine involves injecting the virus into fertile chicken eggs, followed by a period of incubation to enable the virus to grow. The virus is then harvested, killed with formaldehyde, purified and used for preparation of the vaccine. This is a time consuming and highly skilled process, and the synthetic capacity of the various companies involved is only about 300 million doses of vaccine per year, for a world population of about seven billion and rising. This could probably be stretched to 500 million doses for a single strain pandemic.

There is also another vaccine known as Celvapan that is made in small amounts by growing virus in mammalian cells. This is used for vaccinating people allergic to eggs.

One of the problems relating to the present worries over bird flu is that H_5 strains are not good at raising an immune reaction in humans. It is therefore necessary to use more vaccine than normal, resulting in a smaller number of doses being available. Bird flu also causes serious problems for the manufacture of vaccine as it is lethal to chickens, and when injected into fertile eggs, it kills the developing embryo before sufficient virus has been produced for the synthesis of the vaccine. A further problem is that in the case of H_5N_1, it is so dangerous that it requires a laboratory at the highest level of bio-security.

Alternative methods of producing vaccine such as growth of the virus in cell culture are being developed, but are not yet available commercially. Other suggestions are the injection of haemaglutinin rather than whole virus, as this could be genetically engineered and synthesised in microbial cells. A further suggestion is the use of cold adapted flu virus. This is an attenuated, genetically crippled virus that will only grow at the relatively lower temperatures of the nasal passages and not at body temperature. It could therefore be given as a nasal spray, rather than as an injection, greatly simplifying its administration.

One of the latest attempts to make an effective vaccine centres on a viral protein known as the M antigen. The M protein is very similar in a majority of known strains of influenza A. Therefore any vaccine raising antibodies against protein M should approximate to a universal vaccine, thus providing a pro-active protection to most strains of virus instead of a reactive one that can only be prepared after the virus has been identified.

BIRD FLU

Bird flu (H_5N_1) was first described in 1959 when it caused a mild infection in poultry but by 1983 it had evolved into a form of flu that was lethal to domesticated poultry. It is suspected that this evolution took place in poultry that had been subjected to inadequate vaccination against the disease. The natural reservoir of the H_5 group of flu viruses is waterfowl, especially mallard in the UK, and these are the usual source of epidemics in domestic poultry, especially free-range poultry.

In 1996 it appeared in Guandong Province in China and was treated as a fairly minor problem until it spread to the chicken population in the markets of Hong Kong. In May 1997, the first known human case occurred The child involved developed what appeared initially to be a normal respiratory illness with an associated fever, but became steadily worse and died twelve days later. Examination of the virus showed that it did not match any known human flu virus, and it was some time before it was identified as an H_5 type, specifically H_5N_1, in a Dutch laboratory.

All eight RNA molecules are avian, not human, and it is normally only found in chickens and other birds. It was previously unknown for this strain of avian flu to cross the species barrier and infect humans. No definite contact could be shown between the dead child and infected chickens, and the assumption was made that the child had caught it from chicks in a pets corner or playgroup.

In a previous epidemic in Pennsylvania in 1983, millions of chickens had been slaughtered to bring it under control and an H_5 virus also killed a large number of turkeys in the UK in 1991. However, before the Hong Kong outbreak in 1997, H_5 had never been shown to kill humans. Although people in contact with chickens did occasionally test positive for H_5 antibodies, it had been assumed that the disease was asymptomatic in humans. The initial reaction to the poultry in Hong Kong infected with H_5 was that it was an agricultural or economic problem, not one of human disease, and that the first human fatality was a medical aberration. A second case occurred in another child in early November 1997; this child recovered, but more human cases occurred over the next few weeks, a number of them being fatal. By Christmas 1997, there had been eighteen cases across the age spectrum of whom six were dead or later died. Those who died showed very similar symptoms to those dying in the 1918 flu pandemic, such as cyanosis and blood in the lungs. It also targeted a very similar age group with many of the victims being healthy young adults, not the old.

This strain killed a high percentage of people infected, however it could only infect humans in direct contact with chickens, and epidemiological studies showed that it was a totally avian virus caught from poultry by the oral/faecal route. It lacked the one key ingredient enabling it to turn into a human pandemic, it was unable to spread directly from person-to-person. However, the major threat was that the virus might have developed this ability to spread directly, if it had been given time.

On this particular occasion, the entire poultry population of Hong Kong (1.5 million chickens, ducks and geese) was slaughtered during December 1997 to bring the epidemic under control. The mutation rate of the strain involved was very high, the virus appeared to be evolving rapidly, and if the slaughter policy had not been carried out, there would have been a high probability of a human pandemic. The border with China was then sealed to stop more poultry coming into Hong Kong and no chickens were re-imported until the first week of February 1998. Ducks and geese were not re-imported until May 1998 and new rules for the sale of poultry in Hong Kong markets were introduced and enforced. All species of poultry had to be kept separate from each other, so there could be no cross-species contamination and all wooden cages were destroyed and replaced by metal ones that could be sterilised. All poultry was regularly sampled and tested for H_5N_1.

It is unprecedented for an H_5 version of bird flu to attack humans, because the receptor cells in the human respiratory tract (the cells that the virus recognises and can attack) are different to the receptor cells in birds. It was generally considered that for a bird virus to infect humans, it required some human characteristics provided by RNA strands from a human strain of flu. Human flu usually binds to receptor molecules in the nose and throat, whereas H_5 attacking humans binds to receptors deep in the lungs. This means it is more difficult for humans to catch H_5, but when they do, it produces a pneumonia that is likely to be fatal. By early June 2009 there had been 433 cases of bird flu in humans confirmed to the WHO, of these 262 have died, a death rate of over 60%. So far, H_5 binds better to bird receptors than human ones, but reports in 2008 suggest that only two further mutations are needed to enable H_5 to bind to human receptors.

The comment was made at the time that H_5 first appeared in humans that to catch the disease it was, *"necessary to snog a chicken"*. This remark is not as facetious as it might appear. Cockfighting is a popular sport in Southeast Asia and breeders frequently pre-digest food by chewing it, and then force-feed their prize cockerels mouth-to-beak. The existence of prize cockfighting birds also causes problems when infected flocks of chickens are culled, the prize birds have been spirited away and hidden to avoid the authorities carrying out the cull.

The generation of a hybrid virus usually happens via the intervention of pigs as these animals have receptor cells that can recognise both mammalian flu and avian flu. It was thought that in 1957, 1968 and possibly 1918 as well, that a genetic shift between human and bird flu viruses had taken place in pigs. This produced a strain of flu that the human immune system had never experienced before and was therefore capable of causing a pandemic, firstly because it was virulent to humans and secondly because it was easy to transmit.

The major concern is the possibility that if bird flu is capable of infecting humans directly, it could mix with human flu. This could happen if both human and bird flu infected one individual at the same time and this scenario effectively takes pigs out of the equation. If this occurred, then H_5N_1 bird flu could undergo genetic shift, incorporate human genes and turn into a strain that could jump from human to human, thus initiating a pandemic. The most worrying aspect of this possibility is that the double infection would only need to happen in one person, and therefore the more people initially infected by bird flu, the greater the probability of this scenario occurring.

H_5N_1 has already acquired several of the mutations found in the lethal 1918 Spanish flu, and in December 2007 there was a reliable report from China of a father catching the disease from his son. This is the second report of this occurring, an earlier one happened in Thailand when human-to-human transmission was strongly suspected. In both cases, only one person was infected by the initial case, suggesting that although H_5N1 may be acquiring the property of human-to-human transmission, it has not yet perfected it.

One very worrying aspect is that family clusters of bird

flu have occurred on a number of occasions in countries such as Thailand, Indonesia, Vietnam and Pakistan. Single human cases are the first sign that the virus is adapting its behaviour, clusters are the second stage. When clusters appear however, there is a problem of deciding whether human-to-human transmission is occurring, or whether all the sick family members have been infected by a common source. In the cases that have occurred so far, clusters have been restricted to members of the same family, and individuals from outside the family that have come into contact with them have not become infected. This suggests that members of the family became infected by a common source, and available evidence also indicates that in these cases there may be a family genetic susceptibility to the virus.

Once the size of a cluster spreads beyond about twenty to thirty individuals it becomes impossible to contain or control it. Every human infection is a possible mutational event giving the virus a chance to mutate to human-to-human spread and clusters, where some individuals survive, are regarded as extremely dangerous, because it suggests that the virus is adapting to our species.

Bird flu has reappeared on numerous occasions in a wide range of countries since 1997, infecting a number of people, many of them fatally. It was found in chicken flocks in Southeast Asia during the winter of 2003–04, and now appears to be endemic in the populations of a number of wild birds in Asia, Europe and Africa. The recent cases amongst wild birds in Europe have probably been introduced by aquatic birds during migration. The current strain of bird flu is also deadly to ducks, which usually carry it without suffering any ill effects.

In Britain, there has been one major outbreak already at a poultry farm in East Anglia that killed 2,500 birds in February 2007. This led to a cordon with a six mile radius around the farm involved.

The WHO has suggested that poultry workers should be vaccinated, as in a number of cases in Thailand and Vietnam, deaths from H_5N_1 have occurred before a poultry epidemic has been recognised and reported. Vaccination of poultry has been ruled out as the available evidence and computer modelling suggest that imperfect vaccines might encourage more virulent strains of the virus to evolve. Vaccination can also mask the presence of the virus in a flock of birds by suppressing the normal symptoms.

H_5 bird flu is not the only problem, the H_7 family has also caused severe bird flu in Western Europe on several occasions between 2002-4. Each time there were a small number of human cases with at least one known death. In addition, H_9 causes bird flu and a mild form of human flu and the variety circulating in Eurasia at present carries a number of the genes that make H_5 so lethal.

The question of vaccinating poultry has caused considerable controversy. The European Union has directed that there should be no general use of an H_5N_1 vaccine in poultry. It is claimed that it would mask the spread of virus and make it more difficult to contain and monitor. It is also claimed that if the virus is allowed to circulate in vaccinated poultry, it could mutate to a more dangerous form. This is known to have happened on at least one occasion involving an H_5N_2 type. The result is that bird flu epidemics are controlled by culling and creating a quarantine zone around the infected area.

One interesting point is that domesticated chickens have lost a considerable number of their ancestral genes compared with the wild jungle fowl they are descended from. Did the loss of these genes cause them to also lose any ability to combat bird flu?

A further problem with bird flu that has not been publicised widely is that it also attacks other mammalian species. One species that has been attacked badly are tigers in South-East Asian zoos. If this susceptibility extends to domestic cats then there could be the scenario of recommending that all domestic and feral cats were destroyed. The political problems of getting public approval for that measure defy the imagination.

COST OF INFLUENZA

The cost of influenza is very large. In 2004 the research costs, production of vaccine and surveillance were estimated at $283 million, and this was a year when there was no pandemic! The 1957 and 1968 pandemics both killed hundreds of thousands world-wide, and the CDC described them as causing a high rate of social disruption, estimating the economic losses of both of them at $32 billion in 1995 terms. The Forbes magazine in January 2005 estimated the cost of medical care and lost productivity in a major bird flu pandemic as $70-166 billion.

There is also the social cost to be taken into account. In a pandemic infecting some 70% of the population, as the 1918 pandemic is thought to have done, numerous key workers would not be available. Power and water supplies would be seriously disrupted as would transport. It is virtually certain that food and fuel would be in short supply, and there would probably be food riots, necessitating armed police and troops to guard food and fuel convoys and depots.

MEXICAN (SWINE) FLU

This section originally started with the title, "When will the next pandemic occur, and can we control it"? It has been overtaken by events!

In August 2008, the British government published a risk register for various catastrophes that might occur in the UK. Pandemic flu was top of the list being the only catastrophe to score a perfect ten out of ten for severity.

The human species is in denial about emerging diseases and the question is frequently asked, "Will there be another flu pandemic"? The answer to this question is "Yes", it is a case of when, not if. Once this is accepted, the next questions are,

"When will it occur, what type will it be, how bad will it be, how long will it last and can we do anything about it"?

Nobody can predict when pandemics will occur, but if we consider the dates of the last four major pandemics, 1889, 1918-20, 1957 and 1968, it becomes fairly obvious that we were seriously overdue for another one. This arrived in June 2009 when the WHO proclaimed a pandemic of so-called Swine Flu or Mexican Flu (H_1N_1). The two names are based on the facts that the first cases were reported in Mexico and the virus strain involved was first found in pigs. In spite of the alarmist reports that appeared in the press of certain countries, it is not spread by eating pork.

It is fair to say that this pandemic generally took everyone by surprise as the various health and medical organisations were expecting a pandemic of bird flu. In retrospect however, it should have been expected.

Until 1998, a seasonal type of flu had been circulating in pigs in North America. This flu strain was an H_1N_1 descendent of the strain causing the 1918 pandemic (this was deadly to pigs as well as humans). Over the intervening eighty years, it evolved into a mild flu that was relatively stable genetically and only attacked pigs. In 1998 however, this swine flu hybridised with viruses from both humans and birds to produce a triple re-assortment rather than the more usual double re-assortment. The resulting virus, although it is known as swine flu, and contains mainly genes from a pig flu virus, also contains one gene from a human strain and two genes from a bird strain of flu. This produced a virus capable of rapid evolution able to out-compete other swine flu viruses and it has now become the dominant swine flu virus in America.

Initially the problem was seen as a livestock one and routine vaccination of pigs against flu meant that the pigs were not visibly sick. They were however becoming infected and shedding virus particles that would be picked up by humans working on the pig farms. The initial human cases appeared in a Mexican town called La Gloria and three young children died in early April 2009. The disease started to spread extensively two weeks later, at Easter, when Mexicans travel widely to visit relatives for the Easter festivities. From Mexico it spread to the USA and from there to the rest of the world.

By mid-June 2009, there had been approximately 30,000 confirmed cases (and probably a lot more unconfirmed ones) with about 150 deaths, a death toll of approximately 0.5%. It attacks younger people but those over sixty appear to have a high level of immunity. One serious problem is that the type involved is the same as that involved in the 1918 pandemic and it is attacking people in a similar age group, but so far without the terrible death rate.

To date, this swine flu pandemic has been relatively mild in the UK, even although the number of people infected has been the highest in Europe and it has spread considerably faster than predicted. The number of cases peaked in the last week of July at 110,000 and fell to 30,000 during the first week of August. The death rate in the UK to this point was about 0.35%, and most fatalities were people with health problems such as asthma, heart disease or some problem with their immune system. A death rate of 0.35% would have meant about 65,000 deaths, assuming that approximately thirty per cent of the population became infected, which is a fairly typical infection rate. Whilst 65,000 deaths might seem to be a large number, 0.35% is only about one tenth of the death rate of the 1918 pandemic.

The expected number of deaths was downgraded from 65,000 to 19,000 as more evidence became available for the behaviour of this pandemic. A death toll of 19,000 however would suggest 60,000 cases needing intensive care. There are approximately 2,000 intensive care beds available for the treatment of flu and related problems at any one time in the UK. It is therefore probable that a major flu epidemic would shut down virtually every other hospital activity in the UK whilst it lasted.

It was predicted that there would be a second wave of the pandemic in autumn which would be more serious, but the first wave should have created a higher level of herd immunity than will be found in many other European countries. This second wave started in October with weekly figures for swine flu starting to escalate again.

By early January 2010, it appeared that swine flu was probably not going to enter a third phase to become a major pandemic. By the second week of January the UK government was admitting that it had sixty million doses of surplus vaccine on its hands. The pandemic was much milder than first anticipated, and in the UK there were nearly four hundred deaths compared with early predictions of sixty-five thousand. World-wide confirmed cases of swine flu had killed between 13-14,000 people by January 2010.

A major concern was that bird flu is still circulating in numerous countries even although it appears to have disappeared from press reports. If some individual catches a double dose of bird flu and swine flu, then we could see a genetic shift that involved both viruses. If the resulting recombinant virus combined the transmission rates of swine flu with the lethal effects of bird flu, then we would have the ultimate nightmare scenario. As previously pointed out, this only needs to happen once, in one individual.

Even although the swine flu pandemic was relatively mild, there is always the next one and that could be a real threat even if it is five or ten years away. The question of how bad it will be depends to a large extent on the type of flu that appears. The 1918 epidemic killed about 3% of the world's population at that time, and if those figures were projected onto today's population of seven billion, it would suggest over 200 million dead. In the UK, government advisors have suggested a best-case scenario of 50-100,000 dead in a bird flu pandemic, whilst a worst-case scenario predicts half to three quarters of a million dead. The figure of 3% mentioned above, projected onto the present population of the UK, would suggest something of the order of two million dead. If it were bird flu of the type that has occurred in South East Asia over the last few years, and it did not modify its behaviour in a human host, then the effects would be truly catastrophic. The figure of a 60% death rate, mentioned earlier in this chapter, projected onto the present world population would be unimaginable, it would make the Black Death look an also-ran. It would be the Malthusian solution to over-population on a monumental scale. It is naïve to think this could not happen; the assumption is usually made that if H_5N_1 mutates to jump from human-to-human that it would lose much of its lethal nature. There is no guarantee of this.

It should also be pointed out that the treatment of most of those who have survived an attack of bird flu to date has involved the use of high-tech intensive care life support equipment. This is possible when the numbers of those involved is only in the low hundreds. However, the health systems of all countries, even the most wealthy, would be totally inadequate and swamped within hours if H_5N_1 with a fatality rate of 60% became pandemic without modifying its behaviour.

To control a pandemic of bird flu would require unprecedented international co-operation. At present, the surveillance systems are spread very thinly, and this would be a serious problem if a new outbreak occurred in an area where surveillance is minimal, especially if this outbreak coincided with a mutation that allowed the virus to jump directly from person to person. Large numbers of cases could occur in areas of Africa, Russia or South America, before we realise it is there. This is especially true if the outbreak were to start in a war zone, or an area that was politically sensitive, with the local authorities suppressing information, as occurred with the SARS outbreak in China.

Any epidemic that was able to obtain a toehold would probably infect the majority of the world's population within months. As stated earlier, computer modelling suggests that an epidemic in the UK would peak within about fifty days infecting one million people a day at its zenith.

The best way of combating a pandemic would be to slow down its rate of spread, which would allow more time to manufacture an increased amount of vaccine. An annual meeting of the WHO takes place in Geneva, to decide the components of the anti-flu vaccine for the next twelve months. The decision on the components to use is based on strains of flu circulating, as shown by the surveillance systems. Drug companies are informed which strains to use so that they can prepare the appropriate vaccine. Normally very few people bother with flu injections, frequently only 10% of the most susceptible and vulnerable members of the population (sick, old, asthmatics, diabetics and those with heart problems) are vaccinated. However, a pandemic of H_5 would cause serious problems for everybody, which means some seven billion doses worldwide. As mentioned previously, the logistics of producing this number of doses and getting it to everybody in time is impossible. There is also the probability that countries with the capability to produce vaccine would ignore orders from other countries until they had produced sufficient vaccine for their own population as the USA did in 1976.

Production of vaccine for the present swine flu pandemic was fast-tracked. This raises the concern of whether it was adequately tested before use. In this case, the assumption was made that as the vaccine was made using similar techniques to those used for producing seasonal flu vaccines, minimal testing was all that was necessary. Vaccination of people at high risk is probably justified, but it is questionable whether the risk of using a new vaccine, on the whole population, is justified for a virus that is only having a mild effect on the majority of people who become infected.

A few drugs are available for the treatment of flu, these include compounds such as Tamiflu and Relenza that inhibit the enzyme neuraminidase, but these are only effective if given within 24-48 hours of infection. At this point, the question arises regarding the certainty of it being flu as the early symptoms are common to many diseases. These neuraminidase inhibitors work by stopping the release of virus from infected cells. Although they may not cure a sick person, they might stop them passing the virus to a susceptible person, thus slowing the spread of the disease. Their availability also comes into question. The UK government has only stockpiled sufficient Tamiflu for about 25% of the population, and who gets them? Health workers, the police and armed forces and key workers in utilities such as water, power supplies and food distribution are obvious choices, but it is a reasonable gamble that politicians will be at the front of the queue.

One of the problems with Tamiflu however are the side effects. A significant number of those who have taken it report severe nausea and vomiting and it also produces severe psychiatric effects in many patients.

In the UK a National Flu Pandemic Service was created to provide a hotline to a call centre and take some of the pressure off the NHS. There were numerous complaints about this approach. The staff had no medical training and just took callers through a questionnaire; if you ticked a sufficient number of the boxes you got Tamiflu. Such an approach risks missing the symptoms of more serious diseases such as meningitis, especially in young children. It is also open to fraud by people claiming symptoms they do not have and hypochondriacs with colds exaggerating the symptoms. By the end of August 2009, the press were claiming that only one in ten of those contacting the hotline had genuine flu. Handing out Tamiflu on this scale to mild cases raises the risk very considerably of the virus mutating to resistance and there have already been reports of flu strains that have become resistant to the drug. The obvious method of dealing with this problem is to stockpile supplies of more than one drug, for example, Relenza.

THE LAST WORD

It is difficult to improve upon the last paragraph of the British Ministry of Health *"Report on Pandemic Influenza"*, published in 1920. Although this was specifically reporting on influenza, the sentiments expressed could be equally applied to all infectious diseases.

"In the seeming conflict between man and his microscopic competitors, there can never be a time when man is securely master of the universe. Intoxicated by the victories achieved over the plague, over the enteric group, over typhus and over smallpox, we are too apt to suppose that the campaign has ended in our favour. That we have just passed through one of the great sicknesses of history, a plague which within a few months has destroyed more lives than were directly sacrificed in four years of destructive war, is an experience which should dispel any easy optimism on our part".

CHAPTER 16

Malaria and Sleeping Sickness

"Everything about malaria is so moulded and altered by local conditions that it becomes a thousand different diseases and epidemiological puzzles. Like chess, it is played with a few pieces but is capable of an infinite variety of situations".
Lewis Hackett, 1937.

INTRODUCTION

The association between malaria and stagnant water, swamps and marshes that smell of rotting vegetation, was recognised at a very early stage, giving rise to the name that is taken from Italian, *mal'aria* meaning bad air.

Malaria is the most prevalent disease in the world caused by a parasite. It probably kills about three million people annually, a figure matched only by tuberculosis and gastro-enteritis (a catchall phrase for numerous diseases of the gut), although AIDS is catching up rapidly. It also makes a significant contribution to the incidence of many other diseases as it produces a very debilitated and anaemic population who are highly susceptible to infection by other pathogenic organisms. The numbers of people infected are such that it makes a major economic impact on those countries where it is endemic. Although malaria can occur in temperate regions, it is most common in the tropics and subtropics, where climatic conditions are favourable for the mosquitoes that transmit the disease throughout the year.

The natural route for the spread of malaria is the bite of an infected mosquito but it can also be spread by drug addicts

557

sharing needles, or by blood transfusion from an infected donor when blood has not been adequately screened.

An estimated three billion people, nearly half of the world's population, live in areas where they are at risk of catching malaria. The approximate number of people infected worldwide is difficult to estimate, but is thought to be between 300-500 million, and rising on a year by year basis. The majority of those killed by it are children under the age of five[189] and pregnant women in whom it is a frequent cause of miscarriages and stillbirths. It is difficult to estimate these numbers accurately as the disease is so widespread, especially in Africa and developing countries. There are several reasons for this difficulty. The term malaria is frequently an umbrella diagnosis for any disease causing a high fever, especially in the early stages of the disease and in areas where diagnostic medical facilities are poor. It is also common for malaria to mask the presence of other pathogens, and it can confuse the blood tests used in the detection of a number of other diseases, by producing false positive or negative results.

The World Health Organisation (WHO) figures suggest that there are about one million fatalities per year from malaria. Many consider this figure is too low as the WHO accepts the figures produced by various governments at face value. These are frequently kept deliberately low for political reasons and to avoid damaging the local tourist industry. Estimates from various charitable organisations suggest that the true figure is at least three times higher, although it has also been suggested, on several occasions that the figures produced by charities are deliberately inflated to maximise donor sympathy and hence financial support.

The symptoms mimic those of a number of other diseases although symptoms found in young children can differ from those found in adults. Malaria is frequently fatal very quickly

---

189   Many experts consider that malaria is the cause of, or is implicated in, half the deaths of children under the age of five in sub-Saharan Africa.

in children, death occurring within 24-48 hours of the first symptoms appearing.

The onset of the disease normally begins about ten days after infection, although this can vary considerably. It consists of a three-stage process, the first being shivering and joint pains lasting several hours. These are followed by severe flu-like symptoms lasting a varying period of time depending on the type of malaria involved, with a temperature that may rise as high as 41°C (106°F). In the third stage the fever breaks, the victim starts to sweat and then goes into a deep sleep. The process then starts again and the cycle may be repeated a number of times. Attacks occur at regular intervals depending on which form of malaria is responsible and untreated cycles may last up to three months, then disappear for a period of time before reoccurring. The infected person frequently suffers from anaemia due to the large number of red blood cells destroyed. The disease is usually accompanied by enlargement of the spleen, which was recognised by many early medical writers as an important diagnostic sign. This organ plays a major role in destroying infected or damaged red blood cells.

Malaria is caused by a protozoan (Ch 4) belonging to a type known as the Sporozoa. These are non-motile, the whole group are parasites and some of them depend on being carried to a susceptible host by an insect vector. Sporozoans causing malaria are members of the genus *Plasmodium*, the vectors of which are mosquitoes.

Many species of vertebrates, both cold and warm blooded suffer from malaria. Four species of *Plasmodium* are found causing malaria in humans, the symptoms varying somewhat depending on the species of *Plasmodium* responsible. The first is *Plasmodium vivax* causing benign tertian fever (also known as marsh fever or ague) that occurred widely in England during the seventeenth and eighteenth centuries and is probably the most common form. The others are *P. malariae* causing quartan fever, *P. ovale* and the most dangerous, *P. falciparum*, causing malignant tertian fever or blackwater fever (so-called because the massive destruction of red blood cells leads to a dark red urine). *P. falciparum* is the main species found in West Africa, *P. vivax* is widespread throughout the world and is the form occurring in temperate regions, whilst *P. malariae* is found mainly in the Mediterranean and *P. ovale* occurs most commonly in East Africa. The name *falciparum* comes from two Latin words, *falcis* meaning a scythe or sickle, and *pareo* to carry, (the implication being that this is the Grim Reaper). This species causes most of the deaths from malaria in Africa, the majority of these being children. Malaria infections caused by *P. vivax* and *P. malariae* are not usually life-threatening if treated early and in the correct manner. They are occasionally known as benign malarias, this is a contradiction in terms, but when compared with malaria caused by *P. falciparum,* they are relatively mild. Infections with more than one species can occur simultaneously and infection with one does not confer immunity against the others.

The terminology of malaria is confusing. Tertian means every three days, but this counts the first bout of fever as day one, there is then a day of remission followed by another day of fever on day three (which becomes day one of the next bout of fever), so tertian actually means every other day. Similarly quartan is a fever on day one, two days of remission and fever again on the fourth day, whilst quotidian means daily and may be caused by multiple infection of different types of *Plasmodium,* resulting in a more or less continuous fever.

Fifteen to twenty species of *Plasmodium* infect Old World monkeys and apes. Each species of primate has its own spectrum of malarial parasites, each of which is carried by its own species of mosquito. In the New World however, the malarial parasites found in monkeys are the same as those found in humans, suggesting that they came from the same source, and have had less time to specialise and differentiate.

This would dovetail with the fact that malaria was not found in the New World before the sixteenth century.

It is thought that anopheline (see later) mosquitoes capable of carrying malaria were present in the Americas before Columbus arrived, but that *Plasmodium* was introduced by the Spanish. The result was that when malaria was introduced, it spread very rapidly as a vector was already present and the Amerindians had no genetic resistance to the disease. The *Plasmodium* species introduced by the Spanish would probably have been *P. vivax,* the most common form in Europe, but, when the slave trade started in the early sixteenth century, slaves from West Africa would have brought *P. falciparum* with them. The fact that yellow fever did not appear until some time later was due to the absence of the necessary mosquito vector and yellow fever did not become a problem in the New World until the requisite mosquito species had been introduced and had established itself.

Different *Plasmodium* species are also found in numerous other vertebrate species, including birds, each species of *Plasmodium* having its own preferred species of mosquito acting as carrier. These may be transmitted to humans on rare occasions. The specialisation of *Plasmodium*, the vertebrate species they infect, and the specificity of the mosquito species carrying them, suggest a disease with a very long history of infecting vertebrates in the Old World.

The *Plasmodium* carried will also vary depending on the type of mosquito present, for example, one common species of mosquito found in Britain, *Anopheles atroparvus,* can carry *P. vivax* but not *P. falciparum*. The minimum summer temperature required to allow *P. vivax* to complete its breeding cycle is 15°C (59°F), and it cannot develop if the mosquito vector has a body temperature below this figure. The corresponding figure for *P. falciparum* is 20°C (68°F), thus explaining the wider geographical range of *P. vivax*. The summer temperature also affects the length of time required for completion of the life cycle of the parasite, the warmer it becomes the shorter the time required.

Malaria seems to have receded in Northern Europe during the early Middle Ages (Little Ice Age) due to the lower temperatures, but become more serious at the end of the seventeenth century when countries such as England and Scandinavia started to become warmer. In much of Europe, with the exception of parts of Russia, endemic malaria has been virtually eliminated. There are however, occasional cases of autochthonous malaria (originating where found), showing that constant monitoring of the disease is necessary. There are also numerous cases of what is known as airport malaria, that is malaria imported into a country by people travelling from areas where malaria is endemic or epidemic[190].

A number of different species of *Plasmodium* have been examined and their genomes compared which has enabled a phylogenetic tree to be constructed. The trunk of this tree is the genome of the common ancestor that has now disappeared, and whose genome can only be deduced by inference and examination of the genomes of its descendants. Closely related species are branches of the tree that are close to each other; distantly related species are at the tips of branches.

P. malariae is genetically distant to all the other species, and infections of *P. malariae* have been reported as lasting in individuals for forty years, suggesting that this is a very ancient parasite of humans that has entered into a more or less mutual tolerance with the host. *P. vivax* is related to the *Plasmodia* infecting modern day monkeys and apes, suggesting that it only diverged from these species in relatively recent evolutionary time. Genetically, *P. falciparum* is widely separated from both *P. vivax* and *P. malariae,* and is closely related to a number of *Plasmodia* infecting birds, and therefore presumably spread from birds to humans in the recent evolutionary past. Avian

---

190   This is becoming a serious problem as health surveys suggest that up to fifty per cent of people travelling to areas where malaria is found, do not bother to take any precautions against the disease.

malaria is transmitted by mosquitoes of the genus *Culex* not *Anopheles,* and it is possible that *P. falciparum* is attempting the difficult feat of evolving to coexist with a new mammalian host and a new vector simultaneously. A parasite, such as *Plasmodium,* that needs to co-exist with two hosts, is under much greater evolutionary pressure than a parasite that only needs to co-exist with one host. In the absence of treatment, infections caused by *P. falciparum* either terminate naturally after approximately one year, or kill the human host. This suggests that *P. falciparum* is a recent acquisition in which mutual tolerance has not as yet been achieved.

P. falciparum is poorly adjusted to causing disease in humans compared with other types and causes more serious damage. It makes the red blood cells sticky, causing capillary blood vessels to become blocked and then burst either resulting in acute anaemia, or if the parasites are released into the brain causing cerebral malaria. The temperature of the victim may become very high (42°C or 107°F) leading to convulsions, delirium and death. It can also damage the placenta in pregnant women causing miscarriage and destroys the kidneys, producing pigmentation of the urine, hence the name blackwater fever. A significant proportion of children who contract cerebral malaria but recover suffer permanent brain damage. It produces far more parasites in the blood than other forms of human malaria, but if *Anopheles* mosquitoes are exposed to a patient carrying both *P. vivax* and *P. falciparum,* they pick up *vivax* more easily, in spite of fact that there are less of these parasites present in the host.

THE VECTOR

There are a large number of species of mosquito (of the order of 3,000), about one tenth of which are capable of carrying some human disease. The word mosquito is derived from Spanish words meaning, "little fly". Mosquitoes are divided into two main groups, the first are culicines which hold their body parallel to the surface on which they are resting, the second type are the anophelines which rest in a head-down position. As already mentioned, the plasmodia causing malaria in mammalian species are carried by anopheline mosquitoes, whilst plasmodia causing bird malaria are carried by mosquitoes of the genus *Culex* (culicine). *Plasmodium* cannot survive in the wrong type of mosquito, although the physiological or biochemical nature of the barrier is not known. Over four hundred species of the genus *Anopheles* are found; about thirty of them are serious vectors of malaria in mammals, although a number of other species will also carry it.

Mosquitoes are ubiquitous and are found over a wide range of different temperatures and altitudes, each species having its own optimum spectrum of breeding conditions. Relatively minor variables in the environment will change the abundance of one type of mosquito compared with others, making one area free of malaria and others malarial. Numerous factors influence the suitability as a vector. These include population density, flight range (some species will fly considerable distances to obtain a blood meal), feeding preferences, the life span of the female and the preferred temperature range.

Rising temperatures due to global warming will allow the mosquito population to expand its range. It also means they will bite more frequently, and thus one of the consequences of global warming will be a spread of malaria (especially that caused by *P. falciparum*) and other mosquito-borne diseases. This is already occurring and recent reports show that malaria is moving into higher altitude areas on Mount Kenya. Over the last twenty years there has been a rise of 2°C (3.6°F) in the area raising the average temperature from 17°C to 19°C, a rise that improves the survival of *Plasmodium* carrying mosquitoes. The result has been a seven-fold increase in malaria in the area. A research study has ruled out any other factors and the increase in malaria has been attributed solely to the rise in temperature.

All species of mosquito need water to breed, but whilst some prefer gently flowing water, others prefer stagnant water and the level of brackishness is critical for certain species. The eggs are laid on water plants, and develop into larvae that hang onto the underside of the water surface making use of the surface tension. They breathe through tubes that penetrate the water's surface to the air, and the larvae eventually form a pupa and undergo metamorphosis to change into the adult. Only small quantities of water are necessary for mosquitoes to breed and in countries such as Vietnam, water filled bomb craters have caused significant increases in the levels of mosquitoes and malaria.

Some species, known as tree-bole mosquitoes, will normally breed in water-filled holes in tree trunks, but in the absence of these, they will breed in water that has collected in discarded tin cans or old car tyres. As anyone who has attempted it will know, it is virtually impossible to get all the water out of an old tyre, and old tyres being sent for recycling are known to have contributed to the spread of certain species of mosquito to new continents on several occasions. Australia fumigates all old tyres arriving in the country in an attempt to stop this occurring. Container shipping and the baggage holds of aircraft are also known to have contributed to this spread. The major problem in recent years has been the increase in range of the Asian tiger mosquito, *Aedes albopictus,* a tree-bole mosquito, which is extremely aggressive. It will mate with females of other species and these females become sterile as they cannot use the sperm and do not mate again. The result is that the tiger mosquito is replacing other species such as *Ae. aegypti* in many areas. *Ae. albopictus* has been exported from Asia to a number of other countries, and is now found in the Caribbean, South America, the USA and southern Europe. It has recently been found in France and its appearance in the UK in the near future is now regarded as inevitable.

It is only the female mosquito that feeds on blood. The male is a harmless vegetarian (definitely a case of, *"the female of the species is more deadly than the male"* [with apologies to Kipling]). The time of feeding varies depending on the species, some mosquitoes feed at dusk, some at night and others in broad daylight. The female may live several months and lay several batches of eggs. Each female may produce as many as one thousand eggs over her life-time and she needs a meal of blood before laying each batch. It was thought for many years that the female mosquito only fed on blood once during her life, and this was a major cause of the role of mosquitoes in the transmission of various diseases being misunderstood.

Some species will only feed on one host species, others will feed on a wide variety of hosts although they frequently show a strong preference for just one. If the host species is displaced however, they will feed on other mammals, including passing humans. Those mosquitoes feeding on a variety of hosts are more dangerous than those feeding on a single host species, as they have the potential to spread diseases from one host to another, greatly increasing the risk of transmitting diseases found in other species to humans. The Asian tiger mosquito mentioned earlier falls into this category.

Numerous diseases are transmitted by mosquitoes, but malaria is by far the most widespread and most important, and once the female is infected, she is infectious for life. One mosquito, infected by one person, can infect a large number of other people. The Basic Reproduction Number (BRN) is the number of additional infections one infected person will cause. The disease dies out if this number is less than one, but in the case of malaria, the BRN may be as high as one hundred or more. Several factors will influence this number including the density of the mosquito population. A second factor is whether the mosquito bites other species beside humans and this was of major importance in the elimination of malaria from England (see later). The length of time the mosquito survives after becoming infected is also important, obviously the longer it survives the more people it can infect.

The susceptibility of humans to mosquito bites varies widely. Recent research has shown that about twenty per cent of the population receive approximately eighty per cent of the bites. This variation appears to be due to personal odour and there is some evidence that *P. falciparum* may be able to modify the body odour of the infected host to attract more mosquitoes, thereby increasing the infection rate. The antennae of mosquitoes are complex and contain receptors for over seventy different chemicals, many of them occurring in human perspiration.

Research has also shown that the parasite is able to modify the biochemistry of the mosquito by reducing the activity of an enzyme known as apyrase. Apyrase is injected with saliva when an uninfected mosquito bites a victim and stops the blood from clotting, thus allowing the insect more time to feed. When the mosquito is infected with *Plasmodium*, the reduced activity of apyrase means blood clots more quickly and the mosquito cannot get a full meal, so it visits further victims. The result is that the parasite is spread more widely.

Humans are a ground living species and tend to think of territory as two-dimensional space but territory is three dimensional. There are a wide range of organisms and food chains in the rain forest in the vertical dimension and a change of only a few metres in height can produce significant changes, both in the species present, and in their behaviour. This can cause problems, for example, when trees are felled in the rain forest, mosquitoes that normally bite monkeys in the canopy are displaced to ground level where they attack humans such as loggers. Numerous epidemics of a variety of diseases, such as yellow fever, are known to start in this manner. The problem can be caused by primitive farming of the slash and burn type.

This displaces the anophiline mosquitoes carrying *P. ovale* that causes a relatively mild form of malaria, and replaces them with *Anopheles gambiae*. This is a very aggressive mosquito that reproduces in stagnant pools on cleared land and which transmits *P. falciparum*. The result is frequently a huge local increase in the most lethal form of malaria.

LIFE CYCLE OF *PLASMODIUM*

The life cycle of the *Plasmodium* parasite looks complicated, but it is simply a life cycle divided into two parts. A non-sexual phase of multiplication takes place in the blood and liver of humans, and a sexual phase in the body of the mosquito. The mosquito is therefore the definitive host of this parasite (Ch 6).

Any parasite with more than one host has a problem as it has to balance its life style with that of two hosts. From the point of view of *Plasmodium*, it is more important to reach a balance with the mosquito that spreads it. Obviously a delirious mosquito would be of no use whatsoever in the transmission of the disease. This means that the balance between the parasite and the vector is the one that must be stabilised, not the balance between the parasite and human. Although the plasmodium does affect the mosquito in a manner that increases the rate of transmission of the parasite to a new host, it does not matter too much if it is destructive towards the human host. Indeed, for the plasmodium it is a requirement to be as widespread as possible throughout the human body, as the plasmodium should be available to the mosquito wherever it bites the human host. In addition, it does not matter if the human is delirious, it could actually be an advantage, as a delirious human is less likely to swat the mosquito. The same situation applies to many vector borne diseases such as plague, typhus and yellow fever, and generally, vector borne diseases are extremely dangerous ones for the human host.

The infective stage produced in the mosquito is the sporozoite, which is injected when the female mosquito feeds on a human. The sporozoites are motile and swim from the site of the bite to the liver, where they grow inside the liver cells, eventually dividing into multiple daughter cells (merozoites). These are released into the blood where they attack red blood cells. Once inside the red blood cells they grow and divide to form further merozoites that attack new red blood cells when the old one bursts. During this phase, when the red blood cells are examined microscopically they appear to have a ring-shaped structure inside them. The appearance of these structures in infected red blood cells is sufficiently characteristic to be used as a low-tech diagnostic tool.

One unusual feature of the asexual cycle is that the protozoans grow and divide synchronously (all at the same time), and the resulting mass division into merozoites produces the fevers at regular intervals that are typical of malaria. This cycle of events is repeated a number of times, the bursting of the red blood cells coinciding with the outbreaks of fever.

After several cycles of division, some of the merozoites develop into gametocytes that must be swallowed by a female mosquito, when she feeds, before any further development can take place. The gametocytes enter the stomach of the mosquito where they develop into male and female gametes and these fuse to form a zygote that penetrates the wall of the gut and forms a cyst. These grow and divide to form sporozoites that are released when the cyst bursts. The sporozoites released migrate to the salivary glands and at this point, the mosquito becomes infectious. They are injected into a fresh human victim when the mosquito next feeds and the cycle is repeated in the new host. The process is shown in Figure 16.1.

Many forms of malaria are able to survive summers in temperate zones at the outer limit of the viability of the mosquito, and there must have been years when the mosquito population had difficulty in breeding due to the weather. The question therefore arises how did malaria survive in climates such as Scotland, Scandinavia and Russia? There are a number of well-documented outbreaks of malaria in Northern Europe, in the nineteenth century, which occurred before the local mosquito population started to breed.

Figure 16.1. Life Cycle of Plasmodium

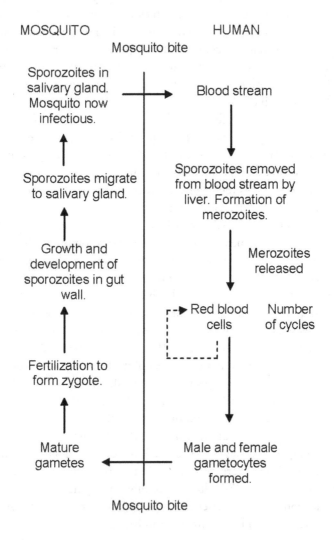

Malarial relapse is a well-known phenomenon and was noted by both Greek and Roman doctors in antiquity with the relapse frequently occurring after the patient had shown no symptoms for many years. Sporozoites entering the body when the mosquito first bites, swim to the liver where they enter liver cells. Most reproduce immediately, going through the cycle already described, but some lie dormant for years. The dormant ones are now referred to as hypnozoites (from Hypnos, the Greek God of Sleep). They are reactivated by shock of various types to the host, common ones being changes of climate and temperature. Hypnozoites are found most commonly in malarias from the temperate zone. They are less widespread in malarias from the tropics, which are carried by mosquitoes that do not need to survive cold weather. They are not found in *P. falciparum* which does not relapse and *P. falciparum* is therefore confined to areas of the tropics and sub-tropics where there is a year round breeding population of mosquitoes able to carry it.

MALARIA AND HUMAN GENETICS

The genetic evidence suggests that malaria probably originated in sub-Saharan Africa, and spread from there to the rest of the world, reaching the Americas in the sixteenth century. The widespread incidence of human genetic diseases, such as sickle cell anaemia and various thalassaemias, suggest that malaria has existed in humans for a very long time in the Old World.

There are a number of different methods whereby humans, descended from Old World ancestors, can have high levels of resistance to malaria. One of these is conferred by the presence or absence of a protein known as the Duffy antigen. This molecule, located on the membrane of the red blood cell, is related to the molecules specifying blood groups and *P. vivax* uses it as a portal into the cell. Most West Africans lack the Duffy antigen, and as a result they have total immunity to malaria caused by *P. vivax,* and an elevated level of resistance to *P. falciparum* compared to Europeans. It has also been claimed that people with blood group O, who lack proteins specifying blood groups, suffer from malaria less seriously than those with blood groups A, B or AB, all of whom possess proteins specifying blood groups.

Another genetic adaptation found widely in West Africa is a disease known as sickle cell anaemia. This was first found in a black student in the USA and was described in 1904 by an American doctor, James Herrick. Other cases soon emerged and it was realised that sickle cell anaemia is a significant problem wherever there is a large population of West African descent. Although the disease was described early in the twentieth century, it has been traced back to at least the seventeenth century in West Africa, and the high percentage of people carrying the gene suggests that it goes back a lot further than that.

Blood samples taken from individuals suffering from this disease contain unusual red blood cells that are sickle or crescent shaped, instead of being round and these individuals have a high level of resistance to malaria. The blood protein haemoglobin (the first protein whose structure was determined) carries oxygen around the body and is made up of four chains, two α chains and two β chains. The structure of the α and β chains are each controlled by two genes in every person, one α and one β gene being inherited from each parent. If the two genes producing the β protein are the same then the person is homozygous for that gene, if the two genes producing the β protein are different, then the person is heterozygous for that gene. Individuals who are heterozygous for the ß gene are referred to as carrying the sickle trait.

Sickle cell anaemia has the distinction that it was the first genetic disease (in 1956) in which the biochemical alteration causing the disease was pinpointed. In an individual with the sickle gene, there is an alteration in the amino acid sequence of the β chain. This causes the red blood cells to take up the characteristic sickle shape instead of the normal round shape. This is especially noticeable in the capillary blood system. Sickling is caused by the abnormal haemoglobin (known as haemoglobin S) precipitating when oxygen levels are low, to produce red blood cells that are very fragile and rupture easily, thus causing the anaemia found in this condition. The mutant haemoglobin carries oxygen less effectively than normal haemoglobin and tissues are not oxygenated adequately which also contributes to the anaemia. Sickle cells also cannot get into smaller blood vessels such as the capillaries and destruction of tissue occurs.

Sickle cell anaemics appear to resist malaria using several mechanisms. Red blood cells containing the sickle gene are very prone to adopting the sickle shape if they become infected by *Plasmodium* species. The infected cells sickle more than non-infected cells and are recognised and removed by the spleen, thereby also eliminating the *Plasmodium*, and producing a significant resistance to malaria. The life span of the infected red blood cells falls from the normal 120 days to about 60 days. There also appears to be damage to the parasite in the presence of the reduced oxygen levels found in the sickle red blood cells.

The genetics of this disease gives rise to several possibilities. If a person is homozygous for the sickle gene, all the β chains will be in the sickle form and a high level of anaemia will be found. This is frequently fatal at a relatively young age in the absence of regular blood transfusions. People heterozygous for the disease have the sickle trait in which fifty per cent of their β chains will be normal but fifty per cent will be sickle chains. However, due to the complicated aggregation process of haemoglobin, only about one to two per cent of their blood cells will sickle in the capillaries in the absence of *Plasmodium*. The person heterozygous for the β gene therefore has a high level of resistance to malaria and the anaemia is reduced to a tolerable level. The individual homozygous for the normal β gene has no anaemia but is at high risk of contracting malaria.

Many homozygotes for the sickle gene will die before maturity (that is, before reaching reproductive age) in the absence of advanced medicine, and therefore there must have been some very strong selective evolutionary pressure to maintain high levels of the sickle gene. This is an example of what is known as balanced polymorphism. In general, deleterious genes are eliminated rapidly, and a gene causing severe morbidity and death would die out within a few generations unless there is a very good reason for its continued survival. The selective pressure in this instance is that heterozygotes show a high level of immunity to malaria. It is an example of a gene that is extremely dangerous in the homozygous state, persisting at a high level in the general population, because there are significant advantages in the heterozygous state. When balanced polymorphisms of this type occur, the number of people in a population having the alternative allele will build up until the advantages and disadvantages to the population equalize.

When the inheritance of the gene is considered, if one parent has the sickle trait then each child has a 50:50 chance of acquiring a single copy of the sickle gene. If both parents have the sickle trait, then the probability is that twenty-five per cent of the offspring will have two copies of the normal gene (homozygous), fifty per cent of the offspring will have one copy of the sickle gene and one copy of the normal gene (heterozygous), and twenty-five per cent will have two copies of the sickle gene (homozygous). The community therefore purchases herd immunity against malaria for fifty per cent of the children of the community, at the expense of twenty-five per cent of the children dying from anaemia and twenty-five per cent being at severe risk of malaria. The situation is shown diagrammatically in Figure 16.2. The statements made in these paragraphs make the assumption that children who are homozygous for the sickle gene die before they reach reproductive age.

Figure 16.2. Sickle Cell Anaemia

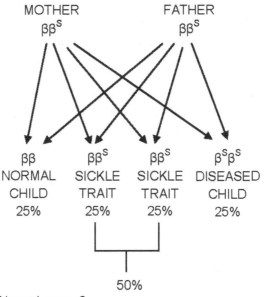

Normal gene β

Sickle gene β^S

Both Parents are Heterozygous and carry the Sickle Trait.

In the case of sickle cell anaemia, if the selective pressure of malaria (especially that caused by *Plasmodium falciparum*) is removed, then the incidence rate of the sickle gene falls. This is seen in the USA where malaria has been more or less eliminated. The incidence rate of the sickle gene amongst West Africans is approximately three times higher than that found in Americans of West African descent even although they are from the same gene pool. In areas where life-threatening malaria is not endemic, the sickle gene becomes the only determinant of morbidity and therefore the frequency decreases. A similar situation exists in West Africa where the sickle trait is noticeably lower amongst those local populations living at high altitude than it is amongst those populations living at or near sea level. This is obviously due to the reduced range of the mosquito and hence, the incidence of malaria being reduced.

Another mutant form of haemoglobin found in West Africa is haemoglobin C. This also involves a change in the β chain and again produces a considerable immunity to malaria, but this time without the problems caused by anaemia. Genetic analysis suggests this mutation has appeared more recently than the sickle mutation, and it is possible that over a period of time (measured in generations) it will replace the sickle mutation as the major adaptation to malaria resistance in the region.

A further mutation conferring significant resistance to malaria is due to a mutant gene for an enzyme known as glucose-6-phosphate dehydrogenase (G-6-PDH). This is one of the most common genetic defects found in humans, affecting over four hundred million people worldwide. A large number of variants of the mutation are found in African, Asian and Mediterranean populations, suggesting that the original mutation occurred in the distant past of human evolution. The enzyme functions by removing molecules known as free radicals. These are highly reactive molecules that take part in random reactions causing cell damage, and cell death, if not removed. Individuals lacking this enzyme have above normal levels of free radicals in their cells and these inhibit the growth of *Plasmodium,* conferring a significant resistance to malaria. Cells with high levels of free radicals are also removed by the spleen more efficiently than normal cells.

The gene for this particular enzyme is carried on the female X chromosome and its behaviour therefore differs depending on whether the individual is male or female. Males only have one copy of the X chromosome and therefore either have the normal enzyme or the mutant form. Females who have two copies of the X chromosome can either be homozygous for the normal gene, homozygous for the defective gene or heterozygous.

The behaviour of G-6-PDH was first discovered during the Korean War in the 1950s. About ten per cent of black soldiers in the US army had an extreme reaction to an anti-malarial drug, primaquine, which caused severe anaemia and death in a small number of cases. Primaquine functions by generating free radicals that attack *Plasmodium,* however, when G-6-PDH is absent, the extra free radicals generated cause cell damage and lysis that in extreme cases can be fatal.

This situation has given rise to a new branch of science known as pharmacogenetics. The pharmaceutical industry has started to take into account the fact that different racial groups and individuals produce varying responses to drugs because of enzyme differences, and what is suitable treatment for one racial group or individual may not be suitable for another.

A similar group of genetic diseases conferring resistance to malaria are the thalassaemias, of which there are several different types, all involving defective synthesis of haemoglobin chains. This group of diseases occur over a wide area from the Mediterranean, through the Middle East into South East Asia. They are named after the Greek word for sea (thalassa), because of the high incidence rate around the Mediterranean. The genetics of thalassaemia are, however, considerably more complicated than those of sickle cell anaemia. Several different types are found; in all of them one of the haemoglobin chains is missing or produced at reduced levels. In those types of thalassaemia where the haemoglobin chain is missing, homozygotes either die *in utero* or shortly after birth. Although the homozygous form of some types of the disease is fatal, the heterozygous form of the disease is usually asymptomatic, and again offers significant resistance to malaria, which until the middle of the twentieth century was a serious problem in the Mediterranean area.

MALARIAL VACCINES

The human immune response to malaria is poor, and one dose of malaria does not give life-long protection against the disease. In addition, infection with one type does not provide immunity against other types. One of the main problems is that the parasite spends its much of its life in different forms inside various organs of the body. These changes in shape and habitat involve changes in the chemistry of the surface proteins that are sufficient to enable *Plasmodium* to avoid recognition by the host immune system. The result is that many of the techniques used for producing vaccines against viruses and bacteria are ineffective when deployed against *Plasmodium*.

There are numerous further problems. Until recently, it was impossible to culture *Plasmodium* in defined media, making test-tube experiments difficult. Malaria is a disease of poor countries, and therefore any vaccine has poor financial prospects for manufacturers and because of the problems mentioned above, the development costs would be extremely high. However, global warming may cause the spread of more dangerous forms of malaria into richer countries making the development of a vaccine more attractive financially.

A number of methods of developing a long-lasting vaccine have been attempted, generally with very little success. Some of these involve making a chimaeric gene by using genetic material from different stages of the parasite, and making a hybrid protein that stimulates the immune system. Attempts of this type have had some limited success, but the main problem is that the parasite is continuously mutating and is a constantly moving target. One of the latest attempts involves using a specific protein based on the outer surface of *P. falciparum* during the merozoite stage (the stage inside the red blood cell). Some parts of this protein stimulate a very strong antibody response from the host, but other parts stimulate a host reaction that hides the parasite from the immune system. The new vaccine takes the whole protein from the parasite, snips out the sections conferring protection, and stitches together the bits that stimulate the parasite killing response. Early trials suggest that there is a limited immunisation produced in suitable patients.

The types of vaccine tested generally fall into one of three groups. The first are the pre-erythocytic vaccines that confer protection in the early stages of the infection, before the injected erythrocytes reach the liver, and would therefore stop the infection developing into full-blown malaria. The second type are the blood stage vaccines that disrupt the replication of the parasite in the red blood cell. These would not stop the infection, but would reduce the number of parasites in the blood system and thereby reduce the severity of the disease.

The third type involves vaccinating people using a protein only found on the parasite when it is in the stomach of the mosquito. If this plasmodium protein is injected into a person, the host produces the antibody and when the mosquito feeds, it picks up both the parasite and antibody circulating in the blood. The concept is that the antibody will neutralise the plasmodium protein when it is produced in the gut of the mosquito and stop the parasite completing its life cycle, thus breaking the malarial chain of events. This does not cure the sick person of malaria, it cures the mosquito and has been called, *"Transmission blocking immunity"*. It does make the assumption that the antibody protein is not broken down in the mosquito gut before it works. Whilst this concept may seem to be extremely convoluted, it does highlight the difficulty in dealing with a parasite that has more than one host and which is also a eucaryotic organism found in a number of different stages in the human host.

HISTORY

A number of ancient manuscripts from India, China and the Middle East describe malaria recognisably. It is mentioned as early as 2,700 BC by the Chinese, around 1,600 BC by the Sumerians and in Vedic literature at about the same time. Classical Greece and Rome suffered badly from malaria and both Hippocrates and Galen described it and recognised that there was more than one form. Hippocrates made it obvious it was widespread and thought it was caused by drinking stagnant water, which was a reasonable hypothesis for the fourth century BC. He also realised that it was seasonal and a problem mainly in late summer and autumn.

Malaria is not mentioned in any Egyptian medical papyri that have been found. However, tests carried out on the mummies of a number of individuals from various periods of Egyptian history (the earliest being about 3,000 BC) have detected antigens produced by *P. falciparum*.

Malaria was widespread in the Roman Republic and Empire. Celsus gave a detailed account of it in *De re medica (ca 30 AD)* and the first century Roman physician, Dioscorides, prepared a tonic of the plant St John's wort *(Hypericum performatum)* in wine as a cure. Some scholars have suggested that the decline of classical Greece was due to malaria and similar suggestions have been made about Rome.

In the sixth to the third centuries BC, a number of areas of Italy were supporting large populations of farmers, but malaria became more deadly over a period of centuries as the Roman Empire grew, possibly due to spread of mosquito vectors capable of carrying *P. falciparum*. By the second century AD, malaria was widespread in the Campagna region around Rome, where a considerable amount of the local food supply was grown, and was a serious problem in Rome itself and much of the Mediterranean. Archaeological excavations on both the mainland and a number of islands, such as Sardinia, have found children's graves containing quantities of honeysuckle. This was used for treating an enlarged spleen, a typical symptom of malaria. Pitting of the skull is also found in children's skeletal remains, this is symptomatic of the severe anaemia that is a common problem in cases of malaria in infants. It is impossible to judge the economic effects of malaria alone, as there were numerous other epidemic diseases by this time, including smallpox. However, in 15 AD, Strabo claimed that malaria in Sardinia was a serious problem and stated, *"The island is unhealthy, it is not profitable to maintain a military presence in the area".* By the fifth century AD, Roman writers are mentioning, *"Zones of pestilence",* and making it obvious that the plains around Rome had been abandoned to disease.

The Huns led by Attila retreated from the gates of Rome in 452, because of an epidemic of fever that has been variously quoted as malaria or smallpox. Fever killed half the army of Frederick Barbarossa, the Holy Roman Emperor, in the summer of 1155 AD, causing Godfrey of Viterbo to write the following words in 1167, *"When unable to defend herself by the sword, Rome could defend herself by means of the fever".*

The Campagna region flooded whenever the River Tiber burst its banks, and malaria continued to be a serious problem most years until Mussolini drained the Pontine Marshes at the mouth of the Tiber in the twentieth century. Rank was no protection against the disease, numerous Popes died from it including Innocent VIII, Sixtus V, Adrian VI and Gregory XV. It also killed many great nobles such as members of the Medici family and various cardinals, who suffered seriously when conclaves were summoned to Rome to elect a new Pope, especially if they were held in late summer.

The problems were not just confined to Rome and the surrounding areas. Malaria forced people to abandon their land in Tuscany in the eighteenth and nineteenth centuries and Edmund Lear commented on the severity of malaria in southern Italy in the summer of 1847.

In early China, malaria was mainly a problem of the south, and may have presented a serious barrier to Chinese penetration and expansion southwards. There are a number of cures mentioned in ancient Chinese writings, and *Artemisia* herbal tea from a recipe over two thousand years old was widely used. This is first mentioned around 170 BC, and is derived from sweet wormwood (*Artemisia annua*). The active ingredient artemisinin (qinghaosu) and its derivatives are receiving considerable interest as modern day alternatives to the quinine based drugs. The Chinese started to research the chemical components of *Artemisia* early in the second half of the twentieth century, but the work was kept secret for about fifteen years under the instructions of the Communist Party. Various rumours reached the West and eventually the plant was found growing on the shores of the Potomac River, a couple of miles from Washington, D.C.

Malaria was also common in England[191], especially in the fenlands, and is mentioned by a number of writers including Chaucer and Shakespeare, who included a reference to it in several plays. In Henry V, Shakespeare wrote that Sir John Falstaffe, *"is so shaked of a burning quotidian tertian that it is most lamentable to behold"*. This might seem impossible as quotidian implies fever every day, whilst tertian implies every other day. It would therefore seem that Shakespeare was using the word quotidian in its secondary meaning of commonplace or trivial. Although malaria obviously occurred in England at the time of Chaucer, it seems to have become more severe by the late seventeenth century.

It is also mentioned by the diarists Samuel Pepys and John Evelyn, and writer Daniel Defoe. Those readers who are feminists or who hold politically correct opinions should perhaps skip the next paragraph written by Defoe, in the early eighteenth century, about the marshy areas of Kent and Essex, and quoted by Rocco (*The Fever Tree*).

---

191   The word malaria was introduced into England by Horace Walpole, the son of Sir Robert Walpole the British Prime Minister, in the eighteenth century after a visit to Rome. It had previously been referred to as ague.

"All along this county it is very frequent to meet with Men that have had from Five to Six, to Fourteen or Fifteen wives; and I was informed, that in the Marshes, over against Canvy Island, was a farmer, who was living with his Five and Twentieth; and that his son, who was but thirty-five years old, had already had about fourteen. The reason, as a merry Fellow told me, who said he had had about a dozen, was this, that they being bred in the Marshes themselves and seasoned to the place, did pretty well; but they generally chose to leave their own lasses to the Neighbours out of the Marshes, and went into the hilly country for a wife: that when they took the young women out of the wholesome fresh air, they were clear and healthy; but when they came into the Marshes amongst the Fogs and Damps, they presently changed complexion, and got an Ague or two, and seldom held it above Half a Year; or a full Year at most. And then, said he, we go to the Uplands again, and fetch another, so that marrying of wives was reckoned a good farm to them".

Another English notable, Sir Walter Raleigh, prayed during his captivity in the Tower that he would not get an ague at the time of his execution as his enemies would claim he was shivering due to fear.

It is claimed that King James I died of malaria in 1625 within a week of being taken ill. There were the usual rumours that he had been poisoned by a Catholic plot to clear the way for his son Charles I who was more sympathetic to the Catholic religion.

Tertian fever or ague was widespread in Europe in the early 1600s and was introduced into the Americas by the Europeans, whilst malignant tertian fever and *P. falciparum* arrived in the tropical Americas with the slave trade. African slaves also brought a number of other diseases with them that require vectors. These became widespread once the appropriate vector became sufficiently numerous to transmit the disease. The most important of these other diseases included dengue fever and yellow fever. Fast ships were essential to avoid too many slaves dying of diseases such as scurvy, typhoid and dysentery during the passage. However, this requirement for fast ships also facilitated the transport of the insect vectors needed to spread many diseases. Whilst the slave trade was reprehensible, to blame the Europeans totally is not acceptable, there was no possibility of this trade continuing to exist without the active participation of local kings and chiefs in West Africa.

In the Americas, malaria became a serious problem. It almost destroyed the Jamestown colony in 1607 and was widespread during the Civil War (1861-1865), when it is thought to have killed more soldiers in the Southern States than were killed in battle. Union troops in malarial areas were given daily prophylactic doses of quinine in whiskey. By the end of the nineteenth century, hundreds of thousands of cases per annum were occurring in the USA. These were greatly reduced by drainage programmes in the early twentieth century although, even as late as 1935, there were approximately 130,000 cases per year causing 4,000 deaths. Drainage of swamps and various other measures had practically eliminated malaria from the USA by 1952.

One of the major problem states until the 1940s (due to the swamps of the Everglades) was Florida where DDT made a large contribution to bringing malaria under control. After this was banned, new insecticides were used as they became available. This level of control comes at a serious cost; the current price of keeping mosquitoes and malaria under control, in Florida alone, is in excess of US$300 million per annum, an amount that is beyond the budget for most countries.

<u>THE DISCOVERY OF QUININE</u>

Rocco gives an excellent account of the discovery and history of quinine. Quinine is derived from the bark of the cinchona tree that grows in South America, and the drug can be extracted by soaking the bark in water. It was first described in Western medicine in the early 1630s by the monk, Antonio de la Calaucha. He wrote that the fever tree that had a cinnamon coloured bark which, when powdered and then dissolved in a drink, cured the agues and tertians. He also mentions that the Inca, who had probably been using it for centuries, took it at high altitudes to stop shivering. This bark became known in Spanish as quina and is reputed to have first been used in western medicine, by the doctor, Juan del Vega, to cure the Countess of Chinchon, wife of the Viceroy of Peru, although there is no documentary evidence to this effect.

It is also mentioned by Bernabé Cobó, a Jesuit priest, who wrote about a *"Tree for the Ague"* in 1639, in his book, *"Historia del Nuevo Mundo"* (History of the New World). He wrote that the bark was powdered and taken in wine, and that samples had been sent to Rome, where it had been used to treat the Pope. The first record of a shipment of cinchona bark to Europe is in 1631.

The Jesuits were well aware of its properties, and for a long time it was known as Jesuit's bark or Jesuit's powder. It was highly valued in Europe from the mid-seventeenth century, and many doctors knew that Jesuit's bark could reduce fever. The name, Jesuit's bark or powder, was unfortunate as it added a religious dimension, which was not a good sales pitch in Protestant England of the seventeenth century, because of the association with papism.

These problems peaked in 1652 when a doctor, Jean-Jaques Chiflet, treated the Archduke Leopold of Austria for fever using Jesuits bark. The treatment initially controlled the fever but it re-occurred a month later. Instead of taking a second dose, the Archduke was so annoyed that he ordered Chiflet to write a book denigrating cinchona bark as fraudulent. This duly appeared in 1653 and was a major success in Protestant Europe, which considered that anything controlled by the Jesuits was suspicious to say the least. The Jesuits responded with their own book, *"Vindication of the Peruvian Powder"*, which countered all of Chiflet's arguments. This in turn was countered by a response from Vopiscus Plempius, a physician who had earlier attacked Harvey for his work on the circulation of blood. Plempius quoted Hippocrates, Galen and Avicenna and pointed out that they had not mentioned powders from

Peru, which is not too surprising considering that Peru was not discovered by the Europeans until the first half of the sixteenth century.

Europe divided into two camps over cinchona bark along religious lines. It also divided the older doctors who still followed classical learning from the younger doctors who were starting to realise that Hippocrates, Galen and Avicenna were wrong over numerous aspects of medicine.

It is frequently claimed that the arch protestant himself, Oliver Cromwell (1599-1658), Lord Protector of England, who came from the fen region of Eastern England, died of the ague after refusing Jesuit's powder. This is somewhat unlikely unless his spleen had been ruptured, as tertian malaria or ague is rarely fatal, and as a fenland farmer, Cromwell would probably have had it for years and had a reasonable degree of immunity. It has also been suggested that he died of septicaemia or kidney stones, and there were the usual conspiratorial claims that he was poisoned. He was replaced as Lord Protector by his son Richard, who was totally incapable of ruling England[192], and whose removal paved the way for the restoration of the Monarchy in 1660.

One of the main advocates of Jesuits bark in England in the seventeenth century was Robert Talbor. Talbor who was born in 1642, was apprenticed to an apothecary in Cambridge where he studied how to regulate the dosage of quinine. In 1670, he opened a shop in London specialising in the treatment of fevers and to publicise himself wrote a tract which opens with the following poem.

> *"The Learned Author in a generous Fit*
> *T'oblige his Country hath of Agues writ:*
> *Physicians now shall be reproacht no more,*
> *Nor Essex shake with Ague as before*
> *Since certain health salutes her sickly shoar (sic)".*

192   He was incompetent to the point that he was nicknamed "Tumbledown Dick". After the restoration of the monarchy, he was allowed to retire to the country and live out his life as a simple country gentleman, indicating that no-one regarded him as a threat.

Talbor states in his book that Jesuits powder produces dangerous side effects, but is safe to use if prepared correctly by a skilful hand (i.e. himself). He also received support from Thomas Sydenham, known as the English Hippocrates, who described malaria very accurately and wrote about cinchona bark in *"Observationes medicae"*, insisting that it was the only effective remedy for tertian fever[193]. In 1717, Bernado Ramazzini, doctor to the Duke of Medina, wrote that, *"Cinchona revolutionized the art of medicine as profoundly as gunpowder had revolutionized the art of war"*.

Malaria was obviously a serious problem in England at this time as when Graunt was checking the Bills of Mortality in the seventeenth century, Agues and Fevers were given as the third most common cause of death after tuberculosis and plague.

John Evelyn mentions in his diary that Charles II had the ague and asked for quincunx. In 1678, Talbor treated Charles II so effectively that he was knighted later that year and the Royal College of Physicians was ordered to admit him to membership as one of the king's physicians, which was not bad for some one who had only trained as an apothecary. The ingredients he used to treat the king were kept secret because of the association with papism. Talbor left for the French court of Louis XIV (the Sun King) shortly afterwards as the Popish Plot was coming to a head in England, and anti-Catholic views were growing stronger and more violent. Louis bought Talbor's remedy for a substantial sum of money, the condition being that that it was not published until after Talbor's death. Talbor died in 1681, and the book, *"The English Remedy"*, was published in 1682. The ingredients were Peruvian bark, lemon juice and rose leaves to mask the taste of quinine, the whole lot being mixed up in wine. Talbor changed the wine at regular

---

193   Sydenham also made the connection between insects and ague noting that, *"agues were very bad when insects swarm"*. This was more than two centuries before Ross discovered the role of mosquitoes in the transmission of malaria.

intervals to confuse other doctors and keep them guessing about the ingredients. By this time, Talbor's brother was selling the cure in England at a guinea for two doses, a huge sum of money at the time.

Brandy was still frequently being used as a cure in the seventeenth century, as also was the catchall cure of mercury. Bloodletting was also used as late as the nineteenth century to cure feverish patients and given the damage caused to blood by malaria, it is difficult to think of a more unsuitable treatment.

The Royal Navy used quinine for the prevention of fever from 1771, though it was not widely used by the civilian population for about another sixty years. Cinchona powder is extremely bitter, and it was usually drunk with alcohol as a palliative. In the British Empire, bitter tonic (tonic water containing quinine) was traditionally drunk with gin, to give the popular drink gin and tonic (G & T).

In 1809, the British army sent a large expeditionary force of 40,000 men to Walcheren in Holland, with the intention of capturing the naval base at Antwerp, as part of the campaign against the French during the Napoleonic Wars. This force suffered severe casualties from malaria after the dykes were destroyed and the area flooded. There were over eight thousand cases of malaria within a month. After the expedition was called off, twelve thousand men were left as the garrison of the island of Walcheren, within a few weeks over half of them had malaria. During the whole campaign, just over one hundred men died in battle and approximately four thousand died of malaria. The appalling army medical facilities caused a considerable scandal and led to a significant re-organisation of the army medical services.

The British army also suffered severe losses in the Caribbean and West Africa. In both areas, it was common for more than half the troops deployed to die within a year from either malaria or yellow fever.

During the nineteenth century, there were numerous attempts to penetrate to the interior of Africa, using the major rivers, the Congo, Zambesi and Niger as highways. These were all unsuccessful because of the expedition members becoming infected with fevers. One typical expedition in 1841, on the River Niger, recorded that some ninety per cent of the Europeans became sick with fever and over a third died, whereas none of the Africans recruited locally became sick and of the Africans who were not recruited locally, about forty per cent became sick but all recovered.

In 1854, William Bakie, a doctor on board a ship exploring the River Niger dosed all members of the expedition with quinine daily and did not lose a single man to fever. He stressed in his reports that this was a prophylactic dose and not being used to cure fevers. Basically, this one expedition opened up Africa to European expansion that until then had been stopped by fever.

Ross (see later) alluded to this when he was writing to Manson. "[Malaria] *is important not only because of the misery it inflicts upon mankind, but also because of the serious apposition it has always given to the march of civilisation. No wild deserts, no savage races, no geographical difficulties have proved so inimical to civilisation as this disease*".

The incidence of malaria started to fall in Northern Europe, especially England, in the late eighteenth and nineteenth centuries, although it was still common in the mid-nineteenth century. This was largely due to changes in farming practices. The species of mosquito that is the most effective vector of malaria in Europe prefers to feed on cattle. If enough cattle are present, then the cycle of infection is broken as the plasmodium causing human malaria cannot develop in cattle. As the level of cattle farming increased, malaria started to disappear; although mosquitoes were still plentiful they were no longer carrying malaria. Malaria continued in the Mediterranean area where it was difficult to produce sufficient fodder crops for cattle because of the lower rainfall in summer and goats were kept more commonly as they can survive on much poorer pasture.

At the same time as this increased farming of cattle took place in England, the fencing of land and a decreased use of common land effectively divided herds into small communities. This reduced the transmission and level of many animal diseases such as rinderpest, brucellosis and bovine tuberculosis, in addition to malaria. Both brucellosis and tuberculosis can be transmitted to humans and around 1750, and unlike France where these changes did not take place, there was a significant improvement in human health in England, leading to a considerable increase in population. This improved agricultural output also produced a significant increase in the wealth of England and funded the technology necessary for the Industrial Revolution to take place. These changes in the distribution of malaria were reinforced by draining marshland for pasture and crops and the increasing availability of quinine.

Major epidemics occurred in Denmark, and in 1831, up to half of the population of some areas of the islands in the Kattegat died. These epidemics also declined after 1862, due to changes in agricultural practice involving cattle.

By the end of the eighteenth century large quantities of cinchona bark were being exported from South America to Europe. The mark-up in prices was huge, twenty to thirty fold if it crossed the Atlantic to Spain and even more when it reached Protestant countries such as England or Holland. The various colonial empires generated a large demand for the powder and by the mid-nineteenth century, the British East India Company was spending over £100,000 per year importing it. This was a vast sum for those days but it came nowhere near satisfying the demand.

South America was the only source of quinine until the 1850s. During the seventeenth and eighteenth centuries it was impossible to visit South America without the permission of Spain, and little was known about the continent as all records were subject to Spanish censorship. In 1735, the Frenchman, Charles-Marie de la Condamine, led a botanical scientific expedition to Peru and in early 1737, he described and drew *Cinchona* in his notebook. These descriptions and drawings reached Europe in 1738, and on the basis of them, Linnaeus put the tree into a new genus. He derived the name *Cinchona* from a misunderstanding of the spelling Chinchon. de la Condamine distinguished three types of *Cinchona* on the basis of the colour of the bark, white, yellow and red; white had no quinine and red had the most[194].

Following a joint Spanish/French expedition that started in 1777, a short monograph on the cinchona tree was published in 1792. The properties of the plant were grossly exaggerated, claiming that the bark cured everything, including smallpox and a host of other diseases. It did however, describe seven species of *Cinchona* and emphasised that not all of them produced quinine.

By the late eighteenth century, the Spanish had started to extract the bark using hot water and sending a paste back to Europe instead of bark. The removal of the bark kills the tree, and by this time it was becoming increasingly difficult to find trees that could be harvested. The Jesuits had initially planted five trees in the shape of a cross for every one harvested, but this early form of sustainable harvesting was ignored after the Jesuits were expelled from the Spanish Empire in 1767. Suggestions that *Cinchona* might grow outside South America were made during the eighteenth century, but not surprisingly, Spain was totally opposed to this idea as it meant the end of their monopoly.

The Spanish empire in South America started to crumble as a result of the Napoleonic Wars in Europe. Peru, Colombia and a number of other countries were independent by the mid-1820s, following prolonged periods of unrest and revolution.

---

194   He also gave one of the first descriptions of collecting latex from rubber trees and using it to make a waterproof covering.

Numerous European countries started to express an interest in growing *Cinchona* outside South America, and in 1852, a reporter, John Royle, working for the British East India Company, wrote to warn that *C. calisaya* forests were being depleted rapidly. Malaria was a serious problem in India for the British in the nineteenth century; it was common to have as many as half the troops incapacitated by the disease and therefore creating a reliable source and supply of quinine was essential. In 1859, a couple of British expeditions managed to obtain *C. calisaya* seedlings and seeds. One led by Richard Spruce went to the Andes and managed to collect specimens that were transported to India where they grew but did not produce quinine. A second expedition led by Sir Clements Markham also managed to get plants out of Peru, but many of them died on the journey to India via London and the rest soon after their arrival.

Charles Ledger arrived in South America in 1836 where he obtained a post as a commodity trader specialising in cinchona bark, and in 1865 an Indian guide, Manuel Mamani, who worked with Ledger brought him a large number of seeds. Ledger sent these to his brother in London who gave some to various parties he thought might be interested, and sold some to the Dutch Consul General. Many of the seeds given away went to India and Ceylon (Sri Lanka) where they did not grow. Those sold to the Dutch were sent to Java, where by 1872, they had formed established plantations, and became the core of the cinchona bark industry.

When the *C. calisaya* trees in Java were mature, they produced about five times as much quinine as the usual *C. calisaya* bark from South America, and following a study, the trees from the seeds provided by Ledger were reclassified as a new species, *C. ledgeriana*. In the first forty years of the twentieth century, these plantations allowed the Dutch to establish a near monopoly on the production and purification of quinine.

The provision of quinine became a major problem in the tropical theatres of war in World War II as Java was the main source. Germany commandeered all the quinine in Holland where it was stored after being sent from Java. The Japanese overran Java soon after they entered the war and the Allies were virtually cut off from a supply of quinine. The Dutch had put an embargo on the export of seeds from Java, but in the 1920s the Americans had arranged for seeds to be smuggled out. These were taken to the Philippines and, by the late 1920s, a plantation of *C. ledgeriana* had been established. This was seized by the Japanese, but not before a supply of seeds had been sent back to the USA where they were germinated and grown. The war was over however before they were sufficiently mature to be harvested.

These problems convinced the Allies that a reliable supply of anti-malarial drugs, that could not be controlled by an enemy, was essential, especially if troops were operating in the tropics. During World War II, the antics of the cartoon characters, Malaria Moe and Anopheles Ann, were used to remind troops in the Pacific that malaria is extremely dangerous and that they should take their medication regularly.

THE DISCOVERY OF THE LIFE CYCLE OF *PLASMODIUM*

French attempts to build the Panama Canal from 1881 to 1888 had been abandoned because of the costs, and as a result of the death of many staff from malaria and yellow fever. When the Americans built the canal that opened in 1914, the first steps in the building work were to control the mosquito population. The control of malaria and yellow fever in the building of the Panama Canal is dealt with in the chapter on yellow fever.

The French physician, Charles Alphonse Laveran, a doctor for the French Foreign Legion, was the first person to show the presence of *Plasmodium* in human red blood cells in 1880, and recognise it as the cause of malaria. He did not make the connection between humans and mosquitoes and was therefore unable to explain how the parasite spread from victim to victim. As a result of this, Laveran was not believed initially by the medical establishment including a number of doctors specialising in malaria. Koch was extremely dismissive of his theories that were not accepted for a number of years.

In the 1890s, an Italian, Battista Grassi, discovered that other vertebrate species, especially birds, also suffered from malaria, but the importance of this discovery was not realised at the time. Grassi suspected that mosquitoes had something to do with the transmission of malaria in birds, but he looked at the wrong genera of mosquito. The plasmodium causing avian malaria could not survive in the mosquitoes he studied. Ross also used birds later for many of his studies.

Ronald Ross (1857-1932), a British Army doctor, discovered the life cycle of *Plasmodium* whilst working in Calcutta. He read an article suggesting that *Plasmodium* might exist in mosquitoes, but the suggestion had been discredited. After several dead-ends studying *Culex* (a genus of mosquito that does not transmit human malaria), and following discussions with Manson (Ch 4), Ross was able to show, in 1898, that the disease was carried by mosquitoes of the genus *Anopheles*. Manson, who had specialised in tropical parasitic diseases including filarial worms, had been able to show that these were found in mosquitoes. Manson's big mistake however was that he believed that mosquitoes only had one blood meal during their lives, and that people contracted filariasis by drinking polluted water that had somehow become contaminated by infected mosquitoes. Alternatively, he considered that the dead contaminated mosquitoes would fall into water where the parasite would be taken up by the developing mosquito larvae, and would appear in the mosquito after metamorphosis.

Ross's crucial discovery was that mosquitoes feeding on the blood of malarial patients form cysts in their stomachs, and that these cysts released sporozoites that migrated to the salivary glands of the mosquito. Those mosquitoes fed on blood from non-malarial patients did not form cysts. The demonstration that the sporozoites could migrate from the stomach to the salivary glands thus explained how malaria could be transmitted from one victim to another. In a key communication, Ross wrote to Manson, *"Malaria is conveyed from a diseased person or bird to a healthy one by the proper species of mosquito, and it is inoculated by its bite"*.

Ross and Laveran were awarded Nobel prizes for medicine for their work on malaria, Ross in 1902 and Laveran in 1907. There was a considerable amount of unpleasantness over these awards as many people considered that Manson and Grassi should have shared the prizes.

CONTROL OF MALARIA.

Malaria is not tropical neither is it under control. It is now contained in the USA and Europe but only by the application of constant and expensive public health measures. Changing patterns of climate and rainfall have increased the risk of catching it in several parts of the world that were once relatively safe.

The record of the World Health Organisation in the area of malaria control is not a good one. In the 1950s, the WHO declared that malaria would soon reach a stage where it would no longer be of major importance. By 1998, there was an estimated minimum of 300 million cases worldwide, and malaria was completely out of control.

There are a number of possible strategies for controlling malaria.

- Destroy the vector. This is possible by the use of several methods. One of these is spraying using insecticides to kill the adult mosquito. This was done widely during World War II using DDT (dichloro-diphenyl-trichloroethane). The programme was very effective until it was realised how toxic DDT was to other wildlife, and in 1969, the WHO decided to discontinue the use

595

of DDT due to environmental damage. The use of other less toxic insecticides such as the pyrethrums is possible. These are naturally occurring and biodegradable but they are considerably more expensive than DDT.

- One method of chemical treatment which is environmentally friendly, is to treat bodies of water containing mosquito larvae with a so-called juvenile hormone, which keeps the larvae in a juvenile state and stops them developing into adults. A further method of the same type is the baiting of traps with sex pheromones (hormones), which attract adults into traps where they can be destroyed.

- In Mexico, it has been found that mosquitoes breed in riverside pools sheltering in the alga, *Spirogyra*. This grows as long strands and its removal by labourers with rakes causes a considerable fall in the number of mosquitoes breeding, and a similar fall in the incidence of malaria.

- Insect vectors can also be controlled by irradiating huge numbers of males to sterilise them (the so-called dud stud solution). These are released into the wild, where they swamp the fertile males during the breeding season. As the female only mates once, if she mates with an infertile male then she cannot mate again, and does not produce fertile eggs, thus reducing mosquito numbers.

- Mosquitoes require stagnant water to breed. Control can be applied at this level in several ways. In many places, the introduction of fish to eat the mosquito larvae not only controls the malaria, but also provides a source of high quality protein. Stagnant water can also be drained, a solution used by Mussolini to drain the Pontine

Marshes around Rome which greatly reduced malaria in the region. This approach does however involve massive changes in the ecosystem, and such methods frequently trigger environmental lawsuits.

- A further control attempt has involved a biological control system using the bacterium, *Bacillus thuringensis,* which produces a toxin lethal to insects but harmless to other species.

- Mosquito larvae hang onto the underside of the water surface by making use of the surface tension then push a breathing tube through the surface. It is possible to kill the larvae by the addition of a thin layer of oil to the water, this reduces the surface tension and the larvae fall to the bottom and drown.

- Control is also possible by preventing the female mosquito feeding. Mosquitoes feed at night and the incidence rate of bites can be greatly reduced by wearing long trousers and long sleeved shirts. The use of screens on windows and mosquito netting around beds reduces the rate of infection considerably, whilst the mosquito nets can also be impregnated with long lasting insecticides such as permethrin. This is a two-step process, it provides the human population with protection against infected mosquitoes and also stops infected people passing *Plasmodium* to non-infected mosquitoes. The use of fans to create a draught is also effective as many species of mosquitoes prefer to feed in still air. Some experts have reservations about the use of nets and consider that, although they may reduce childhood infections of malaria, they actually increase malaria mortality in the long term. In high incidence areas, children under the age of about five catch malaria and some die. As the survivors get older, immunity appears and they start to live with malaria. It has been suggested that the use of impregnated bed nets may interfere with the development of immunity, and malaria susceptibility shifts to the older group, producing an even higher death toll. Whilst it may seem very unsympathetic to suggest it, a percentage of childhood deaths may be the price a society has to pay for a malaria-tolerant adult community.

- Control using drugs is becoming less effective. There are a relatively small number of drugs effective against malaria and resistance to these is rising rapidly. Even those drugs that do work are not very effective because of the multiple stages of malaria in the body. Drugs effective against one stage frequently do not work against other stages.

- A number of trials are being carried out using vaccines. It is too early to be certain about the efficacy of these vaccines, but initial results suggest that some of them may have a partial effect.

- The smell of individuals also appears to be important. Studies show that about twenty per cent of humans receive approximately eighty per cent of mosquito bites. Mosquitoes are attracted by carbon dioxide and various other chemicals produced in perspiration and anti-mosquito creams and sprays containing chemicals, such as DEET (di-ethyl toluamide), are effective at masking human odours. This compound was originally developed by the US army in the 1940s, for use in jungle warfare.

<u>THE ROLE OF DDT IN THE CONTROL OF MALARIA</u>

There have been a number of attempts to kill mosquitoes using chemicals, one of the early ones being a mixture of copper salts (used widely in the 1920s and 30s and known as Paris green), which killed the mosquito larvae. As a preparation of copper, it would have caused considerable ecological damage.

Paul Muller, a Swiss chemist working for Geigy synthesised and patented DDT, originally known as Neocide, in the 1930s, for which he was awarded the Nobel Prize in 1948. It was the most effective insecticide that had been synthesised until then, was cheap to produce, and killed insects for up to a year after application to a surface, unlike other insecticides that had to be reapplied frequently.

DDT was used widely in World War II in a number of spheres for the control of malaria, and other vector-borne diseases such as typhus, and achieved a marked success in these objectives. It was used in North Africa for delousing prisoners in 1943, and also in Sicily, where there was an outbreak of typhus after the allies captured it. In Sardinia, over 250 tonnes were used to control a malaria epidemic in 1946. In Greece, malaria was a major problem in 1942, but was virtually eliminated by 1948 using DDT. After DDT was banned, the mosquitoes returned and are now DDT resistant.

The World Health Organisation was created in 1948 as the health arm of the United Nations, and in 1955 it announced a plan for The Global Eradication of Malaria. From 1958-63, a worldwide programme to eliminate malaria was undertaken, which to a great extent was based on the application of large quantities of DDT. The WHO claimed that malaria would be eliminated by the 1990s, although it had been suggested as early as 1956 that it would only take seven years for mosquitoes to become resistant to DDT.

DDT works by destroying the nervous system of the mosquito and other insects. It is an extremely long-lasting insecticide and is still effective a year after spraying. Mosquitoes rest after taking a blood meal, and the theory therefore was that if all the surfaces that mosquitoes landed on were sprayed, the mosquitoes would be destroyed and the cycle of infection would be broken. Mathematical calculations "proved" that if every house were sprayed in an endemic area, malaria would be eliminated within five years. After that, spraying could be discontinued apart from a few problem areas. However, a series of problems occurred demonstrating that theory is one thing and practice is a totally different matter.

In 1962, Rachel Carson published her book, *"Silent Spring"*, publicising the toxicity of DDT and challenging the assertion that it was safe. She prophesied that the misuse of insecticides in agriculture would lead to widespread insect resistance to these chemicals, and endanger efforts to control malaria and various other insect-borne diseases. The Food and Drug Administration had warned as early as 1950 that the potential hazard of DDT was being under-estimated.

Carson wrote, *"Spraying* [with DDT] *kills the weaklings" "the only survivors are insects that have some inherent quality that allows them to escape harm". "The "control of Nature" is a phrase conceived in arrogance, born of a Neanderthal age of biology and philosophy when it was supposed that nature exists for the convenience of man". "The concepts and practice of applied entomology for the most part date from the Stone Age of science. It is our alarming misfortune that so primitive a science has armed itself with the most modern and terrible weapons, and that in turning them against the insects, it has also turned them against the earth".* It was powerful and emotional prose and the result was that in 1972, the Environmental Protection Agency was formed and one of their first steps was to ban the use and synthesis of DDT in the USA. It is now made only in China and India for use solely against malaria.

DDT was very effective in the fight against malaria, it is very potent, it kills mosquitoes quickly, is cheap to manufacture and use, and remains active for months after spraying. The major problem in the utilisation of DDT was its indiscriminate use by farmers spraying it on crops in large quantities; the general farming consensus was that if a small amount is good, a large amount must be better.

The WHO was (and still is) politically naïve, and like most large bureaucratic organisations it has great difficulty in responding quickly, bending rules and adapting to local conditions. Much of sub-Saharan Africa was (and still is) a war zone and no-go area that was impossible to spray; the WHO could not admit this, or funding would not have been available. Over a period of time, mosquitoes became resistant to DDT as predicted, and more or less simultaneously *Plasmodium* became resistant to chloroquine, the most commonly used anti-malarial drug. The WHO finally admitted it had lost the battle in 1968, and abandoned its mosquito eradication programme in 1972.

Newer synthetic insecticides such as the pyrethrums based on chemicals found in chrysanthemum flowers were developed in the 1970s. These degrade rapidly and are not persistent in the environment, but they are more expensive to manufacture and mosquitoes quickly become resistant to them. A more recent move in this direction has been to spray surfaces with a suspension of fungal spores known to kill mosquitoes, a form of bio-control.

The problems of mosquito control were exacerbated in the 1960s, when the World Bank backed the idea of a Green Revolution to improve Third World economies, by increasing the production of cash crops. Thousands of hectares of land, growing a wide variety of local basic food crops, were replanted into monoculture crops such as coffee, rice, tea and a number of luxury fruits. The growth of many of these crops requires increased irrigation and in the case of rice, paddy fields. Mosquitoes flourished in these and the irrigation canals. When there is plant diversity, an area is also diverse in insect life, there are plenty of predators and no single insect pest is able to dominate the environment. As plant diversity falls, insect predation is reduced and monoculture crops are rapidly destroyed by large numbers of insect pests. The response of farmers is to use more insecticide that kills beneficial insects and damages the food chain up to birds, and a vicious cycle starts. Pesticides such as DDT are used in ever increasing amounts, and resistant mosquitoes and other pest species start to appear.

By 1963, mosquitoes had been more or less eradicated in many countries and malaria had been eliminated from areas such as the USA, Russia, and Europe and greatly reduced in much of the tropics. As far as malaria control is concerned, if malaria is removed from a community and then reappears, resistance has been lost, herd immunity has fallen and the population is more vulnerable than it was previously. One of the problems is that immunity to malaria only builds up slowly, but if an immune individual loses contact with the parasite, they lose their resistance very quickly.

The Indian subcontinent is a classic example of what happened; in 1958, the Malaria Eradication Campaign, backed by the WHO, started using DDT to eliminate mosquitoes. It was estimated that within three years, eighty million cases of malaria had fallen to less than one hundred thousand. By 1965, India was spending one third of its health budget on attempts to control malaria. The programme was disrupted by two wars between India and Pakistan in 1965 and 1970-1 and the cession of Bangladesh (Eastern Pakistan) from Western Pakistan. Spraying was stopped, there was a massive resurgence of malaria in the early 1970s, and by 1977, the number of cases had risen to an estimated thirty million. Communities that had once had a high level of resistance to malaria had now lost their immunity, but lived in areas where mosquitoes returned when the eradication programme stopped. Millions of people became freshly exposed to malaria, and the scale of the problem was increased by the resistance of *Plasmodium* to chloroquine and other anti-malarial drugs.

A similar situation occurred in Sri Lanka (Ceylon), severe malaria outbreaks in the 1930s killed large numbers. DDT was used widely in 1945, and by 1964 malaria had been virtually eliminated from the island; spraying was stopped in the mid 1960s. A civil war started between the Singhalese and Tamil populations in 1983 that did not end until 2009, and malaria is now as widespread as ever.

By the 1960s, it was realised that, *"Eradication does not appear practical in the near future",* the funding dried up and the mosquito eradication programme was reduced. The WHO admitted that it was beaten, and in 1969, officially recognised the failure of the eradication programme. By 1995, the incidence of malaria in many countries was double or treble what it had been in 1961. The mosquito and *Plasmodium* had won in spite of everything that modern science could throw at them.

The result is that the worldwide distribution of malaria today does not look very different to what it was in the middle of the twentieth century, before attempts to eradicate the mosquito. A few countries around the Mediterranean such as Greece, and islands such as Sicily and Sardinia remain free of malaria, but the main difference is that the modern map shows that most malarial countries now have drug resistant malaria and DDT resistant mosquitoes that were not present fifty to sixty years ago.

In an attempt to deal with the problem the WHO sponsored a, *"Roll Back Malaria",* campaign in 1998 which pledged that sixty per cent of African children would be sleeping under mosquitoes nets by 2003. By 2001, the figure was less than fifteen per cent. This again ignores the realities of life. Sleeping under a mosquito net in a hot, humid tropical climate is very unpleasant, and just because people have been given mosquito nets impregnated with an insecticide does not mean they will use them.

Another major problem in sub-Saharan Africa is the rapid rise in urban malaria. By about 2025, approximately fifty per cent of the population will live in cities, and generally an urban population has a lower resistance to malaria than a rural one.

ANTI-MALARIAL DRUGS

One of the main problems of using drugs to combat malaria is that the *Plasmodium* has the same basic cell structure as the human cell, they are both eucaryotic cells. This makes it considerably more difficult to find drugs that show selective toxicity, that is, they will attack *Plasmodium* without having any effect on the human cell.

Modern day medicine is losing the fight against *Plasmodium* which has developed multiple resistance to a number of widely used drugs, even although these drugs were very efficient when they were first introduced.

As mentioned earlier, quinine was the original anti-malarial drug. It reached England in the 1650s and by the last decade of the eighteenth century, Britain was importing about fifty-five tons of *Cinchona* bark per year. There was considerable controversy over its efficacy as it is a natural product and the quality varied widely from batch to batch.

The complicated chemistry of quinine, which is an alkaloid, made it impossible to synthesise commercially. It also produces some unpleasant side-effects such as jaundice, nausea, deafness, headaches and vomiting especially in pregnant women. One major problem with both quinine and some of its derivatives is that they dampen the antibody response to numerous other diseases rendering the individual more susceptible to those diseases. During the 1940s, various synthetic quinine related drugs (proguanil [paludrine] and chloroquine) became available on a commercial scale; these work in a similar way to quinine but with less unpleasant side effects. However, a major problem, with quinine and its derivatives is that once the parasite becomes resistant to one, it recognises the others very quickly and becomes resistant to them also. The result is that the development of new quinine-based drugs rapidly becomes a case of the law of diminishing returns.

Ehrlich (Ch 3) had shown that the dye methylene blue, a derivative of the coal tar industry, had some activity against malaria. This was modified chemically to give mepacrin (atebrin) that became the first synthetic anti-malarial compound. It was made in Germany by I. G. Farben Industries in the 1930s and became the major anti-malarial of World War II. This also produces side-effects, it turns the patient bright yellow and also causes diarrhoea and vomiting. In addition, many troops refused to take it during the war as it was reputed to cause impotence. Mepacrine is more effective than quinine and was used widely in the 1950s to treat quinine-resistant malaria. It was particularly successful in dealing with blackwater fever, the most dangerous form of malaria.

By this time, the malarial parasite had developed wide spread resistance to quinine, and resistance to chloroquine developed rapidly during the 1950s. It is now useless in many parts of the world, although it is still used very widely. In the 1960s, table salt was medicated with chloroquine and another drug, pyrimethamine, to dose entire populations and eliminate malaria. Unfortunately, the parasite rapidly became resistant to pyrimethamine and although chloroquine did better, the combination of chloroquine with salt is not effective. In addition, the uptake of salt by young children, who are the major victims of malaria, tends to be low. The overall result of this programme was to merely increase the rate at which resistance to chloroquine and pyrimethamine developed, and *P. falciparum* is now resistant to chloroquine in virtually all areas where it is endemic.

Mefloquine (lariam) was introduced in the early 1990s. It is now used widely and initially proved to be very effective against malaria that had become resistant to other drugs such as quinine and chloroquine. It rapidly became the drug of first choice for destinations with drug-resistant malaria, and is also used in combination with artemisinin, but this is a very expensive option. Lariam does however cause unpleasant side effects in many people and dangerous ones in a few, especially those with psychiatric problems. From 1995, growing reports of the harmful effects meant lariam became less popular. Resistance to lariam is now also starting to appear in South-East Asia.

A relative newcomer to the malaria battle is malarone, a combination of two drugs, atovaquone and proguanil (paludrine). This combination is extremely effective and acts as a prophylactic, which means that it is effective against plasmodium at the point where the parasite is injected into the body or shortly afterwards. Other drugs tend to act at a much later stage in the development of the parasite, and therefore one key practical benefit is that malarone only needs to be taken during exposure, and for a short period afterwards. Most other drugs need to be taken for at least four weeks after leaving a malarial area.

A variety of other drugs are in use now in attempts to control malaria, the drug of choice depending to some extent on the area involved. In some areas, a combination of sulphadoxine-pyrimethamine (fansidar) is first choice. This is only twice as expensive as chloroquine (which is about the cheapest of the drugs available), but in many areas *P. falciparum* is resistant to it.

Artemisinin, an extract of sweet wormwood (*Artemesia annua)*, has been used for centuries in traditional Chinese medicine. Artemisinin is best given with other anti-malarials such as mefloquine, as artemisinin combination therapy (ACT). The cost however is high, approximately twenty times as high as chloroquine. Although it is a very effective anti-malarial, the cost is a serious factor when the national budget for health is only a few dollars per person per year. Theoretically

ACT should make it more difficult for the parasite to evolve resistance, however people do not follow instructions, especially the poor and illiterate, and frequently revert to a single drug which is cheaper.

Chemically, artemisinin is a very unusual compound containing two oxygen atoms joined together in a manner that is normally unstable. The molecule is now being synthesised worldwide, but resistance to this drug is already being described in the medical literature, especially in Cambodia. Bitter experience suggests that the *Plasmodium* will rapidly develop widespread resistance to artemisinin-based drugs, especially if they are used incorrectly, i.e. as the sole component of the treatment being given. It has been suggested that to circumvent the problem of cost, African countries should be supplied with high yielding varieties of *A. annua* suitable for growth in Africa, which should then be taken as a herbal remedy as used in traditional Chinese medicine.

A recent development in the production of artemisinin has been the elucidation of the genetic code of *Artemisia annua*. This will enable researchers to produce high yielding varieties of the plant thus circumventing the shortage of the drug that is starting to occur.

A new drug Riamet is being marketed by the Swiss company Novatis in combination with the Chinese government. This is a combination of artemether and synthetic drugs, which has not yet been approved by the FDA and is also too expensive for many third world countries. A number of these have threatened to make it, patent or no patent.

A further problem in the use of drugs to treat diseases in general, and malaria in particular, is the increasing problem with counterfeit drugs being produced by criminal gangs in third world countries. These are being sold as the genuine article with packaging that is frequently sufficiently good to fool the companies making the genuine product. It has been estimated that in certain parts of the developing world, over fifty per cent of drugs sold over the counters of pharmacies fall into this category. In spite of a highly efficient surveillance system, they have even appeared in high street shops in Britain on a small number of occasions. These counterfeit products are either totally fraudulent or not of the correct potency, and if used to treat a condition they are ineffective. Worse still, if the requisite potency is not used, they speed up the evolution of resistant strains of the parasite.

A further problem is people purchasing drugs, that can normally only be obtained by prescription, over the internet. Many of these drugs are also counterfeit or not of the requisite strength.

One future possibility for an anti-malarial drug is that *Plasmodium* contains an organelle known as the plastid, and DNA analysis shows that this is related to the chloroplast found in green algae. Plastids were presumably incorporated into the ancestral plasmodium, and are now an essential part of the plasmodium cell. The interest in this organelle is that it contains a metabolic pathway known as the shikimic acid pathway. This is not found in humans but does occur in plants and this pathway is attacked by the herbicide, glyphosphate. This offers a selectively toxic situation and raises the interesting possibility that it may be possible to develop a modified weed-killer that will kill plasmodium in humans.

As a final word on malaria, in recent years a number of charitable organisations, such the Bill and Melinda Gates Foundation, have been pouring large sums of money into the control of malaria and other diseases. Given the results of past attempts to control malaria, although they may well have some success and beneficial effects in the short term, in the long term my money is on the mosquito and *Plasmodium* to circumvent any measures taken to control them.

TRYPANOSOMIASIS

Trypanosomiasis or African Sleeping Sickness is another serious protozoan disease limiting the areas available to man and his domestic species south of the Sahara. The first known reference to it is by ibn Khaldun, a famous Arab traveller of the fourteenth century, who refers to the disease of sleeping sickness killing the ruler of Mali in 1373. There are further accounts in the eighteenth century, one in 1794, mentions that slave dealers could identify victims by their enlarged glands and would refuse to purchase any slave showing the symptoms.

The parasite is a flagellate of the genus *Trypanosomas,* and is carried by flies of the genus *Glossinia* (tsetse fly); several varieties of trypanosome are found causing various forms of the disease, each carried by different species of the fly. The infected fly remains a vector for life (one to six months) and requires a meal of blood each day; it feeds by day, and injects the protozoan when it bites its victim. Sleeping sickness is initially a blood disease, but after a period of time (varying from two months to two years), the parasite crosses into the brain and cerebrospinal fluid. At this point, the symptoms become headaches, lethargy and coma followed by death; once the trypanosome enters the Central Nervous System, the prognosis is very poor.

The protozoan is found widely in wild animals, where it causes very little problem, but domesticated animals are highly susceptible to it, the animal version of the disease being known as nagana or stallion sickness. This probably played a major role in confining the Arabs of East Africa to the coastal areas as it stopped them using cavalry in the interior; neither domesticated horses nor cattle could survive. It also probably curtailed early hunting by humans by restricting areas of settlement.

Sir David Bruce established the epidemiology in the last decade of the nineteenth century, and the organism responsible was demonstrated by Bruce and Count Aldo Castellani in 1903. Dutch and English settlers in South Africa and Zimbabwe (Rhodesia) recognised dangerous areas from practical experience. They made the link between wild and domesticated animals and the breeding areas of the fly, which is bush around water holes and river banks. They understood that avoiding or clearing these areas greatly reduced the problems.

David Livingstone remained free of the disease, in spite of being bitten over a thirty year period which suggests that much of Africa was relatively free of the human form in the mid-nineteenth century. However, major epidemics in the Congo between 1895-1905 killed an estimated half a million people with missionaries reporting numerous villages deserted, whilst twenty thousand died in Uganda in 1901, which also suffered another major epidemic in 1907. Although some control over the disease had been established by the 1960s, since then there has been a significant increase in areas affected due to political instability. Sleeping sickness is now out of control in areas of Uganda and the Sudan. There are an estimated fifty million people at risk of the disease, with 300,000 new cases occurring per year.

The widespread animal reservoirs mean it will never be totally eliminated. Attempts at control include killing the flies using insecticides and traps baited with pheromones, eliminating the game reservoirs near human habitation and the use of drugs. It is not possible to use methods such as sleeping under mosquito nets as the flies bite by day.

Very little research is being carried out on the use of drugs to control this disease. One of the main problems is that although there are a number of drugs that will kill the trypanosomes in the blood, there are very few that will kill them once they have penetrated the brain. Most of the drugs available cannot cross from the blood into the brain.

Laveran (of mosquito fame) showed that rats can be infected with trypanosomes making them a suitable test species, and in 1902, he showed that sodium arsenite was an effective treatment in this species. This led to the development of a number of arsenic containing drugs such as atoxyl and tryparsamide. Both were effective on early stage trypanosomiasis but were highly toxic, blinding a considerable percentage of those treated. A further problem was that the trypanosomes became resistant to arsenic containing drugs very quickly. One relatively non-toxic arsenic containing compound was salvarsan, but this still only cures the early stages and was much more useful against syphilis. In 1903, Erlich found that the dye trypan red cured the early stages of trypanosomiasis and a derivative of this was suramin, which is still used today.

The drug of choice now is eflornithine. This is not cheap, nor is it easy to administer as it requires an intravenous drip for a minimum of fourteen days. It does however cross into the brain and will save people previously regarded as terminal cases. The cost of the treatment however, is roughly $1,000 in areas where the annual income of a family is only a few hundred dollars. There is little or no economic incentive for drug companies to find alternatives as the poor, who are most at risk, cannot afford to pay for them.

CHAPTER 17

Yellow Fever and Dengue Fever

The virus causing yellow fever is a member of the sub-group known as flaviviruses. These belong to the arbo-viruses, a term short for arthropod-borne viruses. Arbo-viruses all need an arthropod vector to carry them from one host to another, for example, an insect, tick or mite. The viruses can be divided on the basis of the type of disease they cause, one group which includes yellow fever, causing haemorrhagic fevers that are frequently fatal. The geographical distribution of the arbo-viruses, and the diseases they cause, is determined by the geographical range of the vector involved.

Yellow fever was shown to be a viral disease in 1927 by a team that included the South African doctor, Max Theiler (1899-1972). Theiler later received the Nobel Prize in Medicine in 1951 for his work on developing a vaccine for yellow fever. A number of laboratory workers developing the vaccine died from accidental "needle-stick" injuries. Theiler also caught the disease, but survived.

Yellow fever is caused by an RNA virus transmitted mainly by the mosquito species, *Aedes aegypt,* and *Ae. africanus,* although other species of mosquito, such as *Ae. albopictus* (the Asian tiger mosquito) have also been implicated, as have mosquitoes of the genus *Haemogogus* in South America. The infected mosquito bites a susceptible person, the virus passes into their blood and the disease develops over a period of about ten days. If the infected person is bitten by a second mosquito, then that mosquito also becomes infected.

The symptoms include fever, chills, joint pains and severe

headaches followed by nausea and projectile vomiting. There is frequently a short period of remission around the third or fourth day, but the virus then attacks the liver and the victim develops severe jaundice about the fifth day, hence the name of the disease. In serious cases, internal haemorrhaging occurs, and the vomit turns black from degraded blood, giving the alternative name of the disease used widely in earlier times, *"the black vomit"* or occasionally the Spanish version, *"vomito negro"*. Yellow fever is also the historical origin of the yellow flag carried by ships to warn of infectious disease on board, producing another name for the disease, *"yellow jack"* as the flag was flown from the jack staff of the ship. The association between yellow fever and ships trading from the tropics was recognised at a very early stage.

Once yellow fever has progressed to the stage of black vomiting it is usually fatal, with death occurring from liver or kidney failure. There are no effective drugs against it even today and therapy is aimed mainly at reducing the fever, controlling the pain and preventing the patient from dehydrating. The mortality rate is about 10-15% for non-immunised adults and considerably higher for non-immunised children. If the infected person recovers they are immune to the disease for life.

The recognition and reporting of the disease are poor due to the similarity of yellow fever to a number of other diseases such as viral hepatitis and malaria. The inadequate medical facilities of many of the regions in which yellow fever is found do not allow the blood tests and serology required to confirm the pathology. The WHO consider that the number of cases reported are probably only 0.1-10% of those actually occurring. The latest figures suggest that there are 200,000 cases and thirty thousand deaths per year. Many countries are reluctant to report cases because of the threat to travel restrictions, quarantine problems and the negative effects on trade and tourism.

Two different epidemiologies are recognised for yellow fever. The first is classical or urban yellow fever, and the second is sylvan or jungle yellow fever. Urban yellow fever consists of a cycle involving a human host and the mosquito, *Ae. aegypti,* with the virus being passed from human to mosquito to human. Established colonies of *Ae. aegypti* are essential for urban yellow fever, and as this species of mosquito has a maximum flight range of only a few hundred yards, eradication of colonies gives an effective method of disease control in cities. It is able to breed in very small amounts of water, such as would be found in discarded tyres or cans and epidemics therefore usually follow extended periods of rain. It must also be warm as *Ae. aegypti* does not survive cold temperatures. Once infected, the mosquito remains infectious for life whilst infected humans are only infectious for about five to six days. The entire disease cycle in humans lasts about ten days (if the victim survives), although this is followed by a long period of lethargy and weakness.

Jungle yellow fever, which was not identified until the 1930s, is mainly a disease of monkeys, although it is also found in a few other species of vertebrate. It is transmitted from monkey to monkey by mosquitoes of a variety of genera. These mosquitoes inhabit the forest canopy and the disease usually stays in the canopy infecting only monkeys. When trees are felled the mosquito comes down to ground level and feeds on the nearest available primate host. The usual victims are lumberjacks or cut and slash farmers working in the forest, however, if these people visit local towns or villages, they can initiate a widespread outbreak of urban yellow fever transmitted by *Ae. aegypti*. The presence of jungle yellow fever in monkeys, living over vast areas of Central America and tropical Africa, means that it will never be possible to completely eradicate the disease in humans. It also suggests that yellow fever was originally a disease of monkeys that has spread to humans.

The only effective method of controlling jungle yellow fever is immunisation of individuals likely to be exposed.

Today, yellow fever is mainly found in rural areas of Africa and Central and South America[195], but it was originally a disease of West Africa, where it contributed significantly to the nickname of the area, *"White Man's Grave"*. The virus and the mosquitoes responsible for spreading it were carried to the Americas by the slave trade in the mid-seventeenth century, and it was a significant epidemiological factor in the New World from the seventeenth to the early twentieth centuries. Some authors have suggested that yellow fever first appeared in South America, and then made its way to Africa, as it was described in the Americas one hundred years earlier than in Africa. However, South American Indians and monkeys are highly susceptible to the disease, whereas West African humans and primates show a high level of resistance. There are also very few species of mosquito in the New World, but a large number of species in the Old World, suggesting that mosquitoes have had a long time to diverge in the Old World, but were only imported into the New World as a small number of species in relatively recent evolutionary time.

The disease therefore existed in West Africa, where it was not recognised, as a childhood infection in an indigenous population with a high level of immunity. There was considerable confusion between malaria and yellow fever from the seventeenth century onwards, and it is possible that it was masked by blackwater fever, the most deadly form of malaria, which is also widespread in West Africa. It is generally so mild in indigenous children in West Africa that it is frequently still misdiagnosed as malaria.

Epidemics occur in Africa at regular intervals and indeed are increasing steadily, both in frequency and the area covered. One of the worst epidemics in the twentieth century was in Ethiopia in 1962, with an estimated one hundred thousand

---

195   Immunological studies show that the African and South American versions of the virus are identical.

cases and 35,000 deaths. This was eventually brought under control by mass vaccination programmes. A series of epidemics have also occurred in Nigeria over the last fifty years or so, and in 1992 there was an epidemic in Kenya, the first in East Africa for twenty-six years.

The risk of the disease is increasing in Latin America, where the numbers of *Ae. aegypti* were greatly reduced in the middle part of the twentieth century by a concerted anti-mosquito campaign in many countries. However, mosquitoes are now recovering in large numbers in South America, and *Ae. albopictus* is spreading rapidly. There was a significant increase of yellow fever in the 1990s with Peru being one of the worst affected areas. *Ae. albopictus* is also spreading throughout the USA, where it first appeared in 1985, and is causing serious concern. *Ae. aegypti* only bites humans and therefore only transmits human diseases such as yellow fever, *Ae. albopictus* however, is an extremely aggressive mosquito which bites a wide variety of vertebrate hosts, and is therefore able to transmit a number of diseases from other vertebrates to human hosts. These include the West Nile virus which is found in birds, and both Western and Eastern equine encephalitis which occur in horses. All three have caused a number of cases and deaths in the USA in the last decade.

The size of yellow fever epidemics in both Africa and South America is related to the size of the vector population, and any factor favouring the breeding of mosquitoes, for example, an exceptionally wet rainy season results in an increased number of cases.

For some unknown reason, yellow fever has never spread to the Indian subcontinent or South East Asia, even though *Ae. aegypti* and a number of other species of mosquito capable of carrying the disease are widespread in these areas. If it did reach a major city in Asia such as Delhi or Calcutta, where there is little or no vaccination against it, the consequences would be serious in the short term, until all the susceptible people could be vaccinated. Some authors have postulated that the reason that it is not found is that South East Asia is already saturated with arbo-virus diseases, such as dengue fever and Japanese encephalitis. The high incidence of dengue fever (see later) may give some protection against yellow fever through cross-immunity, as both are flaviviruses.

There are no long-term human carriers of yellow fever, the victim either dies, or makes a recovery based on the ability of their immune system to combat the disease. If the victim recovers, the virus is eliminated from their body rapidly and the individual is immune for life. Infected humans can only transmit the virus to the mosquito for about five to six days, after that they cease to be infectious. The mosquito, once infected, is infectious for life, which may be as long as six months. When the mosquito bites an infected person, it does not become infectious immediately, but requires a minimum incubation period of about ten days, although this can vary depending on the ambient temperature. This caused considerable confusion during the early stages of research into yellow fever, when it was assumed that the mosquito became infectious immediately after biting an infected individual.

Control of yellow fever is by immunisation, using an attenuated strain of the virus, developed in the mid-1930s. The vaccine available is highly effective and a single injection produces a strong antibody response conferring immunity for at least ten years. It is effective against both urban and jungle yellow fever. Two vaccines were developed against the disease, a French one and an American one, both using live attenuated virus. The American one, designated "17D" after the virus strain used, was attenuated by passing the virus through chicken eggs, whilst the French one was passed through a succession of mouse brains. Both were very effective, but the American one could only be given by injection and was inactivated within a couple of weeks when exposed to heat in the tropics. The French one was considerably more resistant to heat and could also be administered by scarification. This allowed it to be given at the same time as vaccination against smallpox. However, in a number of cases (estimated at between 1 in 100 and 1 in 1,000), it caused encephalitis (which was occasionally fatal) especially in small children, and the use of this vaccine has now been discontinued.

History

The original home of yellow fever is West Africa, where it was so widespread that it was a childhood disease, and most of the indigenous adults were immune to it. In the New World however, it killed hundreds of thousands of whites, New World blacks and indigenous Indians.

It was first recorded in Barbados in the Caribbean and then in Central America when there was a major epidemic from 1647-50. The delay in the establishment of yellow fever in the Americas, following the arrival of Columbus, was the requirement for the correct vector, the mosquito *Ae. aegypti* to establish itself. This species of mosquito is widespread near human habitation, and is capable of existing in water butts on board ship as long as the temperature does not fall below 72°F (23°C). The mosquito is also able to survive in temperate zones during the warm season.

Disease carrying mosquitoes were therefore capable of surviving the voyage from the Old World to the New World, especially after the introduction of the slave trade, as slave ships, by the very nature of their cargo, needed to make a fast passage. The virus would have gone through several cycles of infection on board ship.

Attempts were made to quarantine infected ships arriving in the Caribbean, but were ineffective. The quarantine of ships for a long period obviously had serious commercial implications for the owners, especially when the cargo was a perishable one such as slaves, and they would have done their utmost to avoid it. When an epidemic did break out in port, the population frequently fled from the worst infected areas, but this only served to spread the disease. By the late seventeenth century, yellow fever was widespread with a major epidemic in Brazil in 1685, and epidemics on the American coast in 1668, 1690 and 1691.

Major epidemics also occurred in the southern USA, and on the eastern US seaboard, during the eighteenth and nineteenth centuries. They were an important factor in the decision of the French to sell Louisiana to the nascent USA. The Louisiana Purchase took place in 1803 for $15 million, the French also being in desperate need of money to fund the wars of Napoleon. In 1803, the size of Louisiana was significantly larger than the state is today, and the Louisiana Purchase virtually doubled the size of the then USA.

By this time, yellow fever was widespread in the Caribbean islands and as far north as Bermuda, and caused the loss of many European troops. In 1655, out of fifteen hundred French troops on St Lucia, only eighty-nine survived. Heavy losses were also suffered amongst troops sent by Napoleon to recapture Hispaniola (now Haiti), after the slave revolt led by Toussaint L'Ouverture, (who was referred to as the "Black Napoleon"). L'Ouverture was finally tricked into meeting a French general in 1802, kidnapped and shipped in chains to France, where he died of starvation in the dungeons of the Chateau de Joux in 1803. It is estimated that of the thirty-three thousand French troops sent to Haiti by Napoleon, in an attempt to suppress the revolt, ninety per cent died of yellow fever. The remainder were no match for the slave army and the state of Haiti was declared in early 1804, the first independent black state in the Caribbean.

The Caribbean also had an evil reputation amongst the British Army of the time. Numerous British regiments suffered severe losses from disease and many officers left the army and sold their commissions to avoid being sent there. In 1741, over half of the nineteen thousand British troops attacking Cartagena died of yellow fever, and it has been estimated that the British lost eighty thousand troops in the West Indies between 1793-6 to malaria and yellow fever. It has been suggested that the clearance of the rain forest for sugar plantation in the West Indies would have exacerbated yellow fever by causing a loss of habitat for insect eating birds.

Yellow fever occurred as far north as Boston, and a major outbreak in Philadelphia (the capital city of the USA at the time), was started by French refugees fleeing from the slave revolt on Hispaniola in 1793, and an early account of this epidemic is given by Mathew Carey. It killed more than five thousand out of a population of forty-five thousand in a few months. It started in a working class area and was initially ignored by the authorities, but by late August was a full scale epidemic. There was considerable disagreement amongst local doctors, but many thought the cause was bad air (the miasma theory again). The population was advised to breathe through cloths soaked in vinegar, and to wear camphor sachets around their necks. Sulphur and gunpowder were burnt on the streets to fumigate the air.

There was also considerable argument over treatment, some doctors advocated blood letting and the use of mercury, whilst others wanted to quarantine the refugees but the city was unable to enforce this. Half of Philadelphia's population fled, many of them being ostracised or quarantined at gunpoint when they attempted to enter surrounding communities and other coastal cities. By early September, most of the rich merchants and local authorities (including many of the doctors) had fled, and the local economy had collapsed.

One doctor, Devèze (one of the refugees from Haiti), had considerable experience of treating yellow fever in the French army, and used a treatment of quinine and bed rest. Although this was ineffective, it was considerably more civilised than the blood letting practised by most other doctors. The epidemic finally died out in November when the temperature fell and the first frosts killed the mosquitoes.

The 1793 epidemic caused Philadelphia to create the city's first health department. After another epidemic in 1801, it created the first municipal water system in the USA, and also forced through the introduction of widespread quarantine regulations on the Eastern US seaboard. In spite of these precautions, more epidemics occurred in 1797-9, 1802-3, and 1805.

There were also numerous epidemics in the coastal region of the USA in the nineteenth century, the worst affected city probably being New Orleans. This suffered numerous major outbreaks over a thirty-five year period, the worst being in 1853 that killed over 9,000. In the 1830s and 40s, Florida suffered badly losing a large percentage of its population. The swamps of the Everglades were an ideal breeding ground for mosquitoes.

The disease also travelled up rivers, especially the Mississippi, and in the 1840s it almost caused Memphis, Tennessee, to be abandoned. It reached Memphis again in 1878 this time killing five thousand inhabitants. This outbreak was thought to have started in Cuba as a large number of Spanish troops were sent there in 1876 to suppress a rebellion and this initiated an epidemic lasting three years.

The effect on American trade, investment and commerce from these epidemics and the problems they created was severe, and led to considerable political pressure on the authorities to deal with the situation.

Yellow fever has now been eliminated from the USA, and there have been no new cases since the last major outbreak in New Orleans in 1905 which infected 5,000 people killing 1,000 of them. This has been achieved mainly by control of the mosquito vector. The cost however is vast, it is estimated that the state of Florida alone spends more than $300 million per annum controlling mosquitoes, a sum well beyond the budget of most countries where mosquitoes are a problem. *Ae. aegypti* has re-established itself in the southern USA in recent years, in addition, *Ae. albopictus* that is more tolerant of cold weather and which can also carry yellow fever is found occasionally. Both species are able to carry dengue fever (see later) as well as yellow fever and attempts to eradicate them have been met by environmental lawsuits.

Yellow fever has occurred in Europe especially on the Spanish and Portuguese coasts, with major epidemics in Barcelona in 1800 and 1821. There have also been small outbreaks in France, England and Italy.

The disease was also widespread throughout tropical America, and was an important factor in building the first railway across the Isthmus of Panama between 1851 and 1855, when malaria and yellow fever are estimated to have killed in excess of ten thousand workers. It has also been claimed that one labourer died for every sleeper laid, which would make the number of dead significantly higher than ten thousand.

In 1879, the International Congress of Geographical Sciences voted in favour of constructing a canal across the Isthmus of Panama, and appointed Count de Lesseps, whose French company had successfully built the Suez Canal between 1859-69, to carry out the project. However, they completely under-estimated the magnitude of this enterprise which was a lot more difficult than Suez. Originally a sea level canal was proposed, but at its highest point the Isthmus of Panama is 100m above sea level, and at the start of the rainy season, flood waters can rise as much as 15m per day. There were serious problems with mud slides and it became obvious that a high level canal with multiple locks at either end was required.

There were also severe problems from malaria and yellow fever. It has been estimated that over twenty-five thousand workers died from these two diseases between 1881 and 1889 (some sources claim that the true figure was nearer fifty thousand). The company frequently claimed that the deaths were due to the immoral behaviour of the victims, gambling, drinking and whoring. The epidemics of 1884/5 were the worst ever known. At this time, quinine was still very expensive, and to save money the French did not give the workers any; it was cheaper to replace the workers than buy the drug.

The project collapsed, and in 1889 the Compagnie Universelle du Canal Interoceanique declared itself bankrupt. The project was way beyond the resources of any private company and the political fallout in France from the bankruptcy was enormous. Large number of French shareholders had poured money into the scheme on the basis of the success of the Suez Canal, and the bankruptcy had serious repercussions in the French financial markets. The French government had invested heavily in the project and many of its members were accused of accepting bribes. Ferdinand de Lesseps and his son were both found guilty of fraud. The resulting investigations became political as well as financial and nearly brought down the French government. The scandal also seriously damaged the reputations of a number of prominent French engineers such as Eiffel (of Eiffel tower fame), who had seriously under-estimated the magnitude of the task.

The construction collapsed and the project was taken over by the US government under President Theodore Roosevelt. One of the first changes to be made was from a sea level canal to a series of locks on either side of Lake Gatun. The USA acquired the rights to the Panama Canal Zone in 1903, and the US army built the canal between 1904-1914. The canal opened in August 1914 although the official opening was delayed until 1920 after the end of World War I. Both the Japanese and Indian governments protested about the opening of the Panama Canal, as they considered it would allow yellow fever to penetrate the Pacific. Yellow fever quarantine stations were suggested for Hong Kong, Singapore and the Panama Canal itself.

The American political justification for building the canal was the war with Spain in 1898 over Cuba. After the *USS Maine* was blown up in Havana, it took American warships based in the Pacific ten weeks to go around Cape Horn, and they arrived too late to be of any practical use. Since then all

American warships are built to a maximum size, known as Panamax, that enables them to pass through the canal.

There was a small political problem, Panama was Columbian territory and Columbia would not ratify a treaty with the USA. The USA therefore fomented a rebellion of Panamanian inhabitants that the USA supported, and when it was successful, a treaty was signed with the newly independent state of Panama in 1903. This gave the USA the canal and a strip of land on either side, which became the Panama Canal Zone with exclusive rights to use, occupy and control the Canal Zone in perpetuity. It was as neat a piece of political chicanery and colonialism as any ever carried out by the old European colonial powers.

One of the first steps in building the Panama Canal was to implement the findings of the Reed Commission, and to bring the mosquitoes carrying malaria and yellow fever under control. Practically, the building of the canal only became possible when the transmission of malaria and yellow fever were recognised, and control measures could be implemented.

The epidemiology of yellow fever was first published in 1900 by the US Army Yellow Fever Commission, usually called the Reed Commission, after its leader Walter Reed (1851-1902). During the late nineteenth century, there were a number of theories about the cause and transmission of yellow fever, and in 1881, a Cuban doctor, Carlos Finlay, suggested the involvement of mosquitoes. Finlay was unable to prove his theory, due to his failure to carry out experiments, involving mosquitoes biting humans, that were sufficiently conclusive to withstand scientific criticism. This was before Ross (Ch 16) had shown the involvement of mosquitoes in the transmission of malaria.

Reed noted that soldiers in beds occupied by previous yellow fever victims did not catch it (one of the previously held theories), and therefore it was not transmitted by fomites such as clothing or bedding. He and his associates were able to confirm the initial observations of Finlay and show that yellow fever was transmitted by the mosquito, *Ae. aegypti,* although in earlier work on malaria, Reed had discounted the role of the mosquito. One of the main problems with earlier work on yellow fever was that it had not been realised that the virus is incubated for about ten days in the mosquito before it becomes infective, and is then incubated for a further two to five days in the human before the symptoms appear. By 1900 however, the work of Ross on the involvement of the mosquito in the transmission of malaria had been published, and the realisation had set in that insects were of major importance as vectors in the transmission of a number of diseases. However, the virus was not discovered for another thirty years and the role of wild primates as reservoirs in the jungle yellow fever cycle was recognised about the same time.

Reed tested his theories on a number of human volunteers of whom several died, so also did one of the doctors, Dr Jesse Lazear, one of Reed's team. This was one of the earliest examples of experiments being carried out on volunteers using informed consent. Reed did not volunteer himself as a guinea-pig.

The US Army Yellow Fever Commission was set up after the Spanish-American War of 1898, whilst American troops were occupying Cuba. The Cubans revolted against their Spanish rulers, and the Second Cuban War of Independence from Spain was fought from 1895-1898. At this time the USA was going through a period of aggressive colonial expansionism, and the American press manipulated public opinion towards intervention on behalf of Cuba, which was seen as being in the American sphere of influence[196].

The motivation and political justification for the Spanish American war was a quagmire of intrigue and the cause is still disputed. Cuba was recognised as a source of the frequent yellow fever outbreaks that reached the USA, and just before the war, a yellow fever conference in Alabama recommended

---

196   A cartoon of the time shows Uncle Sam, as an expert fisherman, wielding several fishing rods at once, and simultaneously reeling in Cuba, Puerto Rico, Hawaii and the Philippines.

that the USA should annexe Cuba by force and deal with the yellow fever problem.

The battleship USS *Maine* was sent to Havana, ostensibly to protect American interests during the Cuban War of Independence, and was sunk in Havana harbour by an explosion of unknown origin in February 1898, killing a large number of American sailors[197]. The American administration and press claimed that the *Maine* was sunk by a Spanish mine although there is no evidence to support this theory. It was declared an act of belligerence; America declared war on Spain in April 1898, and the war was over by July 1898. With the usual military incompetence, the war was planned for the worst period of the yellow fever season. Luckily for the American army, the war finished so quickly that it was possible to withdraw many troops before the fever season peaked. There were the usual conspiratorial suggestions that the Americans had blown up their own battleship to provide an excuse for invading Cuba.

During the brief war, American deaths from disease (mainly yellow fever, but also malaria and typhoid) numbered over five thousand and were five to six times the number killed in action. In some areas the number of troops catching yellow fever reached over 85%. One theory destroyed during this period was that black Americans possessed high levels of immunity to tropical diseases. An infantry regiment of Afro-Americans was sent to one hospital to tend the sick and in the space of just over one month, over a third of them died from yellow fever or malaria. Large numbers of Spanish troops also died from various diseases.

Following the ratification of the peace treaty, fifty thousand American troops occupied Cuba from 1898-1902. The Surgeon General of the American army (George Sternberg) ordered

---

197   The topmast of the *Maine* is now at Arlington cemetery in Washington, D.C. The sinking of the *Maine* gave rise to the American battlecry for the war:

Remember the *Maine*,
To hell with Spain.

various sanitary measures to be carried out in Cuba as he was convinced that the island was the source of most of the epidemics on the eastern US seaboard. He also believed that yellow fever was caused by dirty living conditions, and could be reduced by improvements in hygiene. Although these were not sufficient to control yellow fever, epidemics of typhoid that are spread by contaminated drinking water and generally unsanitary conditions were reduced significantly. Sternberg did have the advantage that it was a military occupation, martial law was declared, and any civilian objections to his measures were over-ruled. Yellow fever however, reappeared in the summer of 1899, and in 1900, Sternberg ordered the Yellow Fever Commission to be established.

An army doctor, William Gorgas (who had survived an infection of yellow fever), implemented the health and hygiene measures in Havana. He attempted to vaccinate troops by allowing recently infected mosquitoes to bite them and produce a mild dose of yellow fever. This was unsuccessful because of the time it takes for the virus to mature in the mosquito. He eventually broke the chain of infection by isolating the victims in buildings with mosquito screens, so that mosquitoes could not bite them and become infective, and covering ponds with oil so the mosquitoes could not breed. The result was the virtual elimination of yellow fever from Havana.

In 1904, the USA restarted work on the Panama Canal, and Gorgas was appointed as Chief Sanitary Officer to the Canal Zone with the full support of the President, Theodore Roosevelt. His first job was to control diseases such as malaria and yellow fever. Initially there was a great deal of hostility to his ideas, and he had considerable problems with civilians who would not obey orders and army generals who did not believe mosquitoes spread disease. With the support of Roosevelt however, he was able to enforce his measures, which initially included covering ponds and cess pools with oil to kill the mosquito larvae and screening all standing water supplies. He then fumigated all the living quarters where there had been a case of yellow fever using burning sulphur. This was eventually extended to the whole of Panama City and all the towns along the canal. Gorgas also insisted on the labour force sleeping under mosquito nets, and obtained a supply of enough quinine to ensure that every worker could be given a regular dose as a prophylactic.

The results were extremely effective, and by 1906, yellow fever had been virtually eliminated from the Canal Zone, with no cases occurring from 1907 onwards. By the time the canal was finished in 1913, the incidence rate of malaria had fallen to less than ten per cent of what it had been in 1906. Only two per cent of the workforce were hospitalised, compared with over thirty per cent when the French were attempting to build the canal. Gorgas was promoted to general and given an honorary knighthood by King Edward VII.

The Italian bacteriologist, Sanarelli, had previously identified the bacterium *Bacillus icteroides* as the cause of yellow fever. However, the Reed group following Koch's postulates were able to show that this bacterium could only be found in thirty per cent of fatal cases of yellow fever. *B. icteroides* has now been shown to be the bacterium *Salmonella typhimurium,* an organism causing severe and frequently fatal gastro-enteritis, and occasionally producing symptoms similar to those of typhoid. Sanarelli's mistake can be easily understood when yellow fever, typhoid and dysentery were occurring simultaneously.

Dengue Fever

Dengue fever or breakbone fever probably evolved from yellow fever, but is less dangerous. The name dengue comes from a Spanish word for affectation, and dengue fever was also known as dandy fever, so-called because those recovering from it moved very carefully, and developed a mincing gait to avoid severe pain in their joints. The disease produces a fever, headaches and severe joint pains lasting about a week. It is caused by a flavivirus very similar to the yellow fever virus, and is carried by mosquito vectors of the genus *Aedes,* the main one being the urban mosquito *Ae. aegypti,* although it is also carried by the tiger mosquito, *Ae. albopictus.* There is some antigenic overlap with yellow fever and an infection with one is thought to give some protection against the other.

It was first described in 1779 in the USA by an American doctor, Benjamin Rush[198], who gave it the name breakbone fever, and also in the Dutch East Indies at the same time. It is found in South America, South East Asia and Africa. The WHO estimates there are approximately fifty million cases a year, several hundred thousand of which will turn into the more dangerous haemorrhagic form with about twelve thousand of those being fatal. This figure may be a considerable under-estimate as there are serious problems of distinguishing it from malaria and other fevers, especially in areas where medical facilities are poor.

Dengue fever was frequently mistaken for yellow fever which entailed a quarantine, so it became commercially necessary to distinguish between the two. In 1897, an epidemic in the Gulf of Mexico reached the south eastern USA, causing a major row over whether it was yellow fever or dengue fever.

A new form of dengue fever appeared in Manila in 1953 known as dengue haemorrhagic fever. Dengue fever is unusual in that there are four distinct serotypes of the disease. Infection with one of these is rarely fatal and produces a life-long immunity for that serotype only. However, it also generates an increased probability of a severe reaction if the victim is infected with a second, different serotype. All the victims had had an initial mild form of dengue fever that sensitised them. The antibodies to the serotype causing the first infection then attacked the different viral serotype causing the second infection, and the host macrophages engulfed them. However, instead of the macrophage destroying the virus, the virus took over the macrophage and used it to gain access to all the organs of body, sending the immune system into overdrive. This created a high fever, anaphylactic shock, severe

198   One of the signatories of the Declaration of Independence.

haemorrhaging and death. This form of dengue fever is more dangerous than the normal form, causing death in 5-15% of cases, especially in children. Obviously there are serious implications for the development of a vaccine if vaccination against one serotype predisposes a population to a more serious outbreak of a different type.

Because of the four different serotypes, it has not been possible as yet to make an effective vaccine. The virus synthesises all its proteins as one long piece, which is cut into specific sections by an enzyme. One strategy for vaccine production is to use an altered enzyme that cuts the parent viral protein in different places, to produce a virus that can still reproduce but only poorly compared with the wild type. It is hoped that this might make an effective vaccine as the altered virus would be incapable of causing the disease, but would be sufficient to activate the host immune system as protection against a future attack by the wild type.

Dengue fever spread widely due to World War II; there was disruption to mosquito spraying and in addition, bombing created craters that filled with water forming ideal mosquito breeding grounds. There were rapid troop movements and massive human migrations over long distances, with densely populated refugee camps and PoW camps, all creating ideal conditions for the spread of the disease, and causing a mix of the four different serotypes. The Korean and Vietnam wars also created further opportunities for the virus to expand its territory.

Dengue fever is still a serious problem, there were major epidemics in Cuba in 1970 causing severe economic problems, and another one in 1981, causing several hundred thousand cases and it appears to be increasing its range in the West Indies. There were also epidemics in Delhi in 1982, which caused an estimated one and a half million cases, and again in 1996 in Delhi when over four hundred died.

CHAPTER 18

HIV and AIDS

Several new diseases, many of them caused by viruses appeared in the twentieth century. The most dangerous of these for several reasons was the Human Immunodeficiency Virus (HIV), a member of a group of *retro*-viruses known as lentiviruses (slow viruses). They are known by this name as they usually take a very long time to produce any symptoms. It is already obvious that HIV has changed, and is going to continue changing the pattern of human life, demographics and behaviour for a considerable time to come.

HIV causes AIDS (Acquired Immune Deficiency Syndrome). As this is a deficiency of the immune system, unlike other diseases, it has no constant specific symptoms. Once the immune system is compromised, a wide range of opportunistic diseases can occur and the acronym AIDS is a catch-all term for these symptoms and diseases. The modern definition of AIDS is when a person tests positive for antibodies to HIV, has one of these opportunistic diseases and/or a CD4 T-lymphocyte count of less than 200/µl of blood. The number in a healthy person is approximately five times this figure (one µl is one millionth of a litre).

AIDS first became apparent in homosexual men in the USA in 1981, indeed the disease was initially known as GRIDS (Gay Related Immune Deficiency Syndrome). A number of homosexual men started to develop unusual medical conditions that included Kaposi's syndrome (a rare form of skin cancer normally only found in Africans), a rare form of pneumonia caused by the protozoan *Pneumocystis carinii* known as PCP, unusual protozoal brain infections, tuberculosis and severe infections of the fungus *Candida albicans*. The final stage in many cases was severe dementia. The most common of these opportunistic invaders is tuberculosis which is also the most important for the public health of the general population, as this can be transmitted to a person who is not compromised immunologically.

It rapidly became obvious that HIV and AIDS were also causing serious problems in those people injecting drugs on a group basis using shared hypodermic needles. Later still it was found that it could be transmitted by heterosexual sex, the use of contaminated blood products and mother-to-baby transfer.

The UN figures for 2007 estimated that approximately thirty-three million people were living with AIDS and that there were two million deaths and nearly three million new cases in that year. Half of all new infections were people under the age of twenty-five. A number of other sources consider that the total numbers living with AIDS is significantly higher, usually in the region of forty to forty-five million, although one or two sources suggest that the figure may be over fifty million. These figures are up from an estimated eight million in 1990. The recent reduction by the UN in the estimated numbers of those infected has been due to improvements in the statistical models used, and the extrapolation of figures from these models. However, the stigma of the disease in many rural and traditional communities, in countries such as India, makes it very difficult to obtain accurate figures. Since it first appeared there have been approximately twenty-five million deaths, with more than two-thirds of these occurring in sub-Saharan Africa, which also has approximately three quarters of the cases.

SCIENCE

HIV is only found in humans, it is spread by sex (both heterosexual and homosexual), intravenous drug use and contact with infected body fluids, including blood, semen and breast milk. It can pass from mother to child during pregnancy, childbirth or by breast-feeding.

Structurally, HIV is an RNA *retro*-virus (Ch 4) that contains genetic material in the form of two identical strands of RNA surrounded by a lipoprotein envelope. The target of HIV is a type of white blood cell containing a surface protein known as CD4. In addition to CD4 there must also be another protein, either CCR5 or CXCR4, on the cell surface. These act as co-receptors for the virus which must lock onto both the CD4 protein and either one of the other two before the cell can become infected. The more usual co-receptor is CCR5 and this has important consequences as seen later. Cells containing these receptors include the helper T-lymphocytes and macrophages whose functions are crucial to the immune system (Ch 7). The helper T-lymphocytes play an important role in activating the β-lymphocytes that produce antibodies and stimulate the macrophages to attack invading micro-organisms. Therefore when the helper T-lymphocytes and macrophages are destroyed by HIV, the ultimate result is the total collapse of the immune system.

Once the cell has become infected, the viral RNA acts as a template and is copied to form a single stranded DNA molecule known as c-DNA (copy-DNA) using a viral enzyme called reverse transcriptase. The c-DNA is itself copied to form double-stranded DNA. This is integrated permanently into the genome of the host cell where it may become latent (effectively a state of hibernation) for a long period of time. This integration is carried out by a viral enzyme known as integrase. Depending on the individual involved and the strain of the virus causing the infection, the latent period may be less than one year or as much as ten years. Eventually, the DNA is activated and starts to produce new viral RNA molecules, protein corresponding to the viral coat is synthesised and the components are assembled into new virus that can then attack the appropriate host cells.

All *retro*-viral reverse transcriptases are prone to making mistakes when copying, but the reverse transcriptase from HIV is the most inaccurate known. The result of this is the formation of a very high number of mutants that are subjected to extreme pressure by the immune system of the infected individual[199]. The vast majority of viruses are destroyed, but those that survive are the ones able to evade the immune response and show resistance to any anti-*retro*-viral drugs that are being taken. HIV is the most rapidly mutating virus known, and as the immune system of each individual varies slightly the virus population in each infected individual varies. This degree of variation increases the longer the person has been infected, forming a star burst effect in which the virus at the distal point of each ray differs genetically from the virus at the distal point of every other ray, producing a type of population sometimes known as a quasi-species.

Infected CD4 cells attract non-infected CD4 cells and these fuse to form giant multinuclear complexes known as syncytia; each infected cell may bind up to fifty non-infected ones. Once syncytia are formed, the fused cells rapidly lose their immune function and die.

Initially there is a very strong immune response from the infected individual and in the early stages of the infection, this destroys about one billion (10^9) virus particles per day. However, the number of helper T-cells and macrophages that are destroyed by the virus exceeds the number of new cells produced by the immune system, even though the immune system makes new cells extremely rapidly. The result, over time, is a decline in the number of helper T-cells and macrophages, and the progress of the disease can be followed by determining the number of helper T-cells and macrophages in the blood of the patient.

---

199   The number of virus particles produced is about ten billion (10^{10}) per day in an individual who is not receiving treatment.

HIV attacks the body in a totally different manner to other pathogens. In other diseases the pathogen challenges the immune system to produce antibodies, HIV destroys the immune system, thus destroying its capacity to produce antibodies. The best simile is to compare the pathogen with an invader attacking a castle. Other pathogens attack the castle walls trying to batter them down whilst the defenders try to shore them up and if the defenders can shore up the walls for a sufficient length of time, the invader goes away. HIV however, tunnels under the castle walls, undermining them until they collapse.

There have been suspicions recently that long term HIV infections can also damage the ability of the immune system to recognise the difference between self and non-self, thus causing low level auto-immune problems (Ch 7).

When a person is infected with HIV, the course of the infection involves three stages. During the primary stage, the virus replicates very rapidly and frequently produces flu-like symptoms that may last for several weeks. There is a very high virus count (load) in infected individuals and during this period they are highly infectious, a dangerous situation as the infected person is frequently unaware at this stage that they have the disease[200]. HIV tests, most of which measure antibodies in the blood or saliva, are initially negative as the antibody level does not become detectable until about six weeks after an individual has become infected. The second stage is asymptomatic and may last from a few months to ten years or more; during the early stages of this phase the rise in the antibody level reduces the virus count in the blood and the infected person becomes less contagious. The virus count might rise again temporarily if the individual becomes infected with another disease making demands on the immune system, and if this occurs they may become more infectious. The virus continues to replicate and in the later part of the second stage

---

200   Estimates in 2005 suggested that the number of undiagnosed cases in the USA was three hundred thousand, whilst figures for 2009, claim that there are twenty-one thousand similar cases in the UK.

there is a rise in the virus load, and a fall in the count of cells containing the CD4 protein until it reaches a figure of less than 200 cells per micro litre (µl) of blood. At this point the individual becomes infected with one of the opportunistic pathogens mentioned earlier, and the disease enters the tertiary and final stage, AIDS.

Medical practice used to delay combination therapy until the CD4 cell count dropped below 200/µl. It was not started sooner as the unpleasant side effects of the early anti-*retro*-viral drugs were so severe and patients were taking in excess of twenty tablets a day. Now however, using combinations of newer drugs that cause less severe side effects and only need to be taken a couple of times a day, treatment is started when the CD4 cell count falls to 350/µl which reduces heart, liver and kidney problems.

There are two forms of HIV, HIV-1 and HIV-2, HIV-1 being the more dangerous and accounting for over 95% of AIDS cases throughout the world. HIV-2 closely resembles a virus found in the sooty mangabey (a West African monkey), and it is generally confined to localised areas of West Africa. Although it also causes AIDS, it is a much milder form than that caused by HIV-1.

Three major strains of HIV-1 are found, M (major), N (new) and O (outlier) of which O is restricted to West Africa. N was discovered in Cameroon in 1998, is very rare, and possibly represents a recent infection from a chimpanzee. The most important group is M and this contains nine different sub-types (clades) labelled A-K, plus a number of intermediate types, the predominant type varying from country to country. Sub-type C is the most dangerous causing about fifty per cent of cases and is the one found predominately in Africa and India.

It is possible to get a super-infection of two different sub-types indicating that infection by one type does not necessarily confer immunity against a second type. The possibility of infection by two different sub-types means that new sub-types will almost certainly evolve over a period of time in a manner analogous to the evolution of new strains of influenza (Ch 15). The fact that one sub-type does not necessarily confer immunity against others and the evolution of new strains makes the development of an effective vaccine extremely difficult.

HIV-1 is similar to a virus known as SIV (simian immunodeficiency virus) found in chimpanzees and several variations of SIV are found in different populations of chimpanzees. The one corresponding most closely to HIV-1 is found in a sub-species of chimpanzee (*Pan troglodytes troglodytes*) living in southern Cameroon. This borders the Congo and Gabon, the countries where AIDS first appeared. Some researchers have suggested that there is genetic evidence that the SIV found in these chimpanzees is a genetic hybrid of two distinct SIVs found in different species of monkey. One of these is the red-capped mangabey and the other is the greater spot-nosed monkey. Chimpanzees are known to hunt these two species, and it is thought they became infected with both these SIVs more or less simultaneously. These hybridised and the hybrid SIV was capable of infecting humans when chimpanzees were hunted in their turn for bush meat.

The number of different sub-strains of HIV-1 suggests that the virus may have jumped from chimpanzees to humans on several occasions. Although we share approximately 98.4% of our DNA with chimpanzees, obviously something in the remaining 1.6% allows HIV to infect us and cause AIDS, but not chimpanzees. The discovery of what this factor is could provide a useful guide to the development of new methods of controlling HIV in humans.

It is possible that once it had entered the human population the virus was then transferred between people by the repeated use of non-sterile needles in local hospitals. This practice is well known to occur in many African hospitals where hypodermics are at a premium, and sterilising equipment is non-existent. A survey in 2009 claimed that medical procedures using dirty needles were responsible for one in five of the HIV+ cases in Africa, many of these cases being related to the anti-malarial programmes. There is also a widespread belief in rural Africa about the efficacy of injections and in many countries, untrained injectionists travel from village to village giving the sick injections of vitamins and poor quality antibiotics, in many cases using non-sterile needles. It has also been pointed out that there was a large programme in the 1950s in an attempt to eradicate yaws (Ch 14). This involved mass injection of antibiotics, frequently under non-sterile conditions. This type of sequential transfer is known in microbiology as serial transfer and is a well-known method of selecting new mutants in the laboratory. As the virus passed through successive human hosts it would have been subjected to attack by their immune systems, which would have honed its deadly potential with each successive transfer.

As already mentioned, there are a number of different sub-types of HIV and these strains behave differently, some appear to be much more virulent than others. Because of the different sub-types, it is possible to plot the evolution of the virus mathematically and estimate when it first appeared in humans. Early calculations suggested that the first cases probably occurred in the 1930s, but more recent work suggests that it may have infected humans as long ago as the last decade of the nineteenth century. Stored blood samples taken from people dying from unknown diseases as early as 1959 have tested positive for HIV and the genetic patterns found are the ones predicted, suggesting that the mathematical calculations applied to the evolution of the virus are correct.

At present there is no effective vaccine or cure of an HIV infection. Attempts to control the disease using drugs prevent further progress of the infection but they do not eliminate the virus from the body. The most effective measures at preventing

HIV infection have focused on changes in sexual behaviour such as the use of condoms, and providing clean hypodermic needles for injecting drug users.

A number of different drugs are available for treatment and these are divided into various groups depending on the way they attack the virus. One group inhibits the reverse transcriptase of the virus and stops the synthesis of c-DNA; this group can be sub-divided into two sections depending on the chemistry of the drug used and its precise target and mode of action. A second group known as protease inhibitors inhibit the viral enzyme, protease, that is essential for the maturation of the virus. A third group of newer types of drugs are known as entry inhibitors. These block the receptor proteins on the surface of a susceptible cell and prevent HIV from entering the cell. As the virus must enter the cell to replicate, no entry means no replication. One of these entry inhibitors is the drug, maraviroc, that blocks the CCR5 protein. The FDA requires anyone given this drug to undergo pharmacogenetic testing to determine which co-receptor is being used and the drug is only given to a patient in whom the virus is attaching to CCR5.

Newer drugs are undergoing testing, one group are known as integrase inhibitors. These are drugs that inhibit the enzyme integrase that the virus needs to insert the DNA that it has copied from its RNA into the genome of the host cell. One point that should be made is that drugs attacking the obvious and easy targets have already been synthesised and are in use. Finding drugs that attack fresh targets is becoming increasingly difficult.

It is essential to use combination therapy to treat AIDS. This is a cocktail of drugs from different groups in an attempt to minimize the problems of drug resistance as the virus replicates and mutates so rapidly. The combination of three or more drugs is known as Highly Active Anti-Retroviral Therapy (HAART), and its use has produced a marked fall in the mortality rate from HIV infections in the industrialized world since it was first introduced in 1996. The cost of this combination therapy is high, as much as £16,000 per year in the UK and recent figures for the USA suggest costs of $27-28,000 per year. It is not only the cost of the drugs, the patient also has to have their viral load monitored regularly. These figures have been increasing steadily as more sophisticated drugs become available and will continue to do so. If the viral load starts to increase, it means the virus is becoming resistant to the drugs being used, and it is necessary to change the drug combination making up the cocktail. It is estimated that one in five HIV+ individuals will develop drug resistance over a period of five to six years. The sums mentioned above are obviously much too high for the general public in the developing countries, where HAART is confined to the richest groups. The use of HAART also requires a hospital system with a sophisticated level of technical expertise.

Combination therapy does not eliminate HIV from the body, however it does stop viral replication, giving the immune system time to recover which enables it to counter opportunistic diseases. The virus does persist in a latent state in some of the T-cells and it can re-activate if the drugs are stopped. It is therefore necessary to take the drugs without a break for life. Many of the drugs used are highly toxic and can have extremely unpleasant and severe side effects that tempt a significant number of patients to have a holiday from taking them. However, if HAART treatment is stopped for any reason the viral load increases and the patient runs a severe risk of developing a drug-resistant strain of the virus; they also become more infectious again. With some of the earlier versions of drugs, almost thirty per cent of patients undergoing therapy were forced to stop treatment because of toxic side effects. Later versions have improved but a considerable number of patients are still forced out of their drug programme.

Recently a number of HIV +ve individuals, who have been receiving chemotherapy for a long period of time, are showing signs of early onset dementia and other signs of senility such as bone and muscle weakness. There is some disagreement between doctors and scientists over the cause of this premature senility, some think it is caused by the virus whilst others think it may be caused by the long term exposure to the anti-*retro*-viral drugs.

Many of the drugs used must also be taken under specific conditions, some need to be taken before food, others with food. The number of tablets required each day also means it is easy to forget one unless a highly organised regime is followed. One type of drug regime is known as Post Exposure Prophylaxis (PEP). This is a four week course of drugs which is started immediately after known exposure to the virus caused by rape or a needle-stick injury to a health care worker. The treatment is usually effective, but the side effects are extremely unpleasant including diarrhoea, vomiting and serious fatigue. In addition to taking the drugs to combat HIV, any patient in whom the diseases has progressed to AIDS will also need to take drugs to combat any opportunistic disease that has been caught.

In 1984, after the virus causing AIDS had been found, the US Secretary of Health stated that there would be a vaccine available within two years A quarter of a century later, that can only be described as one of the most unfortunate remarks ever made. Numerous attempts at producing a vaccine, using methods tried and tested for other diseases, have failed abysmally, and we are probably not much closer to a vaccine now than we were then. All that can be said with any degree of certainty is that we now have a better idea of what does not work. Recent pronouncements on the subject by the WHO suggest that an effective vaccine is probably at least still fifteen years away.

A recent study in 2009 claimed that a vaccine trial carried out in Thailand had been successful. The vaccine consisted of two vaccines that had been used in previous trials used together in combination. Although it was claimed that the trial was effective, the efficacy was only marginal and there was controversy over the statistical significance of the results.

EPIDEMIOLOGY

One of the major problems of dealing with HIV is that the monitoring of AIDS cases provides no information on the current situation of HIV infection, it tells you what was happening between approximately one and ten years ago. As a result, if the number of HIV+ individuals is monitored, a fall in numbers with HIV does not necessarily mean the rate of infection is falling. It may mean that more of those with AIDS are dying; more deaths than new infections means that the number of those living with HIV falls, even although the number of newly infected individuals may be rising sharply.

The virus is not very hardy and does not survive for long outside the body. In sexual terms it is relatively difficult to become infected as it cannot penetrate an unbroken surface and needs lesions around the genitals, anus or mouth. Transmission of HIV is therefore greatly facilitated by the presence of other STIs, especially those causing ulcers such as herpes, chlamydia and syphilis. As HIV attacks the white blood cells (T cells) that concentrate at the site of infection of an STI, this means that the virus has a bigger target if one of these diseases is also present. It has been estimated that the probability of an individual catching HIV during unprotected sex increases fourfold when the non-infected individual has another STI of the type mentioned above.

Initially the virus showed two distinct epidemiologies although the distinction between these is becoming blurred. The first to be recognised was outside Africa where initially transmission was mainly through homosexual sex and injecting drugs on a group basis. This is now changing and transmission on a heterosexual basis is now becoming more frequent. The second type of epidemiology was in Africa where transmission of HIV was virtually exclusively through heterosexual sex.

In 1981 there were reports of clusters of unusual cancers occurring in homosexual men in California, and the following year it was suggested that these were caused by an infectious agent that was being transmitted sexually. Later in 1982, there were reports of transmission by blood transfusion and cases of mother-to-child transmission during pregnancy started to appear. It also became obvious that injecting drug addicts sharing needles were becoming infected.

One major problem when considering the epidemiology of AIDS is that many people becoming infected do not fit into one discrete box, such as sex worker, injecting drug addict, homosexual, heterosexual or bisexual. One of the major sources of confusion with many HIV control programmes in the past has been due to the fact that medical staff and researchers have not made due allowance for this fact; for example, many injecting drug addicts of both sexes are selling sex to buy drugs.

Drug injection is a major risk, using a hypodermic needle to inject drugs, after it has been used by a person who is HIV+, virtually guarantees getting the disease as the virus bypasses the protective barrier of the skin. Further problems with injecting drugs are found, heroin impairs the immune system by depressing T lymphocytes, and taking heroin facilitates contracting other diseases. Numerous cases of injecting drug addicts catching malaria are known where they had not been exposed to mosquitoes and hepatitis B is also spread by injecting drugs. This cannot be treated and the virus is known to initiate liver cancer in some cases.

Glasgow was the first place to use needle exchange, that is, providing injecting drug addicts with clean hypodermic needles on the basis that it is a lot cheaper to provide clean needles than it is to treat AIDS victims. The plan worked and was copied in a number of countries, such as Australia, England and Holland. During the 1990s, in those cities with needle exchange programmes, HIV rates fell; in those without, it rose. In the USA, clean needle exchange programmes are not used as politicians claim it encourages drug taking. The statistical evidence however shows that it reduces HIV and does not increase drug use.

The other major group in which AIDS was found in the early 1980s were homosexual men. Many doctors refused to treat them, those that did were frequently ostracized by the rest of the medical profession. The attitude to AIDS in the early 1980s was to distinguish between innocent victims (those acquiring infection through contaminated blood products and children who caught it from an infected mother), and the perceived guilty perpetrators of the disease i.e. those who had caught it through homosexuality, promiscuity and drug taking. These were considered to be life-style choices and therefore this type of behaviour leading to AIDS was deemed to be voluntary. In 1988, the US Surgeon General stated, *"People get AIDS by doing things most people do not do, and of which most people do not approve"*. This is still a widely held attitude in many communities and societies.

Many homosexuals, especially when AIDS was first discovered, frequented bath houses with a view to casual sex. One of the most notorious cases involved an Air Canada steward who was HIV+ and who claimed to have had over three hundred homosexual encounters in a two year period. Many men also play both roles, passive and active, and this results in a faster spread of the disease than if men only play one role. There is a weak immune response in the anal area and as the anal lining is not very thick, it is more likely to be damaged during sex thus allowing the virus to enter the body. One study has shown that women who have anal sex are significantly more likely to be infected by a HIV+ partner than women who only have vaginal sex, and homosexual men who only play the passive role are more likely to be infected than men who only play the active role.

A number of the early cases of AIDS in the developed world were caused when people were given blood transfusions with contaminated blood. It was realised quickly that this was a serious problem and by 1983, most European countries and the USA were carrying out heat treatment of blood to destroy HIV. An infected blood bank acts as a mega enhancer or amplifier of the disease. One major contribution to the problem in the USA was drug addicts selling their blood to bloodbanks for money to buy drugs. This problem did not arise to the same extent in the UK as blood donation has always been voluntary, all you get is a cup of tea, a biscuit, an invitation to the next blood donor session and a buttonhole pin after donating a certain number of pints. The sale of blood by drug addicts was banned in the mid-1980s in most of the industrialised world, but it still occurs in the developing world, where it acts as a major amplifier of HIV infection.

There were a number of countries that did not treat the blood donated to blood banks until relatively late. A court case in France in the mid-1980s alleged that approximately 4,500 people, many of them haemophiliacs, had been given HIV infected blood. A large number died and it was claimed that France had blocked an American test for HIV contaminated blood to give a French company working on a similar test time to catch up. The French authorities cleared the American test for use one month after the French companies' test came online. Other European countries were testing blood in 1983, France did not do so until 1988. A similar situation occurred in Japan where companies were selling blood contaminated with HIV throughout much of the 1980s. The Japanese did not start to heat-treat blood until 1988, by which time a large number of haemophiliacs had contracted AIDS.

One major scandal involving China was covered up for a number of years and not revealed until 2001. In the early 1990s, Chinese peasants in the province of Henan were selling blood to medical supply companies who were using unsterilised equipment. The blood was mixed and treated in bulk, the red blood cells were removed and the company only kept the plasma. The unwanted portion of the blood was then re-injected into the peasants, who had donated blood, so that they could donate again more quickly. It only needed one case of HIV+ to initiate a massive epidemic. The central government closed the programme in 1996, but then covered up the appalling consequences until 2001. Compulsory mass screenings carried out identified approximately thirty thousand cases as a direct result of the programme, although several sources claim that the number of cases was in the hundreds of thousands. By 2002, the Chinese authorities admitted there were a million cases of AIDS in China, although AIDS activists suggested that there were one million in Henan Province alone and that the Chinese authorities were suppressing the true figure. UN reports also suggest the real figure is significantly higher, and estimate that there could be at least ten million infected in China by 2010.

A number of children born to HIV+ mothers are infected and usually succumb to AIDS rapidly. Children are very difficult to treat, the liver is immature and cannot cope with toxic drugs and they also have immature immune systems which means they succumb more quickly than adults. Approximately one in three pregnant women who are HIV+ will pass the virus on to their child during pregnancy, during birth or by breast-feeding, with the majority of infected children catching it during pregnancy. The number of children infected can be reduced considerably by treating the mother with drugs such as AZT (Azidothymidine). Although the side effects are severe, it has the advantage of being one of the cheaper anti-*retro*-viral drugs available.

The epidemiology of AIDS in Africa differs from that found in the developed world. Drug taking usually consists of chewing or smoking the drug, and injecting drugs is a relatively minor activity. Much of traditional African society also disapproves of homosexuality and, in Africa, AIDS is spread mainly by heterosexual activity. The pattern of heterosexual partnerships however is somewhat different to that found in many other parts of the world, and this has a major influence on the rate at which HIV spreads. In much of Africa, sexual relationships tend to be of a type known as webs or nets (multiple partners), whereas in much of the rest of the world relationships tend to be chains or strings (single partners).

For example, in a chain, if an HIV+ male has one partner, he will only infect one woman; even if he is a serial monogamist, he will only infect one woman at a time, and she will not infect anybody else if she is also in a monogamous relationship. In a net however, if an HIV+ male has an official wife in town, and a girl friend (known as a bush wife) in every village he visits on business, whom he only sees once every few weeks, then he is going to infect several women. If he is only seeing the bush wife once a month, and she has several other boyfriends whom are visiting her as well, and if each of these has an official wife in town and bush wives in other villages he is visiting, the net or web of infection becomes very large very quickly. If the wife of male number one also has boyfriends visiting her whilst husband is away, and is part of one or several other networks, then the size of the net increases dramatically. The available data shows that these networks are a common arrangement in much of sub-Saharan Africa, possibly as a descendant of the custom of polygamy. The more partners that both men and women have, the quicker the virus spreads. It is also customary in some traditional African societies for a woman to marry the brother of her dead husband as a form of social security. If the husband died of AIDS, then his wife is obviously going to introduce it into the brother's family.

There is also a problem of men in well paid jobs, who are living away from home (for example, workers in the gold and diamond mines), with access to prostitutes, and when this is combined with a visit to the home village several times a year, the result is lethal. HIV has been shown to move along truck (trade) routes in Africa, a situation reminiscent of the movement of epidemics along sea trading routes in medieval Europe. The whole problem is exacerbated in Africa by a very strong anti-condom culture amongst the male population who insist on a skin-on-skin experience when having sex.

There do appear to be groups of individuals who have a natural resistance to HIV. A small but significant percentage of Caucasians possess the mutant gene CCR5-Δ32, which has already been described (Ch 9). The gene codes for a membrane protein that HIV requires to enter the susceptible cell in a majority of people; possession of a single copy of the gene slows down the rate of HIV infection, whilst possession of two copies appears to result in total immunity in these individuals.

Resistance was also described in a small percentage of prostitutes in Kenya and Uganda in 1992. These women, who statistically should have contracted AIDS within a certain time, were still healthy many years later, as were their daughters who were also prostitutes. This suggests that the resistance has a genetic basis and examination of their blood samples showed they had contracted the virus, but that infected cells were being recognised and destroyed very quickly by super-efficient killer T-cells.

Over a period of many generations, it is reasonable to predict that both of these types of resistance will spread throughout the human gene pool. The speed with which this type of resistance spreads does depend on the method by which the disease is transmitted and the severity of the disease.

One problem that is now happening in the developed world is that the number of cases of HIV is increasing in the older age group. In 2008 new cases amongst the over fifties in the UK were approximately double those of five years earlier. Many older people who have recently divorced or separated meet a new partner and do not bother about using a condom as the woman is over child bearing age.

HISTORY

AIDS appeared in the medical dictionary in the early 1980s and was officially given this name in 1982. It was initially known as GRIDS, and also as the "4H disease" because the four groups who appeared prone to it were Haitians, homosexuals, drug (heroin) users and haemophiliacs. As mentioned earlier, HIV is thought to have first infected humans in the Congo in the late nineteenth century. It is not known why it appeared to spread so suddenly after about seven or eight decades of obscurity, but it is possibly because of the massive movement of people due to the numerous civil wars, caused by various groups attempting to gain control of the mineral wealth of the area. The seventy to eighty year time span between the earliest suspected cases and the recognition of AIDS, also coincides with the development of cities in countries such as the Congo, a rise in high risk behaviour and the movement of large numbers of people from a rural to an urban environment. Sexual promiscuity tends to be a lot higher in urban conurbations than it does in villages where everyone knows everyone and nobody's business is private. The genetic diversity of the virus suggests that HIV was widespread (an estimated one hundred thousand cases) in the Congo by 1960, but took another twenty years to become recognised. In 1985, a wasting disease (known locally as Slim), which had been occurring widely throughout Africa, especially Uganda, for a number of years, was identified as AIDS.

Many early cases of HIV were found in Haiti. Genetic examination followed by mathematical analysis suggests that virtually all the HIV strains circulating outside Africa in the early stages were descendants of the strain circulating in Haiti. HIV probably arrived in Haiti in 1966 and had been carried there by one person from the Congo, where many Haitians were working at the time. It circulated in Haiti for several years then jumped to the USA around 1969, again it is thought to have been carried there by one person. It remained undetected in the USA until the early 1980s, not being recognised, until it reached homosexual groups when epidemiologically significant clusters of unusual diseases became obvious.

The documentation of much of the early research on HIV is confused because of the controversy between French and US laboratories with accusations and counter-accusations flying in both directions. The HIV virus was reported in May 1983 by Luc Montagnier of the Pasteur Institute, and in April 1984, Robert Gallo of the CDC in Atlanta announced that the cause of AIDS had been found. It rapidly became obvious that the French and American viruses were the same, and it was widely alleged at the time that the work of the Pasteur Institute was deliberately held up until an American researcher was ready to publish. Gallo claimed priority and it took three years of bickering and the intervention of Presidents Reagan and Mitterand before it was agreed that Montagnier and Gallo were co-discoverers of the virus. In spite of the agreement of the two presidents, the Nobel Prize Committee obviously agreed with the French version of events, as they awarded the Nobel Prize in Medicine in 2008 to Montagnier and his co-worker Francoise Barre-Sinoussi for their work on HIV. The comment of a member of the committee was, *"there was no doubt as to who had made the fundamental discoveries".*

By 1985, serological tests to detect the virus had been developed, although many of the early ones gave very inaccurate results when used on patients suffering from other diseases such as malaria. This problem with so-called "sticky serum" gave rise to some widely varying and highly inaccurate figures for HIV+ levels in much of Africa during the late 1980s and 1990s. The quality of current HIV test kits are also very variable and the most sensitive ones still give a positive result, even when blood is HIV negative. It is also necessary to refrigerate many test kits which is a major problem in some parts of the world where AIDS levels are high. A further problem is the very high cost of many diagnostic systems in countries where the per capita spend on medicine is only a few pounds a year. Some of the later test kits make use of PCR (polymerase chain reaction) technology. This copies the viral RNA and enables the virus to be detected after very recent infection, before antibody production commences.

By 1982, AIDS had been found in Europe, Central Africa and the Caribbean and by 1985, it had become a pandemic with a fatality rate of one hundred per cent, no vaccine and predictions of tens of millions infected worldwide. It has already caused and will continue to cause massive demographic changes, especially in Africa and a number of other developing areas.

There are numerous rumours about the origin of HIV that range from the reasonable to the bizarre. This is a common reaction when any new disease strikes a population, and mirrors the human behaviour of previous centuries when new pandemics such as plague, syphilis and cholera arrived on the scene. A similar situation probably happened when most new diseases started, but these three examples are probably the best documented.

It is difficult to trace the source of HIV. US law requires hospital records to be kept for five years only, and when HIV appeared, many US and European hospitals deliberately destroyed files and computer records to avoid litigation over the use of contaminated blood products and transfusions. In addition, tracking contacts amongst the homosexual and drug addict populations, which is where the disease first became prominent, is virtually impossible. Many are dead, others are of no fixed abode, and many of the homosexual population had multiple unknown partners. Therefore many of the clues that might have helped trace the focal point of AIDS have been lost or deliberately eliminated.

Where did HIV come from? As mentioned earlier, the suggestions range from bizarre to reasonable. One suggestion was that it came from outer space; this of course totally begs the question of how it got into outer space in the first place, how it survived the intense UV radiation of outer space and how it could have survived the heat of re-entry. Other suggestions are divine retribution on homosexuals (strongly supported by many fundamentalist religious groups), the CIA suggested it was a KGB plot to destabilize the USA and the KGB suggested it was genetic engineering by the USA to destroy communism (this technology was not available when HIV first infected humans, but one should never let a fact get in the way of a good story). Further suggestions were a US plot to destroy the black population of the USA (sub-sets of this scenario are the use of the anti-HIV drug AZT to poison the black population, and forcing them to use condoms which are genocidal). Another sub-set of this was that it was introduced by BOSS (the South African Bureau of State Security), at the time of apartheid, to reduce the black population of Southern Africa. Other suggestions are that smallpox injections activated ancient but small scale HIV infections, this totally ignores the fact that smallpox vaccination had been carried out for about a century before AIDS appeared. Homosexual newspapers blamed the CIA for releasing African swine fever virus into Cuba to destabilise the economy whilst US veterans groups blamed the use of dioxins, such as Agent Orange, used as a defoliating agent in the Vietnam War. A final suggestion was that it was the mutation of a pre-existing virus caused by nuclear testing. The believers in the conspiracy theory had, and are still having, a field day.

There are two sensible theories for the origin of HIV. The first of these relates to the use of cells from the kidneys of monkeys used in tissue culture to make polio vaccine. It was suggested that these cells were carrying SIV (the Simian Immunodeficiency Virus) which is similar to HIV, and that this mutated to HIV when injected into humans given the vaccine. Most of the stocks of the original polio vaccine have been used or destroyed, but a surviving sample found recently did not contain SIV and this hypothesis is now regarded as untenable. It has also become obvious over time that HIV had appeared in the Congo decades before a polio vaccine became available. The generally accepted explanation is that given earlier, it was the SIV virus carried by chimpanzees that infected hunters when chimps were killed and butchered for bush meat.

The spread of AIDS was then helped by a number of human activities that have already been documented in the previous section.

AIDS is very different to previous pandemics. It attacks the human immune system in a unique manner that negates the experience we have gained in controlling other diseases using methods such as vaccine production. It is a viral disease as opposed to a bacterial one such as syphilis, which means that the number of drugs capable of combating it is strictly limited. There is no vector that can be eliminated compared with diseases such as bubonic plague and typhus. The virus is extremely unstable and mutates rapidly compared with other viral diseases such as yellow fever and this has made the preparation of a vaccine impossible to date. There are no obvious symptoms in the early stages compared with smallpox, and there is a very long incubation period compared with flu. These last two factors allow the HIV+ individual to infect numerous other victims, either intentionally or unintentionally, before their condition becomes obvious. All these factors combine to make AIDS an extremely dangerous disease, probably the most dangerous disease that the human race has encountered to date.

Possibly one of the most frightening aspects of AIDS is that it could have easily remained undiscovered or unrecognised for another 5-10 years if any of following factors had altered:

- if HIV took longer to produce recognisable disease symptoms
- if the immunodeficiency of AIDS caused an increase in more typical infections instead of unusual infections, for example, normal pulmonary pneumonia instead of pneumonia from *Pneumocystis carinii*
- if it had been widespread in the general community instead of clustering into certain groups i.e. homosexuals and injecting drug addicts, which produced recognisable epidemiological patterns at an early stage
- if it had not occurred at an early stage in the USA which has a well developed disease surveillance system.

The important point is that any disease anywhere can rapidly become a problem worldwide in these days of rapid travel, and viruses and bacteria do not recognise national borders or customs posts.

It will probably adapt to humans over time (many scientists consider a reasonable time scale would be several hundred years), but will cause massive demographic changes before the human population and HIV stabilise. It is filling the vacuum left by the elimination of smallpox (see Malthus, ch 10) and probably an even more depressing thought is that there could well be another disease of a similar type waiting its turn on the central stage.

In August 2009, a French research group reported that a woman from Cameroon living in France, since 2004, was infected with a previously unknown strain of HIV related to the SIV strain found in gorillas. It is not known how widely this strain is circulating but it is replicating rapidly in the patient although it has not progressed to AIDS. The woman involved claimed she had had no contact with gorillas or bush meat, which if true means she must have contracted it from another human source. The research group stated, "[it] *highlights the continuing need to watch closely for the emergence of new HIV variants particularly in western central Africa".*

The discovery of this new variant means that we could be missing new strains of HIV because existing tests are biased towards detecting medically important strains already in circulation. The existing tests may not detect new strains if they are sufficiently different genetically to the older strains.

Transmission of *retro*-viruses from other primates to humans is not limited to HIV. When people living in Cameroon (the point of origin of HIV), who have been exposed to the blood of non-human primates are tested, over one per cent tested positive for antibodies to the Simian Foamy Virus (SFV). This is also an RNA *retro*-virus that can insert DNA copies of the virus into the genome of the host; it causes cells to fuse to form syncytia that look like foaming bubbles. It has not yet been linked to any specific disease but a number of experts have suggested it may predispose individuals to other viral diseases. Does this sound familiar?

THE POLITICS OF AIDS

Pisani has written an excellent account (*The Wisdom of Whores)* of the politics of the HIV epidemic that should be compulsory reading for all doctors, teachers, NGO and charity workers and all those involved with the disease. It may seem a rather cynical comment to make, but many doctors and scientists consider that the bureaucracy of HIV and AIDS has spread even more relentlessly than the disease itself.

The following section is distilled from Pisani's book and reiterates many of the points she makes. The politics of HIV/AIDS is a medley of sex, drugs and political correctness, with finance, ideology, various political and religious groups and powerful lobbies and spin groups controlling governments, charities, and non-governmental organisations (NGOs). There are a large number of organisations defending or trying to enlarge their empires, WHO, UN World Bank, UNESCO, various NGOs and charities, and the World Council of Churches to name a few. Some of them have very little to do with HIV and AIDS, but they all want a slice of the funding being poured into HIV and AIDS.

The politics of AIDS also raises the very serious question of whether science can remain detached and objective when it is funded by governments, big business, large rich charities and NGOs, who each have their own political (and frequently religious) agenda. It raises the equally important point that science that works in the laboratory frequently does not translate into the public domain of election winning policies, and practical and sensible public health practices that work on the ground. The brutal fact is that when it comes to subjects such as sexually transmitted diseases, especially HIV and AIDS, as a generality, most politicians and the public would prefer not to know.

The political correctness employed frequently defies what many individuals would consider to be common sense. Whilst most people would have a range of epithets to describe homosexuals, prostitutes and drug addicts depending on the company they are frequenting, the following example is taken from Pisani who quotes a UNAIDS document entitled, *"Men who have sex with Men". "While we use the term "men who have sex with men" here it is within the context of understanding that the word "man"/"men" is socially constructed. Nor does it imply that it is an identity term referring to an identifiable community that can be segregated and so labelled. Within the framework of male-to-male sex, there are a range of masculinities, along with diverse sexual and gender identities, communities, networks and collectives, as well as just behaviours without any sense of affiliation to an identity or community".* Many people reading this statement would find it risible if it were not such a serious subject, and most teenagers would regard it as totally incomprehensible. As a piece of politically correct speak, incomprehensible to the general public, one would have hoped it was unique, but Pisani quotes numerous similar examples.

Political correctness has also stopped many of the most basic principles of public health being applied to the AIDS epidemic. Many countries have mandatory reporting of diseases such as syphilis and the tracing of contacts, whom are then offered treatment. This is frequently not done with HIV and AIDS as it risks offending the homosexual lobby, yet it is probably the most effective method of tracking, treating and controlling a sexually transmitted disease.

What causes AIDS? About two thirds of those infected with HIV live in Africa, south of the Sahara desert, and virtually all of the HIV in Africa is spread by sex between unprotected heterosexuals when one partner is HIV+. However, many people, including a large number of African politicians and many aid workers, claim that HIV is spread by poverty, under-development and gender inequality. A UN official report of 2004 blamed poverty, social instability, sexual violence, low stature of women, large migratory labour forces and ineffective leadership (in Africa). This is politically correct rhetoric that ignores the scientific facts. There is plenty of poverty and gender inequality in North African countries, but HIV levels are low. In sub-Saharan Africa, both South Africa and Botswana are amongst the highest in terms of per capita income and female literacy, however they are also two of the highest countries in percentage terms for HIV+ individuals. In South Africa and Botswana, HIV is more prevalent in richer households than poorer ones, and also amongst literate women compared with illiterate ones. In African countries such as Mali and Sierra Leone, there are low rates of HIV even though these countries have a low per capita income.

Life expectancy has fallen drastically in those countries worst affected, for example in Botswana, by 2006, it had fallen from sixty-five to less than forty years. In many African countries, death certificates, if they are issued, do not require

AIDS to be stated as a cause of death and the subject is frequently taboo in the local culture making it very difficult to establish the true extent of the disease. Ignorance is a major factor in the spread of HIV Many people are not aware that it is a sexually transmitted disease, witchcraft is frequently blamed and condoms are culturally unacceptable in many traditional societies. There is also a widespread belief that AIDS can be cured by having sex with a young girl who is a virgin.

Many African leaders consider it is not nice to talk or write about sex so they blame something else. In 2001, Kofi Annan, the UN Secretary General, spoke at considerable length to African leaders on the subject of AIDS and the need to combat it. He did not mention sex once. Similarly, Thabo Mbeki, the South African President until recently, consistently denied HIV caused AIDS and one of his health ministers advised people to eat garlic, beetroot and lemons as a cure. In 2007, a second Health Minister, who publicised the facts and declared that HIV and AIDS was a national emergency, was sacked. After one conference in Durban, over five thousand scientists and doctors signed a statement declaring that the evidence that HIV caused AIDS was obvious and overwhelming; a spokesman for the South African government declared the conference statement was rubbish. One presidential spokesman justified refusing to treat pregnant HIV+ women with AZT to stop their children catching the virus, by saying that the mothers were going to die anyway and, *"we don't want a generation of orphans".* The traditional African way of dealing with orphans is adoption by the extended family. However many communities and families are over saturated with orphans and grandparents are looking after children because the parents are dead from AIDS. There are at least nine million cases out of a population of forty-five million, but South Africa did not start to distribute anti-*retro*-viral drugs until AIDS activists went to court to force the issue. The amounts being distributed are still only a fraction of what is required. It might have been thought that the situation would improve when Mbeki ceased to be President of South Africa, but the new President, Jacob Zuma, admitted to having unprotected sex with an HIV+ woman, but claimed it was not a problem because he had a shower afterwards. If African politicians, the media and religious leaders deny HIV causes AIDS, what chances have uneducated peasant farmers got?

In South Africa about thirty per cent of pregnant women are HIV+, in Botswana an estimated eighty per cent of university students are infected, and in Swaziland forty-three per cent of all adults are infected. In Zimbabwe, the officially recognised incidence of AIDS is twenty per cent, the few doctors remaining in the country claim it is considerably higher than this and an estimated twenty-five per cent of children are orphans mainly because of AIDS. In spite of these figures, it is still politically correct to insist that HIV is spread by poverty, not sex.

The increasing mortality of young adults means that there is a smaller skilled work force causing lower productivity, and it also means there is a reduction in the tax revenues that governments can raise with significant knock-on effects for public expenditure on the infrastructure. The cost of AIDS is huge. Between 1996 and 2006, the number of people with HIV rose approximately forty per cent, but spending on HIV in developing countries rose 2,900%. By 2007, $10 billion per year was being spent on HIV prevention and treatment in developing countries, much of it was being misspent and not targeting the right problems. Prevention is a lot more effective and cheaper than treatment, but helping communities stay disease free does not raise the political profile the way helping people who are already ill does, and does not provide the same feeling of moral superiority.

The USA has laws channelling a very large proportion of aid dollars donated by the US back into the purchase of American products. However, goods made in the USA frequently cost significantly more than the same thing made locally. There are also bureaucracy, shipping costs, customs tariffs and local bribes; it adds up to a lot of wasted financial aid. Drugs, such as antibiotics, have to be approved by the FDA in the USA, even though they are not going to be used in the USA. American aid dollars cannot be used to buy cheap generic preparations of drugs from a local supply. To quote Pisani in just one example, in East Timor, locally obtainable penicillin derivatives used to treat syphilis cost $1.50 per dose for a preparation that is temperature stable. Because of the buy American policy, it has to be ordered from the USA at over $70/dose for a formulation that must be kept between $4\text{-}8^0C$ in tropical countries subject to frequent power cuts. When all the costs are added up, the product is frequently 100x more expensive than if a generic product were purchased locally. If this had been done it would save a lot of money that could be used elsewhere and would also put money directly into the local economy. The UK does not require aid money to be spent in the UK, the general attitude of UK charities is get it locally if it is available, get it cheap and if it works, fine.

In addition to the above problems, a number of the American NGOs and charities have their own religious agenda, and aid frequently comes with religious conditions in the small print. Over forty per cent of charitable donations in the USA are made to faith based organisations and a number of these charities, in particular Catholic based ones, oppose the use of condoms which are also opposed by many Muslim preachers. This is extremely unfortunate as, in spite of what the Pope and senior cardinals state, condoms are very effective, especially if used properly on every occasion, at reducing the rate of transmission of all sexually transmitted diseases, including HIV. The conditions attached to charitable aid, especially that channelled through the churches, frequently preclude supplying and promoting the use of condoms.

The stupidity of this policy can be seen by examining the situation in Thailand in the early 1990s, when the country was threatened with a serious epidemic of HIV. The Thai authorities targeted the sex industry with a campaign promoting a one hundred per cent use of condoms. By 2003, the number of new infections had fallen to 19,000 per year from a peak of 143,000 per year in 1991. Nobody is claiming that condoms are the only answer to HIV but they are extremely effective as part of a package of measures.

A further major problem is the level of corruption in many African countries where the sums of money being poured into AIDS treatment by various donors is a veritable honeypot for corrupt officials. Epstein documents numerous scams in her book *"The Invisible Cure"* and points out that many of these scams are caused by politically correct ideology and inadequate supervision of aid funds.

A further problem is, what happens if (when) donors stop giving money? Until a cure is found for HIV infection, anti-*retro*-viral drugs are like puppies, they are for life, not just Christmas. What happens when some other good cause arrives on the scene or just a plain old fashioned credit crunch causes donors to tighten their belts?

There are also many arguments amongst NGOs and aid agencies, whose anti-*retro*-viral drugs are treating whose AIDS, whose condoms reduced AIDS transmission in which country? All of them claim it was the work of their organisation. This might seem irrelevant to the local donor who dropped a small coin into the charity collecting box on flag day, but it is not just a hypothetical question. The charity needs to be able to demonstrate to fund raisers, spin doctors and politicians that it was their agency that was effective so that they continue getting public support and taxpayers' dollars, pounds or euros. The lobbyists will also have a financial interest, they will be creaming off a percentage of the funds raised to pay their salaries, overheads and advertising.

The recent earthquake in Haiti is a classic example of these problems of duplication of effort. Within a few days of the earthquake there were six major charities soliciting donations in the same newspaper on the same day. Whilst all no doubt had excellent motives, the fact remains that six banks of phones had to be manned, six groups of administrators had to be paid and it is a reasonable bet that not one of the charities had much idea what the other five were doing except in very general terms.

It is politically incorrect to ask questions and demand answers about many of these things. The fact is that to quote Pisani, *"it is politically incorrect to talk about the AIDS epidemic like it is. It is racist, it is homophobic, it is perceived to denigrate sex workers, it upsets aid donors, it upsets people who already have AIDS, it upsets those in high risk groups, it upsets religious groups and most importantly it upsets politicians who would prefer to sweep these problems under the carpet where they cannot be seen".*

WHAT ARE THE SOLUTIONS TO THE AIDS EPIDEMIC?

The blunt answer to that question is that there are not any at the present moment. There are no drugs that will cure it and there is no effective vaccine available. Even optimistic observers would not envisage an effective vaccine making an appearance within the next ten years. There have been too many false dawns in the past.

Given the above facts, the best courses of action are to take certain simple measures to prevent the transmission of HIV, and try changing people's behaviour. Trying to persuade people to give up sex is obviously not an option, in spite of what George W. Bush said. Bush decided that sexual abstinence was the answer to AIDS, *"it works every time"*. To say that approach is naïve is a serious understatement; try telling that to some teenage soldier just back from six months in Afghanistan and high on a cocktail of alcohol and testosterone. Under Bush, one third of US AIDS charity went into *"Abstinence until Marriage"* programmes, presumably due to pressure from the religious right wing of American politics.

Efforts need to be made to persuade people to give up risky sex, such as reducing casual sex encounters and taking sensible precautions such as using a condom at all times. Colin Powell, US Secretary of State under Bush, had a more pragmatic approach to condoms, *"My instinct is to keep kids from getting a disease, not to save them from moral turpitude".*

There is a great need for educational programmes for young people on the dangers of casual sex, especially when inhibitions have been lowered by alcohol or illicit drugs. In the UK, when AIDS first appeared in the late 1980s there were publicity programmes such as the TV campaign *"Don't Die of Ignorance"* showing tombstones with an epitaph. Many parents objected to this claiming that it caused anxiety in children and young adults. The answer to that is a simple question, would you prefer your children and teenagers to be frightened or dead? Anti-HIV publicity has been phased out, and AIDS levels in the UK are rising.

Massive educational and publicity programmes that pull no punches are required, people, especially young adults and teenagers, need to be told that HIV kills. Publicity programmes do work, in Uganda, at its peak in 1991, HIV was infecting fifteen per cent of the population. A massive publicity programme entitled *"Zero Grazing"* started in 1986. This promoted the use of condoms and made everybody aware of the danger of casual sex. The incidence rate of AIDS fell to less than half that rate over the next fifteen years. The programme was stopped in the 1990s because of political pressure from various aid agencies.

Unfortunately, the use of drugs to control AIDS in the developed world means that people are becoming less afraid of it, which results in them getting careless. In the five years between 1989 and 1994, rectal gonorrhoea halved. In the ten years between 1995 and 2005, it quadrupled, as did syphilis with a concomitant rise in AIDS. Gonorrhoea is frequently considered as the marker disease for STIs. The effects are unpleasant and become obvious relatively quickly compared with many other STIs, causing the infected person to visit the doctor or health clinic at an early stage, which results in data being more reliable. If gonorrhoea cases quadrupled, it is a reasonable assumption that all other STIs have also increased significantly and the available data confirms this.

In the case of injecting drug addicts, needle exchange programmes should be used to provide clean needles, addicts should be encouraged to start methadone treatment and effective drug treatment programmes should be encouraged in prisons, which are one of the main amplifiers of AIDS. The heat treatment of blood donated to blood banks and used for transfusions is an obvious precaution, and all injecting equipment and catheters should be sterilised. HIV+ mothers should be treated with the appropriate drugs to reduce the risk of infecting their child, and should use formula milk to avoid problems of breast-feeding.

The statistical data shows that HIV spreads less rapidly in countries where a large percentage of men have been circumcised. The evidence indicates circumcised men are six to eight times less likely to contract HIV than uncircumcised ones, however circumcision does not slow down the rate of transfer of syphilis. This would suggest that there is a biological reason rather than a cultural or behavioural one. The reason is that the Langerhans cells on the inside of the foreskin are attacked by HIV, and removal of these during circumcision removes a major target for the virus. Although men can still become infected, the rate of transmission is slowed significantly. Male circumcision on a large scale would be a very effective method of reducing the rate of transmission and the spread of AIDS, but promotion of this measure would inevitably involve major cultural, religious and practical issues.

The US government, again under pressure from the churches, required US aid channelled through charities to pledge opposition to prostitution. This again is an extremely naïve approach as closing red light districts drives prostitution underground where it is more difficult to control. A far more effective measure would be to legalise prostitution, collect taxes and enforce regular and frequent medical check-ups for all sex workers.

Several African countries have controlled HIV effectively. Senegal started a prevention programme before HIV reached a critical mass and was able to control the problem by regulating prostitution, treating women for other STIs and promoting the use of condoms. HIV prevalence in Senegal has remained at a low level, around one per cent.

Many countries register people suffering from syphilis and ask questions about their sexual partners, then medical teams or social workers track them down and offer tests and treatment. No-one complains about this, but when a number of countries used the same methods in the early stages of the AIDS epidemic, there were numerous complaints about human rights, especially from the homosexual lobby. As a result, mandatory testing and contact tracing were rejected in many countries, and the basic principles of public health and epidemiology were overridden in the name of political correctness. The introduction of these measures would contribute significantly to our knowledge of the way AIDS is spreading and provide information that would be of considerable use in its control.

Free Drugs for Africa?

Many charitable groups working with AIDS patients in the developing world consider that the industrialised world has a moral duty to supply the latest anti-*retro*-viral drugs either free or at cost, and regularly lobby governments for this to be carried out. If it is not done, there is frequently the threat to use generic versions of the drugs in question before the patents expire on the original versions.

There are several aspects to these suggestions. Firstly, many anti-*retro*-viral drugs must be taken under regular medical supervision with regular monitoring of the viral load. They also have to be taken for life and if their use is not followed correctly, there is a high probability that the strain of virus involved will rapidly become resistant to the drug being used. This requires relatively sophisticated groups of patients who understand the risks of breaks in treatment and who are prepared to stick with the drug regime long-term. This level of drug awareness is unlikely to be found in a rural community relying on traditional doctors and faith healers. A number of doctors and scientists have emphasised this point very strongly. There is also the problem of a lack of trained medical staff in much of the developing world, especially Africa, who can provide the appropriate level of supervision and monitoring of viral loads.

The supply and transport infrastructure are also important, much of rural Africa becomes impenetrable during the rainy season and there is a high probability of disruption of the supplies of drugs due to extreme weather conditions or various wars. There is also the problem of corruption that is endemic in much of Africa. This will almost certainly cause drugs to be held in customs or somewhere along the supply chain until an appropriate bribe has been paid.

The scientific conclusion therefore is that if anti-*retro*-viral drugs are supplied freely or cheaply in bulk to Africa, they will almost certainly be misused. The result will be that HIV will mutate to resistance to these drugs even faster than it is doing at present.

The other major problem is the question of patents. When a drug is patented, the patent runs for twenty years; this is from the time the drug is first patented, not from the time it comes onto the market. Typically, once a patent has been granted, the drug goes through the development process and various trials for ten to fourteen years before becoming available for public use. The company developing the drug therefore usually has, on average, about eight years to recover their costs and make a profit.

The cost of developing a major new drug is obviously variable depending on the drug, but a typical figure would be between $500 million and $1 billion. For every hundred drugs discovered at the bench top, only one or two will survive the various tests to make it onto the market. The cost of the ones that fail will vary; those rejected at the bench top stage may only cost a few million pounds, those rejected at the final stage III trials may cost nearly the full amount quoted above. The one or two successful drugs have to generate sufficient profits to cover not only their own development costs, but also the costs of the ninety-eight or ninety-nine that failed. In addition, the successful one must generate dividends for the shareholders in the company. It is all very well for charitable groups to claim that shareholders do not matter, if sufficient shareholders sell their shares because the dividend is not good enough, the drug company collapses and so do any new drugs in the pipeline.

It is therefore worth remembering that before purchasing generic drugs, the companies making them are piggybacking on the research efforts and costs of the companies that first produced and patented the drugs in question. Secondly, generic drugs produced after patents have expired are old technology, the micro-organisms causing the disease may well have become resistant to the drug in the eight years it has been available to the public. It is also worth remembering that in some cases, the only alternative to a brand name drug under patent may be no drug at all.

IMMIGRATION AND HIV IN THE UK

Some people may find the comments made in this section unpalatable or politically incorrect, however, the figures quoted are taken from the 2008 report on *"HIV in the United Kingdom"* and can be found on the website of the Health Protection Agency, a Quango (quasi-autonomous non-governmental organisation) using officially published government figures for various diseases.

At the end of 2007, 56,556 people living in the UK had been diagnosed as HIV+ and there were a further estimated 20-21,000 who were unaware of their condition, giving a total of approximately 77,400. The corresponding number of diagnosed cases for 1998 was 17,911 and for 2006 it was 52,083. The 2007 figure is therefore an increase of 8.6% on the 2006 figure and more than triple the 1998 figure. A recent editorial in *"The Lancet"* accused government ministers of *"an appalling failure to tackle HIV"* and of having *"no creditable strategy to diagnose and care for those living with, but unaware of, HIV in Britain".*

Approximately seventy per cent of the 56,556 individuals known to be HIV+ are receiving anti-*retro*-viral treatment; this approximates to 39,600 and if the cost of treating these is £16,000 each, then the total is about £634 million per year. The true figure will be considerably higher than this, as the calculation above does not include the thirty per cent of HIV+ people not receiving drugs. The CD4 cell count of these has presumably not yet fallen to the point where they need treatment but there will still be the cost of monitoring their viral load at regular intervals. The calculation also makes the assumption that all those being treated are receiving first line drugs; those individuals receiving second line drugs will cost the NHS considerably more. The corresponding figures for 2001 and 2002 were £165 million and £345 million.

The sum of £634 million quoted above is of course just the figure for 2007. Because anti-*retro*-viral drugs are for life, the cost in 2008 would be the same as that for 2007 plus the cost of treating any new cases diagnosed in 2008. This also makes no allowance for inflation or the higher costs of any new drugs that became available during this period.

In 2007, 7,734 new cases were diagnosed in the UK, of these 4,887 were men. The data indicates that approximately 55% of the new cases were infected through heterosexual activities, 41% through homosexual activities, 2.5 % were injecting drug addicts and 1.5% were mother-to-child infections. There were 4,260 new heterosexual cases and of these an estimated 3,300 (77.5%) were probably infected outside the UK; 2,850 of the 4,260 cases were black Africans (67.9%) and an estimated 90% had acquired HIV abroad, mainly in sub-Saharan Africa.

The figures of the Health Protection Agency suggest that the number of new homosexual HIV infections for 2007 was

3,160, of which about 82% were thought to have acquired the disease in the UK. This figure is approximately 20% up on the previous year, which might seem surprising as most homosexuals are well aware of the risks of HIV infection. It may be that the development of drugs capable of arresting the development of AIDS has led to them taking deliberate risks by having unprotected sex with partners known to be HIV+, an act known as "bare backing". It has been suggested that in some homosexual circles, one is not part of the community unless one is HIV+, and being HIV+ is a statement of belonging to the group. Many people probably have considerable difficulty in understanding the mindset of someone who deliberately courts infection by such a dangerous virus.

The Health Protection Agency takes great care to avoid the use of the word immigrant and does not state how many of the approximately 3,880 (3,300 heterosexual and 580 homosexual) people who caught HIV abroad were immigrants. Instead it uses euphemisms such as, *"probably caught outside the UK"* and *"probably caught in sub-Saharan Africa"*. It is a reasonable assumption that most of these cases are immigrants especially if they caught the disease in countries such as Zimbabwe. The figure of 3,880 as a percentage of 7,734 new cases is 50.2%. This tallies closely with figures for the number of HIV+ immigrants in the 1990s and the early part of the first decade of the twentieth-first century, when we were rather less politically correct about such matters and the word immigrant was used.

If the figure of 3,880 cases caught abroad is multiplied by the cost of treatment (£16,000) per person per year, the figure obtained is in excess of £62 million. This again is just the figure for new cases in 2007; they would also have needed treatment in 2008 and 2009 and so on. The same sort of figures will apply to those who caught the disease abroad and brought it into the country in 2008, and those who caught it in 2009 *etcetera*. If we assume that an HIV+ person has an average life expectancy of twenty-five years after contracting the disease abroad, then the cost of treatment for such a person is £400,000 in today's figures.

The cost of HIV treatment is increasing on a year-by-year basis, and recently some 13% of Primary Care Trusts in the UK are starting to limit access to the latest drugs available on the grounds of exceeding their budgets.

Numerous countries screen immigrants for infectious diseases such as HIV and tuberculosis, the UK does not. A UNAIDS statement in 1998 stated that, *"There is no public health rationale for restricting liberty of movement or choice of residence on the grounds of HIV status".* It should be pointed out that the UN does not pick up the bill for treating HIV+ immigrants arriving in the UK, the British tax-payer does, and the amounts mentioned earlier in this section add up to a lot of hip and knee replacements or cataract operations.

It is not just the costs of treating HIV. As mentioned earlier in this chapter, HIV is in many ways a unique disease acting in a novel manner. As such, over a period of generations it will probably be a greater threat and risk to the UK than that posed by various terrorist groups. A major function of elected politicians is to defend the UK from real and perceived threats. They are not doing a very good job of defending the UK against HIV and AIDS.

Arguments against testing immigrants in the past have included the length of time required to carry out tests, the confusion that these would cause at point of entry and also the fact that the earlier tests measured antibodies which did not appear in the infected person for about six weeks. The more modern tests for HIV can produce results within an hour and before antibodies appear. There is nothing to stop these tests being carried out by an accredited doctor in the local British Embassy before a prospective immigrant leaves their home country.

It has also been suggested that immigrants contribute a lot to this country even if they are HIV+. At a cost of £16,000 per year to treat an HIV+ person, the infected immigrant must have the skills to hold down an extremely well paid job to pay sufficient taxes to cover that figure.

CHAPTER 19

Schistosomiasis (Bilharzia)

"A nasty thing, the schistosome,
It turns your bladder into home".
(with apologies to the Institute of Biology)

Schistosomes or blood flukes are metazoan parasites that have two hosts, one a vertebrate and the second a freshwater snail usually of the genus *Bulinus*. The WHO estimates that they infect approximately 200 million people worldwide and cause about 200,000 deaths each year, making them the second most important parasitic disease after malaria.

The adult fluke, the form found in humans, is about one centimetre long and the name schistosome means split body. This relates to the fact that they exist in pairs and the male has a split in its body in which the smaller female travels. In the vertebrate host they live in blood vessels in the intestine, bladder, liver and various other organs. The female produces hundreds of eggs per day that pass out from the vertebrate host in the faeces and urine and enter a body of fresh water in which the snails live. Once they have entered the water, the eggs hatch to form larvae known as miracidia that have a few hours to find a suitable snail host. They enter the snail and commence a phase of asexual reproduction to form large numbers of highly mobile larvae with forked tails called cercariae. These are released into the water and on finding a vertebrate host they bore through the skin, make their way to the liver, mature, pair up and migrate as a unit through the blood vessels. The disease is therefore spread by activities such as washing, swimming and fishing in infected water. In the absence of any treatment the adult flukes may live in the body for as long as twenty years.

Several important species of schistosome are found. As the name suggests *Schistosoma japonicum* is found in China and Japan and inhabits the blood vessels of the intestine and liver, *S. mansoni* is also found in the blood vessels of the intestine whilst *S. haematobium* inhabits the walls of the bladder. *S. haematobium* and *S. mansoni* are the species found in Africa. Although *S. mansoni* was carried by the slave trade to Brazil, Venezuela and some of the Caribbean islands, it has not have spread further into the Americas due to the lack of suitable carrier snails. A fourth species *S. mekongi* is found in South East Asia. There are numerous other species infecting a wide range of animals, both domestic and wild.

Schistosomes were discovered in 1851 by Theodor Bilharz whose name gave rise to the alternative name of the disease, but their life cycle was not elucidated until World War I by Robert Lieper. The disease has a complex epidemiology and the organisms can usually infect a wide range of vertebrate hosts but only a small range of aquatic snails.

The adult worms do not cause a serious problem but their eggs possess spiny hooks that lodge in tissues of the host such as the liver, spleen, genitals, lungs and brain causing inflammation and bleeding. Post mortem examinations have shown eggs in virtually every organ of the body. The infected tissues frequently calcify and scar severely and heavy infections may cause bladder cancer and liver failure. The species found in the bladder may also cause the formation of kidney stones and secondary bacterial infections of the urinary tract. In the case of *S. haematobium*, early symptoms are blood in the urine and Egypt was known as, *"the land of the menstruating men"*. In the case of heavy infections, the host may suffer from severe anaemia that renders them more susceptible to infections by other micro-organisms.

Although the adult flukes are large compared with other micro-organisms that infect us, they are able to evade the immune system of the host. The outer surface of the fluke is covered by a membrane, known as the tegument, which is able to capture host proteins. Amongst the molecules captured are the proteins specifying blood groups and these camouflage the fluke, so that even although the fluke is present, the host immune system cannot recognise it. Although the adult fluke is invisible to the host, it is the host immune reaction to the eggs that produces many of the symptoms associated with the disease. This invisibility of the adult has made the development of a vaccine impossible to date.

Infections were probably low level in hunter-gatherer societies as is the case in primates other than humans at the present time. Human contact with infected water would have increased as farming in river valleys increased and it would have spread from these foci. The first known infections have been found in the Nile Valley and dated to pre-dynastic Egypt. Infections also occur in a number of mummies from the New Kingdom and it is widespread in modern Egypt, with most village children probably infected. It has been suggested that the penis sheaths shown in some Egyptian tomb wall paintings were worn to stop infection by schistosomes. Although the Egyptians would not have been aware of the cause, the loss of blood in the urine would have led them to assume that the problem entered the body by the same route, hence the penis sheaths worn as protection.

Traditional irrigation systems of the Nile Valley consisted of flooding large areas every year in summer, allowing the floods to subside and planting crops in November. Schistosomes were present at low levels because the snails died as the soil was allowed to dry out, and the human/fluke contact was lost. This type of agriculture was practised for centuries and levels of *S. haematobium* are still low where traditional agricultural methods are used. In the nineteenth century, agriculture changed in the Nile Delta. Deep canals were cut and permanent irrigation was started to allow large scale production of cash crops, such as cotton, that require large volumes of water. Under these conditions schistosomiasis increased tenfold and became even higher when the Aswan dam was finished.

A similar situation was found in China. Schistosomiasis caused by *S. japonicum* was present at low levels in the Yellow River Valley about 3,000 BC when millet, rice and barley were farmed. It appeared on a large scale when the Yangtse Valley was settled and will probably get considerably worse now the Three Gorges Dam is finished.

Schistosomiasis became widespread amongst communist Chinese troops preparing for an attack on the Nationalist held island of Formosa (present day Taiwan), in the late 1940s, to the extent that the attack was cancelled[201]. The territorial integrity of Taiwan was then underwritten by the USA, leading to a long period of confrontation between the Chinese and Americans and ultimately to President Krushchev's famous comment to Chairman Mao, *"the US is a paper tiger,* [but] *it has nuclear teeth"*.

Schistosomiasis has never become established in the Indian subcontinent or the USA because the necessary species of snails are absent.

Attempts to control of the disease take place at several levels. The first of these involves controlling the snail population with chemicals known as molluscicides whose success is very variable, some of them, such as copper sulphate, having undesirable ecological side-effects. The second method is treatment of the infected person with a drug known as praziquantel, This has been available since the 1970s and a single dose is usually sufficient to cure an individual. Unfortunately as the immune system does not recognise the schistosome, re-infection is very common and reports are starting to suggest that the fluke may be becoming resistant to the drug. As praziquantel is the only really effective drug against most species of *Schistosoma*,

---

201   *Schistosoma* became known as *"The fluke that saved Formosa"*.

resistance was an almost forgone conclusion and the only real surprise is that it has taken so long to develop.

The third method of control is clean water and effective sanitation. Obviously if effective sanitation is available, infected urine and faeces will no longer pollute the water-course and the snails will no longer become infected.

There may be one positive effect of infection by *Schistosoma*. Research on experimental animals shows that *Schistosoma* provides a significant level of protection against auto-immune diseases such as various forms of colitis (Ch 7).

CHAPTER 20

The Problems of the Twenty-First Century

It is obviously impossible to forecast with any degree of certainty which diseases will be prevalent in the twenty-first century. It is however a biological certainty that there will be pandemics in this century, indeed the first has already occurred. It is possible to make some predictions based on the known behaviour of diseases that have caused problems in the past. It is also salutary to remember that HIV was not recognised as a serious problem until the ninth decade of the twentieth century. We therefore have to face the very real possibility that some presently unrecognised micro-organism or virus might cause a major pandemic in the future.

It is important to distinguish between localised epidemics and truly global pandemics. Whilst diseases such as cholera and typhoid will cause epidemics that might well spread over considerable areas, the effects will be confined to countries where the water supply is not safe to drink. Similarly, diseases such as malaria or yellow fever requiring an insect vector will be confined to areas where the insect can flourish. Thus, although malaria may spread over a very wide area and infect extremely large numbers of people, it is debatable whether it can be considered a truly global pandemic. A similar situation is found with syphilis and AIDS; although both are widespread across the world, both could to a considerable extent be brought under control by taking sensible precautions and using safe sexual practices.

Diseases with the potential to become truly global pandemics are those spread by droplet infection, that is, the infected person coughs or sneezes out infectious particles that are breathed in by a susceptible person. Of the diseases mentioned in this book, the ones that have, or have had, truly global potential are all spread by droplet infection. They are smallpox, measles, influenza, tuberculosis and the Black Death (if one accepts the premise that it was not bubonic plague). Of these, smallpox, measles, influenza and possibly the Black Death are viral diseases. Tuberculosis is a bacterial disease but it does possess one property in common with viral diseases in general, it is extremely difficult to treat using antibiotics.

It is therefore reasonable to predict that any global pandemic in the twenty-first century will have some or all of the following attributes:

- it will be spread by droplet infection
- it will probably be caused by a virus
- if caused by a virus, it is more likely to be an RNA virus rather than a DNA one because the mechanism of reproduction of RNA viruses is not subject to proof reading, and therefore large numbers of mutations are more likely
- it will be difficult to treat using presently available drugs
- there will not be an effective vaccine available in the short term.

There is also the distinct possibility that it may be caused by contact with some rare animal species as a result of humans moving into a new environment such as jungle that has been recently cleared.

The problems caused by infectious diseases are most obvious in the developing world, and a report in the USA in 1992 suggested six major causes for the emergence of diseases and considered that the problems the human race is faced with are as follows:

- Breakdown of public health measures
- Economic development and land use

- International trade and travel
- Technology and industry
- Human behaviour
- Microbial adaptation

Other causes such as climatic changes and terrorism using biological weapons can be added to the six listed above. All of these could initiate the appearance of, or influence the behaviour of any future pandemic.

BREAKDOWN OF PUBLIC HEALTH

Public health measures fall into a number of areas, however, the public health measures that have probably contributed more to the improvement of general health than any others are immunisation (Ch 7) and the provision of clean drinking water alongside the efficient disposal of sewage (Ch 12).

In spite of the fact that it has been known for about one hundred and fifty years that polluted drinking water is a major source of a number of dangerous and highly contagious diseases, approximately one sixth of the world's population does not have access to safe drinking water and about forty per cent do not have an efficient sewage disposal system. A supply of clean piped water is the exception in many countries; water has to be brought from a well or stream by hand over considerable distances, the quality is frequently poor being contaminated either biologically and/or chemically, and the amount is inadequate. In many places, it is a case of drinking polluted water or dying of thirst.

Safe drinking water and the adequate disposal of sewage and other waste is always of primary importance in an emergency. Public health measures are at their most vulnerable following economic collapse or disruption caused by major events such as war, drought, floods, volcanic eruption or earthquakes that can destroy the infrastructure over a considerable area and create large numbers of refugees. Typically, starving people in famine situations move large distances to find food and water and congregate at the few places where these are available, usually either state warehouses or food aid distribution centres. The increase in movement spreads the disease over a greater distance, and the concentration of a starving population into a small area greatly increases the probability of an epidemic occurring as the few facilities available are overwhelmed. Under these conditions where public health measures have broken down, the first diseases to appear are nearly always water-borne ones, especially cholera.

Widespread immunisation of children has also played a major role in combating diseases and brought many diseases such as polio under control. One disease, smallpox, has been completely eliminated. However the controversy and loss of public confidence over the MMR vaccine in the UK has led to a reduction in the number of children immunised. Present immunisation figures are significantly below those necessary to control measles. As a result there have been several outbreaks of measles in the UK during the last fifteen years or so, and problems of immunisation in a number of countries mean that we are seeing the re-emergence of diseases, such as diphtheria, that had been more or less eliminated in many countries.

Other public health measures are also of importance. The incidence of diseases such as tuberculosis in the UK has been reduced by better diets, better housing, improved working conditions and pasteurisation of milk. Outbreaks of food poisoning can be controlled by measures such as the inspection of different types of food and rigorously following up problems such as parasite infestation.

The US report mentioned above concluded that the threat of emergence of new infectious diseases was a real one, and that the public health authorities in most countries were incapable of dealing with the problem adequately. This inadequacy falls into several areas. In wealthy countries with an aging population, public health medicine is the poor relation compared to other aspects of medicine, for example, heart surgery and research into problems such as arthritis. Political infighting within governments frequently takes place driven by available budgets. Obviously, within a fixed budget, if more money is spent on public health then there is less available for other aspects of health care, and if more is spent on health, less is available for other high spending areas of government expenditure such as education and defence.

There is also a serious lack of isolation facilities for dealing with more dangerous diseases such as Ebola. Even in a country the size and wealth of the USA, the number of isolation units of a sufficiently high standard available to deal with a major outbreak of Ebola or Marburg disease is low. This lack of facilities covers both the civilian and military authorities.

To give an idea of the problem, there are only five adult ECMO beds for the population of the UK, that is, over sixty million people. ECMO stands for Extra Corporeal Membrane Oxygenation and is basically a machine that takes over the functions of the body for a person too sick to carry it out for themselves. It is obvious that in a pandemic of bird flu attacking the lungs, five beds are not going to be of much use.

Public health is virtually non-existent in some under-developed countries, especially in the cities, where large shanty-towns have developed to deal with the population influx from rural areas. Occasionally the lack of, or failure of public health measures are exacerbated by sheer stupidity or ignorance, as was the case in Lima in the 1990s, which created the present cholera epidemic in South America (Ch 12).

Public health measures can occasionally go wrong in a spectacular manner. A classic example was the attempt to bring malaria under control using DDT to eliminate the mosquito vector. This is discussed in some detail in Chapter 16.

ECONOMIC DEVELOPMENT AND LAND USE.

A major problem of the twenty-first century will be the use of land, agriculture and the economic problems associated with it. It is impossible to separate these problems from those of population size, the use of resources and the politics of birth control.

The world population at the end of World War I was approximately 1.5 billion (1.5×10^9), at the end of World War II it was 2.5×10^9, and by the year 2000 it was over 6×10^9. The present figure is about seven billion and rising. This represents an increase of nearly 500% in just over ninety years. Demographic projections by the UN in 2009 estimated this figure will rise to over 9.1 billion by 2050. This represents a seriously unstable system, and although many sources claim that fertility rates are already falling in most countries, it does not alter the fact that a world population of over nine billion people represents a massive extra demand on already strained resources. It is also worth pointing out that if the next pandemic is transmitted by airborne infection, then the denser the population, the more rapidly it will spread.

The US National Academy of Sciences and The Royal Society of Great Britain stated in 1992 that if population forecasts of this size are accurate, then science and technology would not be able to prevent either irreversible degradation of the environment or continued poverty for much of the world's population. A Royal Society paper in 2009 stated that, *"slowing population growth is essential if the poor are to be lifted out of poverty and if the next generations are to live in a biologically sustainable economy"*.

The politics of population size are complicated by the use of resources of that population and the carbon footprint that it produces. If the use of resources and the carbon footprint per head of population are calculated, the most over-crowded country on the planet is the USA. It is estimated that if all the world's population lived at the level of the average inhabitant of India, the world could support approximately 15 billion people. However, the world could only support about 1.5 billion living at the level of the average citizen of the USA.

Probably the best example of too large a population destroying the available resources is Easter Island. Diamond gives an excellent account of the collapse of the Easter Island civilisation in his book *"Catastrophe"*. The size of the population and their demands on the available resources were such that over a period of about six hundred years they turned a thriving ecosystem into a more or less barren wasteland in which the final stages of the tragedy were civil war and cannibalism. To quote Diamond, *"it is the closest approximation we have to an ecological disaster unfolding in complete isolation. It is a salutary education in the mismanagement of resources"*.

There are numerous other examples of populations severely damaging their environment leading to the collapse of that society, but Easter Island is the most comprehensive and is an object lesson for all of us as we sail through space on a planet with finite resources.

The present world population figures are already a severe burden on the environment in many countries, and those countries with the most rapid growth in population are frequently those with the greatest environmental degradation. There have been huge ecosystem losses in the Amazon, much of Africa, the Philippines and parts of Asia. When the ecosystem is severely damaged, a small number of species able to adapt to these changed conditions quickly become the new dominant species. The result is a less flexible ecosystem and it may be many years before biological diversity returns, if it ever does.

The incidence of Lyme disease in the North Eastern USA is a classic, relatively straight forward illustration of this situation. During the eighteenth and nineteenth centuries forest was converted to farmland by settlers, and apex predators such as wolf, bear and cougar were virtually eliminated. Over a period of time, much of the farmland was allowed to revert to forest following changes in agricultural policies and subsidies, and this resulted in a large increase in the deer population as there were no apex predators to cull them. Deer carry ticks harbouring the spirochaete, *Borrelia burgdorferi,* that causes Lyme disease and a significant rise in the incidence of this disease has occurred in the local human population using the forest for recreational purposes.

There is also the problem of urbanisation, which can be demonstrated using the figures for the population of France. In 1939, 35% of the French population was rural, by 1980 it was less than 10%; in 1970 there were two million farms, by 1985 there were less than 900,000 and the number is still falling. It is estimated that in 1800, ninety-eight per cent of the world's population were farmers and villagers, now fifty per cent (and rising) live in cities, some of them megacities (defined as a city with a population of greater than ten million).

In the 1950s there were only a few megacities, London and New York being two examples. Both of these had developed relatively slowly in nations affluent enough to afford adequate water and sewage treatment, and which could afford reasonable housing, transport and general infrastructure. There were over twenty-five megacities by 2000, Mexico City being the biggest with a population of over thirty million. Many of these cities are in the under-developed countries of Africa, Asia and South America where poverty is already extreme, and they create a huge strain on the public health systems of the countries involved. Many cities are also growing rapidly, partly due to the high birth rates and partly due to population migration, and greatly outstripping the available taxes and revenues needed to provide the necessary infrastructure. Using Mexico City as an example, many areas have to be supplied with water by tanker on a daily basis as the water supply and distribution networks are totally inadequate. Even megacities such as Tokyo with an estimated population of twenty-three million are hard pressed to deal with all the problems, and if these problems were to be exacerbated by a major earthquake (which is long overdue for the Tokyo region), then it is difficult to imagine the scenario that would ensue. The last major earthquake in the Tokyo area in 1923 killed an estimated 125,000 people, at a time when the population density was much lower than at present.

A further problem relates to natural resources and their distribution. If the population is growing, it is obvious that resources will be divided more thinly, for example, the water flow of a river may need to be divided between more people. To quote one source, "*Oil is expensive but there are a number of alternatives, water is less expensive but there are no alternatives*". Recent calculations suggest that within twenty years, half of the world's population will live in areas where there is a shortage of fresh water.

Numerous examples are found. In the Middle East, Israel is extracting 10-20% more water than is renewed annually, much of this water coming from deep aquifers. As a result the water table is falling rapidly, sucking in seawater and causing salination of wells. The population of Israel is expected to increase by fifty per cent by 2020 over its year 2000 figure. Even allowing for improved management of water, there will be an increased water requirement of at least 25% by Israel which, given the political and religious problems already existing between Israel and its neighbours, will almost certainly exacerbate an already tense situation.

The damming of rivers that pass through more than one country is another example. The damming of the Euphrates by Turkey is causing considerable unease in other countries such as Iraq through which it passes, whilst the damming of the Indus and attempts to reduce the water flow have caused major tension between India and Pakistan, creating an extremely serious political situation given that both sides have nuclear weapons.

The problems even occur when there is no second country involved. In Australia, it is necessary to tap into aquifers formed 80,000 years ago to obtain sufficient water to sustain the tourist population of the Ayers Rock area, and the extraction of water in the catchment area of the River Murray means this no longer reaches the sea. A similar situation is found in the USA. The extraction of water from rivers such as the Colorado and Rio Grande means they also no longer reach the sea. Indeed in the USA, the extraction of water for cultivation (including lawns and golf courses) in states such as California, Arizona and Texas is leading to considerable tension between various states and agricultural and urban requirements. There is a cynical comment in the south-western USA that it is the only place where water flows uphill (towards the money).

Even in traditionally wet countries such as the UK, the extraction of water is such that many rivers in the south of England[202] are drying up in the summer or running at such low levels as to be an ecological catastrophe. In addition, the number of cases of Water Boards in the UK that are being subjected to fines, for allowing sewage to pollute rivers, is rising rapidly indicating that the present sewage treatment infrastructure is incapable of coping with the volumes involved. Many beaches have also been removed recently from the list of approved beaches for recreational purposes because of problems of pollution by sewage. It has recently been suggested that the population of the UK will rise by ten million over the next twenty years, mainly due to immigration, and if past trends are continued, the majority of these will move into the south east of England. The availability of water and sewage treatment facilities in the south is now such that an increase in numbers of this magnitude would overwhelm the present infrastructure, constituting a major argument against further immigration into the UK. These are objective assessments, unlike education and health where the figures can always be manipulated by

---

202   Rivers such as the Kennet and the Lee which are both tributaries of the River Thames are both drying up. The cause is the extraction of excessive amounts of water by Thames Water to supply new homes in the Thames Valley. The situation has become so bad that the Environmental Agency is applying for permission to reduce or cancel several hundred permits allowing companies to extract water. The problem is not confined to the Thames Valley, shortages are also occurring in rivers in North Yorkshire and in rural areas along the River Dart.

the government in power to present the appearance of an increase in productivity. The supply of fresh water and sewage treatment cannot be manipulated, they are either adequate or they are not.

The amounts of water involved are huge. It has been estimated that to prevent disease, 30-50 litres water/day/person is necessary depending on the heat. This contrasts with the amounts used in the UK which is approximately 140 litres (31 gallons) /day/person, and the amount used in the USA which is a massive 410 litres (91 gallons)/day/person. These figures do not include industrial usage. If this is included, the figure for the USA rises to over six thousand litres (approximately 1,350 gallons) of water per person per day. This figure may seem high, but calculations suggest that it takes 120 litres of water to produce enough coffee beans to make one cup, 3,000 litres to make one cotton shirt and a massive 8,000 litres to produce one beef burger.

In countries such as the UK where the availability of land for reservoirs is limited, this has led to considerable recycling of water. Whilst this is laudable, it does raise considerable practical problems of purifying water so that it is acceptable for further use, and the problem is not just the bacteriological one outlined in chapter 12. One serious consequence is the appearance of breakdown products of the birth control pill that is causing unforeseen effects such as distortion of the sex ratios in some aquatic and amphibious vertebrates.

Other resources beside water will also become more thinly spread as the population rises. The area of arable land available per person will fall significantly by 2050, the figures varying depending on the location and the demographic model used. The pressure on the land available will result in a reduction in the area of forests, and the increasing use of fertilisers in agriculture will cause increasing pollution and eutrophication of aquifers, lakes, rivers and seas. Many of these problems are already occurring and others are only a matter of time. As has already been pointed out in Chapter 12, phytoplankton blooms are a source of diseases such as cholera, allowing them to undergo rapid mutation.

There are considerable differences of opinion regarding the severity of the problems caused by over population. One extreme suggests that there is not a world wide food shortage, just inefficient food distribution. The other extreme suggests that population limits should be enforced using the Chinese model, i.e. four grandparents, two parents, and one child. One factor that may help in correcting the large increase in population is the cultural desire of many families in certain countries to have boys. Ultra-sound scans of pregnant women followed by a termination if the foetus is female are leading to a considerable imbalance of the sexes in some countries such as India and China.

The problem of over population is not helped however by fundamentalist and extremist religious leaders in certain countries exhorting their followers to have large families, because different religious groups are trying to "outbreed" them.

As the Nobel Prize winner H.W. Kendall stated, *"If we do not halt population growth with justice and compassion, it will be done for us by nature, brutally and without pity - and will leave a ravaged world"*.

INTERNATIONAL TRADE AND TRAVEL.

International trade and travel were also identified as being major factors in the spread of disease. There are numerous historical examples of diseases being carried to other countries, two of the earliest are the Plague of Athens (Ch 8) and the Plague of Galen (Ch 10). A more recent example is the transport of bubonic plague to the USA from Asia around 1900. Previously, sailing ships had been so slow that the disease had died out before reaching the Americas. It is now endemic in the ground squirrel population of the USA (Ch 9). Another example is the present epidemic of cholera in South America thought to have been caused by a ship flushing its bilges (Ch 12).

The speed of modern air transport means that it is possible to transport sick but asymptomatic passengers and deliver them to their destinations long before health authorities realise there is a problem. The spread of SARS from China to Hong Kong and Toronto in 2002 was an example of this (Ch 6), and demonstrated how quickly a major pandemic could spread.

It is not just the transport of sick people that might be a problem. In 1967 there was an outbreak of a disease in Marburg in Germany that became known as Marburg Disease. This was caused by a filovirus producing a severe haemorrhagic fever (very similar to that caused by the Ebola virus) that killed seven of the thirty-one individuals infected. Research showed that the virus was carried by African green monkeys that had been imported from Uganda for work on a polio vaccine. Since then, there have several small outbreaks and two large ones, the first in the Congo (1998-2000) that involved 154 cases of whom eighty-three per cent died, and the second in Angola in 2004 involving 163 cases of whom over ninety per cent died. Recent research has suggested that the natural source of the virus may be bats.

TECHNOLOGY AND INDUSTRY

These can also contribute towards the spread of disease. The bulk processing of food and centralized distribution networks are very important economically, but significantly raise the risk of food poisoning over a wide area if the processing system goes wrong. There is also the question of what happens if a major epidemic, such as influenza, cripples the distribution network. Distribution networks in developed countries work on the basis of just enough and just in time. This has led to the concept of, *"three meals from anarchy"*. The number of meals from anarchy varies from three to about ten depending on the source, but the principle is that if the distribution network were to fail or be compromised, then most families could only exist for a few days on the food available in the house. It is no use claiming that there is plenty of food in the freezer, if the distribution network crashes because of a major epidemic, it is a reasonable expectation that the power systems will also fail, and without power, no water will be pumped, no sewage will be treated and no electricity will be available so the food in the freezer will last about three days.

The problem is not just the delivery of food but also other necessities. How long could the local hospital continue to carry out operations without oxygen and anaesthetic gases being delivered? A few days is probably an optimistic estimate and this is just one example.

Other examples of technology influencing diseases include Legionnaires disease that is spread by droplet infection caused by aerosols from air conditioning and through shower systems. The recycling of air on aircraft has also been pinpointed as a contributor towards diseases spread by droplet infection. This air will be recycled frequently during a long flight, and if one passenger aboard the plane is suffering from a disease such as active TB, then everyone on the plane will be exposed to it.

The use of medical technology also increases the spread of disease. There have been a number of cases of AIDS caused by blood transfusions where the donor was infected. Individuals have also been infected by diseased transplants and the sharing of needles amongst drug addicts is notorious for spreading HIV, hepatitis and malaria.

Further problems are caused by major building projects such as dams, for example the building of the Aswan dam in Egypt has caused a considerable increase in schistosomiasis in the area and the building of the Three Gorges across the Yangtze is expected to create similar problems (Ch 19). The Aswan dam has also caused large increases in the mosquito-borne, viral disease Rift Valley fever in Egypt since the dam was completed in the 1970s.

Further aspects of technology involve war. The bombing of Vietnam during the 1970s caused a vast number of craters to be formed which, when they fill with water, are ideal for the growth of mosquitoes. The result has been a significant increase in the transmission rate of malaria and other mosquito born diseases.

It is probable however that the two most potent factors in the transmission of disease are human behaviour and microbial adaptation.

HUMAN BEHAVIOUR

Human behaviour in terms of living in large cities has already been discussed in Chapter 5, but there are numerous other aspects of our behaviour that also influence diseases and their spread. Many human activities act to amplify diseases for example, multiple partner sex, brothels and homosexual bathhouses have all been shown to have played, and are still playing, a major role in the transmission of HIV and various other sexually transmitted diseases. Syringes being reused are probably the most effective amplifier of all as they bypass the body's safety features. This is done for both genuine medical reasons and for drug taking purposes. In one Ebola epidemic, five syringes were being used on 3-600 patients per day without being sterilised, and being sharpened on a whetstone between injections when necessary. There have been similar problems in the former USSR where the breakdown of state resources has meant widespread reuse of non-sterile syringes. The same problem occurs with drug users injecting drugs such as heroin on a group basis using shared syringes.

Further amplifiers are blood banks and transfusion centres where the blood has not been treated correctly to destroy various pathogens. Both HIV and hepatitis B are known to have been transmitted to haemophiliacs by this route.

Any place where people congregate can act as an amplifier. Schools, universities and army barracks are well known amplifiers of diseases such as chickenpox, glandular fever and meningitis. Prisons, especially in countries such as Russia, have become notorious for the amplification of AIDS and TB. Hospital wards can also act as amplifiers, one case of active TB in a ward full of transplant patients who are compromised immunologically, could cause widespread TB amongst the other patients.

Further problems are caused by improvements in our medical technology. Our technology now allows us to keep alive children suffering from genetic diseases such as cystic fibrosis until they reach child bearing age. As such diseases are caused by a double copy of the defective gene (Ch 5), this means that when people suffering from the disease reproduce, the defective gene will be passed onto the next generation. Such a policy repeated over a number of generations will cause considerable attrition in the human gene pool. In the event that public health systems break down, these people will be amongst the first to be challenged by micro-organisms.

A further problem is that in the event of a major pandemic there is a distinct possibility of some supra-national organisation such as the WHO, the UN or the European Union being appointed to oversee operations. Unfortunately the senior bureaucracy of such organisations is riddled with failed, incompetent and/or corrupt politicians sidelined by their national governments for political reasons. The prospect of EU bureaucrats attempting to control a major pandemic in Europe does not inspire one with confidence.

Microbial Adaptation

The final problem that was highlighted in the US study was microbial adaptation. Micro-organisms have a short generation time and are able to evolve rapidly. The bacterium of the gut, *Escherichia coli,* is able to divide about every twenty minutes under optimal conditions and will produce a random mutation approximately once in every million cells. Whilst this might seem like a large number, if one bacterial cell is present at time zero and is dividing under optimal conditions, then over a million cells will be present in less than seven hours. Bacteria are also not a fixed species and can undergo genetic change very rapidly. *Escherichia coli* O157 is a classic example. It first appeared as a problem in the USA in the early 1980s and searches of culture collections have failed to detect it earlier than the late 1970s. It is a strain of *E. coli* that has acquired additional virulence genes from distant relatives through horizontal genetic transfer. One of the main virulence factors is a toxin called verotoxin or shiga-like toxin acquired from the food poisoning bacterium, *Shigella*. The toxin produces severe damage to the large bowel and causes kidney failure in young children and old people. This strain of *E. coli* has caused a number of outbreaks of food poisoning since it was first found, that have included numerous fatalities.

Humans also put micro-organisms under extreme genetic pressure from the widespread misuse of antibiotics and force them to exist at the limit of their capability. Such pressure favours the micro-organism which mutates rapidly and that mutation may be detrimental to human health. The more encounters we win against micro-organisms the more pressure we put on their genetic capabilities, thus increasing the probability of a catastrophic epidemic.

The conclusion accepted for many years by microbiologists was that the evolution of the host and pathogen relationship leads to a moderation of virulence, that is the pathogen does not kill off the host too quickly because if the host dies, the pathogen has to spread to a new host or die itself. Computer modelling has shown that this is not necessarily correct. A pathogen that is only transmitted slowly to a small number of new susceptible victims will move towards a more benign relationship with the host organism. However, a pathogen that is transmitted rapidly and effectively to a large number of susceptible victims can afford to become more deadly.

<u>TERRORISM</u>

The problems of using micro-organisms for terrorist purposes were considered in the chapter on "The History of Microbiology".

<u>CLIMATE CHANGE</u>

The question of climate change is an extremely controversial one. The majority of scientists accept that climate changes are occurring, although a few do not agree. Amongst those who think that climate change is already occurring, there is considerable debate about why it is changing, how quickly it is changing, how much it will change, what effect it will have on the human species and what we can do about it.

Global warming will influence several aspects. A rise in temperature will increase the range of a number of species of insects that carry diseases and we can therefore expect an increase of many diseases, yellow fever and malaria probably being two of the most important. This situation is already occurring with malaria in the mountains of Kenya.

Secondly, an increase in the surface temperature of the oceans will cause changes in weather patterns leading to floods in some areas and droughts in others that will obviously influence agriculture. Flooding will increase the probability of water borne diseases, whilst drought will lead to increased migration.

The rise in temperature will also cause a rise in sea levels through two factors, the first is obviously the release of water from the Greenland and Antarctic ice caps and the second is thermal expansion of the sea as the temperature rises. How far sea levels rise will obviously depend on how far the temperature rises, but sea levels rose approximately seven inches during the twentieth century. Whilst this might not sound very much, if the average height of a country is only one or two metres above sea level then seven inches is a significant rise. A number of low lying countries such as many Pacific islands, parts of Holland and much of Bangladesh would be subjected to increased flooding leading to massive migrations. Many other countries, including the UK, would lose considerable areas of land if there were significant rises in sea levels leading to a large rise in the population per square mile. The strain on power supplies, water supplies and sewage disposal would be increased, raising the probability of water-borne diseases occurring.

CONCLUSION

The increase of infectious diseases has been very rapid in a short evolutionary time and is linked more to our social development than our evolutionary development. There is a strong tendency especially in the developed countries to ignore epidemics as undesirable things that occur in faraway places. Ignorance however is a destructive luxury, the speed of modern travel means that epidemics that occur in developing countries can be in London, Paris or New York within a matter of hours, as microbes do not recognise artificial human boundaries such as borders and customs posts. No country is self sufficient and closing borders is neither an option nor is it a solution.

Disaster planning by governments usually assumes that any disruption is local, for example, Hurricane Katrina devastating New Orleans. However in this age of rapid transport, pandemics will attack us everywhere more or less simultaneously. Many plans for pandemics assume there would be a low mortality rate based on the relatively mild flu epidemics of 1957 and 1968. This assumption will have been reinforced by the mildness of Mexican flu of 2009. If bird flu became pandemic and did not modify its behaviour then these assumptions are obviously totally inadequate.

A major problem is that our response to any new disease must always be reactive. By the time we are aware of a new disease or a variation on an old one, it is already reaching epidemic status. This raises a serious problem about being able to produce an effective vaccine to a new disease in the middle of an epidemic. In reality, the chances of producing a vaccine to a new disease sufficiently rapidly to stop an epidemic in its tracks are virtually zero. Many big companies are pulling out of vaccine production as there is very little profit in the vaccine market, especially in the developing world, and in the developed world, especially the USA, there is the problem of litigation if anything goes wrong.

As Margulis has stated, *"Nature is not benign and the survival of the human species at the expense of every other species is not pre-ordained"*. Every civilisation in the past has collapsed sooner or later. Could our civilisation survive a catastrophic pandemic or would it also collapse? We think we are different to every other species and every other civilisation that has gone before and consider our civilisation is now so complex and integrated that it is immune to collapse. However, instead of becoming more resilient, our society is becoming more vulnerable due to its complexity. Mathematical studies on complexity suggest that once a society has developed beyond a certain point it becomes unstable, and even small problems can destroy it. These studies show that as networks become more tightly integrated they transmit shocks rather than absorb them.

History shows that what happens in a major pandemic depends to a large extent on the complexity of the society involved. The Black Death in Europe from 1347-50 killed about one third of the population. The population was largely a rural one and most communities were self sufficient for the basic commodities. Although the initial impact was severe, life returned to a similar pattern relatively quickly. However when severe epidemics with a similar death toll to the Black Death attacked the Western Roman Empire from the end of the second century AD, over the next two centuries the empire collapsed. The system was more complex with a centralised authority and large urban populations that were not self sufficient in food.

If industrialised society does fail, the most vulnerable will be the urban masses. Those most likely to survive would be subsistence farmers. There is a proverb, rags to riches to rags in three generations. *Homo sapiens* may find that a variation on this theme is, dirt farmer to urban citizen to dirt farmer in five hundred generations.

FURTHER READING

General Reading

Baker, R. Quiet Killers. 2007, Sutton Publishing.

Cartwright, F. F. & Bidiss, M. 2000, Disease and History. Sutton Publishing.

Dobson, M. Disease: The Extraordinary Stories behind History's Greatest Killers. 2007, Quercus.

Kipple, K. F. Plague, Pox and Pestilence: Disease in History. 1997, Weidenfeld & Nicolson.

Loudon, I. (Ed). Western Medicine; An Illustrated History. Chapters 2-7, 1997, Oxford University Press.

Moalem, S. Survival of the Sickest. 2007, Harper Collins.

Chapter 1

Carmichael, A. G. Sweating Sickness. The Cambridge World History of Human Disease. 1993. Ed. Kipple, K. F. Cambridge University Press.

The Forgotten Apostle. New Scientist, 4th August 2007.

Karlem, A. Plague's Progress, a social history of Man and Disease. 1995, Victor Gollancz, London.

Leavitt, J. W. Typhoid Mary; Captive to the Public's Health. 2000, Beacon Books.

Zimmer, C. What is a Species? Scientific American, June 2008, pp 48-55

Chapter 2

Ball, P. The Devil's Doctor: Paracelsus and the World of Renaissance Magic and Science. 2006, Heinemann.

Cartwright, F. F. & Biddiss, M. Disease and History. 2000, Chapter 1, Disease in the Ancient World. Sutton Publishing, Stroud.

Keay, J. The Spice Route; A History. 2005, John Murray.

Loudon, I. (Ed) Western Medicine; An Illustrated History. 1997, Oxford University Press. Chapters 2-5

Lyons, J. The House of Wisdom; How the Arabs Transformed Western Civilisation. 2009, Bloomsbury, London ,Berlin, NY.

Masood, E. Science and Islam, a History. 2009, Icon Books.

Mayor, A. Greek Fire, Poison arrows and Scorpion Bombs, Biological and Chemical Warfare in the Ancient World. 2004, Overlook Ducksworth Woodstock London.

Nunn, J.F. Ancient Egyptian Medicine. 1996. British Museum Press.

Pain, S. The Pharaohs' Pharmacists. New Scientist, 15th December 2007, pp 40-43.

Wilson, S. Formula for Success. Family History, January 2005, pp 30-32.

Woolley, B. The Herbalist, Nicholas Culpepper and the Fight for Medical Freedom. 2004, Harper Collins.

Chapter 3

Alibek, K. & Handelman S. Biohazard, 2000, Delta New York.

Barnaby, W. The Plague Makers, the Secret World of Biological Warfare. 1997, Vision.

Cole, L.A. The Eleventh Plague, the Politics of Biological and Chemical Warfare. 1997, Freeman.

de Kruif, P. The Microbe Hunters, 1926, Republished 1996 Mariner Books.

Loudon, I. (Ed) Western Medicine; An Illustrated History. 1997. Chapters 6, 7. Oxford University Press.

Lucretius. On the Nature of the Universe. Translated R. E. Latham. 1951. Penguin.

Walsh, C. T. & Fischbach, M. A. New Ways to Squash Superbugs. Scientific American, July 2009 pp 32-39.

Chapter 4

Buchsbaum, R. Animals without Backbones. 1951, Penguin.

Desowitz, R.S. Tropical Diseases. 1997, Harper Collins.

Hamilton, G. Welcome to the Virosphere. New Scientist, 30th August 2008, pp 38-41.

Lapage, G. Animals Parasitic in Man. 1957, Penguin.

Zuk, M. Riddled with Life. 2007, Harcourt.

Chapter 5

Diamond, J. Guns, Germs and Steel. The Fate of Human Societies. 1997. Jonathan Cape, London

Dillehay, T. D. The Settlement of the Americas. 2000, Perseus Books.

Dobbs, D. The Silt Road. New Scientist, 4th March 2006, pp 44-47.

Heckenberger, M. J. Lost Cities of the Amazon. Scientific American, October 2009 pp 44-51.

Jones, D. Going Global. New Scientist, 27th October 2007, pp 36-41.

McNeill, W.H. Plagues and Peoples. 1976, Anchor Press/ Doubleday New York

Mithen, S. After the Ice. A Global Human History 20,000-5,000 BC. 2003, Wiedenfeld & Nicolson.

Nicholls, H. Taming the Beast. New Scientist, 3rd October 2009, pp 40-43

Oppenheimer, S. Out of Eden: The peopling of the World. 2003, Constable & Robinson, London.

Pringle, H. Follow that Kelp. New Scientist, 11th August 2007, pp 40-43.

Spinney, L. Where are the bodies? New Scientist, 8th November 2008, pp 40-43.

Stix, G. Traces of a Distant Past. Scientific American, July 2008, pp 38-45.

Storck, P. L. Journey to the Ice Age. 2004, University of British Columbia Press.

Vavilov, N.I. The Origin, Variation, Immunity and Breeding of Cultivated Plants. 1951, Ronald Press Co.

Ward, P. What will become of *Homo sapiens*? Scientific American, January 2009, pp 54-59.

Wood, M. In Search of the Dark Ages. 1981, BBC Books.

Chapter 6

Hotez, P.J. A Plan to Defeat Neglected Tropical Diseases. Scientific American, January 2010, 74-79.

Karesh, W.B. & Cook, R.A. The Human-Animal Link. Foreign Affairs. July/August 2005, pp38-50.

McKeown, T. Origins of human disease. 1988, Oxford University Press.

Wolfe, N. Preventing the Next Pandemic. Scientific American, April 2009, pp 60-65.

Chapter 7

Garëon, N. & Goldman, M. Boosting Vaccine Power. Scientific American, October 2009, pp 52-59.

Giles, J. Hard to Swallow. New Scientist, 26th January 2008, pp 37-39.

Hamilton, G. Filthy Friends. New Scientist, 16th April 2005, pp 34-39.

Kaplan, M. Just What the Doctor Ordered. New Scientist, 11th July 2009, pp 42-45.

Orwant, R The Cure that came in from the Cold. New Scientist, 19th March 2005, pp42-45.

Wood, P. Understanding Immunology. 2001, Pearson Education Ltd. Harlow UK.

Chapter 8
Thucydides. History of the Peloponnesian War. Translated by Warner R. 1954, Penguin Classics.

Chapter 9
Gottfried, R. S. The Black Death: Natural and Human Disaster in Medieval Europe. 1983, Robert Hale.

Gummer, B. The Scourging Angel: The Black Death in the British Isles. 2009, Bodley Head.

Kelly, M. A History of the Black Death in Ireland. 2001, Tempus Publishing Ltd, Stroud, UK.

Keys, D. Catastrophe: An Investigation into the Origins of the Modern World. 1999, Ballantine Books, New York.

Naphy, W. & Spicer, A. The Black Death: A History of Plagues. 2001, Tempus Publishing Ltd, Stroud, UK.

Rosen, W. Justinian's Flea: Plague, Empire and the Birth of Europe. 2007, Cape.

Shewsbury, J.F.D. A History of Bubonic Plague in the British Isles. 1970, Cambridge University Press.

Scott, S. & Duncan, C.J. Biology of Plagues. 2001, Cambridge University Press

Ziegler P. The Black Death. 1969. Collins.

Chapter 10

Crosby, A. W. The Columbian Exchange: Biological and Cultural Consequences of 1492. 1972. Westport, Conn. USA.

Glynn, J. & Glynn, I. The Life and Death of Smallpox. 2004, Profile Books

Wood, M. Conquistadors. 2000, BBC Books.

Chapter 11

Carmichael, A. G. Leprosy: Larger than Life. In Plague, Pox and Pestilence; Disease in History. 1997, Ed Kipple K. F. Widenfeld & Nicolson.

Dormandy T. The White Death: A History of Tuberculosis, 2000, New York University Press.

French, R. K. Scrofula. The Cambridge World History of Human Disease. 1993, Ed. Kipple, K. F. Cambridge University Press.

Johnston, W. D. Tuberculosis. The Cambridge World History of Human Disease. 1993, Ed. Kipple K. F. Cambridge University Press.

Chapter 12

Furlow, B. To Your Good Health. New Scientist, 3rd December 2005, pp 47-49.

Hempel, S. The Medical Detective: John Snow, Cholera and the Mystery of the Broad Street Pump. 2006, Granta Books, London.

Halliday, S. The Great Stink of London. 1999, Sutton Publishing.

Johnson, S. The Ghost Map. 2006, Penguin, London.

Rogers, P. Facing the Fresh Water Crisis. Scientific American, August 2008, pp 28-35.

Chapter 13

Bell, D.A. The First Total War: Napoleon's Europe and the Birth of Modern Warfare. 2007, Houghton, Mifflin Harcourt.

Crowley, R. Empires of the Sea: The Final Battle for the Mediterranean, 1521-1580. 2008, Faber.

Harden, V. A. Typhus. 1993 in The Cambridge World History of Human Disease. 1993, Ed. Kipple K. F. Cambridge University Press.

MacKenzie, D. Let them eat Spuds. New Scientist, 2nd August 2008, pp 30-33.

Póirtéir, C. (Ed) The Great Irish Famine. 1995, Mercier Press.

Zinsser, H. Rats, Lice and History. 1934, republished by Papermac, 1985.

Chapter 14

Arrizabalaga, J., Henderson, J. & French, R. The Great Pox. The French Disease in Renaissance Europe. 1997, Yale University Press.

Cruickshank, D. The Secret History of Georgian London. 2009, Random House.

Chapter 15

Barry, J. M. The Great Influenza: The Epic Story of the Deadliest Plague in History. 2004, Viking New York.

Crosby, A.W. America's Forgotten Pandemic: The Influenza of 1918. 1989, Cambridge University Press.

Davies, P. Catching Cold. 1999, Michael Joseph, London.

Garrett, L. The Next Pandemic. Foreign Affairs. July/August 2005, pp 3-23.

MacKenzie, D. The Predictable Pandemic. New Scientist, 2nd May 2009, pp 6-7.

MacKenzie, D. An End to Flu. New Scientist, 22nd August 2009, pp28-31.

MacKenzie, D. The Bird Flu Threat. New Scientist Supplement, 7th January 2006.

Osterholm, M.T. Preparing for the Next Pandemic. Foreign Affairs. July/August 2005. pp 24-37.

Chapter 16

Harrison, G. Mosquitoes, Malaria and Man: A History of Hostilities since 1880. 1978, John Murray.

The Cambridge World History of Human Disease. 1993. Ed. Kipple K. F. Cambridge University Press

Nicholls, H. Ending the Nightmare. New Scientist 25th August 2007, pp 35-37.

Rocco, F. The Miraculous Fever-Tree. 2003, Harper Collins, London.

Spielman, A. & d'Antonio, M. Mosquito: the Story of Mankind's Deadliest Foe. 2001, Faber & Faber, London.

Chapter 17

Cooper, D. B. & Kipple, K. F. Yellow Fever. The Cambridge World History of Human Disease. 1993. Ed. Kipple, K. F. Cambridge University Press.

Nowak, R. A Plague on Plagues. New Scientist, 30th May 2009, pp38-41.

Parker, M.. Panama Fever: The Battle to Build the Canal. 2009, Hutchinson.

Chapter 18

Aldhous, P. HIV's Killing Fields. New Scientist 14th July 2007.

Epstein, H.. The Invisible Cure: Africa, the West and the Fight against AIDS. 2007, Viking.

Garrett, L. The Lessons of HIV/AIDS. Foreign Affairs July/ August 2005, pp 51-64.

Marx, V. Cut! New Scientist, 19th July 2008, pp 40-43.

Pisani, E. The Wisdom of Whores. 2008, Granta Books, London.

Steinberg, J. The AIDS Denialists. New Scientist, 20th June 2009, pp32-36.

Chapter 19
Skelly P. Fighting Killer Worms. Scientific American, May 2008, pp 72-77.

Chapter 20
Ananthaswamy, A. Going, going. New Scientist, 4th July 2009, pp 28-33.

Brown, L.R. Could Food Shortages bring down Civilisation? Scientific American, May 2009, pp 38- 45.

Diamond, J. Collapse: How Societies choose to fail or succeed. 2005, Viking Press.

Garrett, L. The Coming Plague: Newly Emerging Diseases in a World out of Balance. 1994, Farrar, Strauss & Giroux, New York.

MacKenzie, D. Are We Doomed? New Scientist, 5th April 2008, pp 32-35.

MacKenzie, D. The End of Civilisation. New Scientist, 5th April 2008, pp 28-31.

MacKenzie, D. What Price more Food? New Scientist, 14th June 2008, pp 28-33.

Pearce, F. The Parched Planet. New Scientist, 25th February 2006, pp 32-36.

Rogers, P. Facing the Freshwater Crisis. Scientific American, August 2008, Pp 28-35.

Salyers, A. A. & Whitt, D. D. Revenge of the Microbes: How Bacterial Resistance is undermining the Antibiotic Miracle. 2005, American Society of Microbiology Press. Washington.

Tainter, J. The Collapse of Complex Societies. 1998, Cambridge University Press.

INDEX